The Little Handbook of Palliative Care

Dr. Tan Seng Beng

PARTRIDGE

To order additional copies of this book, contact
Toll Free 800 101 2657 (Singapore)
Toll Free 1 800 81 7340 (Malaysia)
orders.singapore@partridgepublishing.com

www.partridgepublishing.com/singapore

I would like to dedicate this little handbook to all doctors, nurses and medical students.

May this book be a guide to relieve suffering of palliative care patients and their family caregivers.

May it help all who read it and lead them to the path of enduring happiness.

Contents

Part III: Symptom Control – Non-Pain Symptoms

Part IV: Management of Death and Dying

Part V: Psychosocial and Spiritual Care

Part VI: Self-Care

Foreword

by Professor Dato' Dr Christopher Boey Chiong Meng

It is my great honour to write a foreword to this important book on palliative medicine by Dr Tan Seng Beng who has been a friend and colleague for many years.

The dignity and preciousness of life is the fundamental starting point of all effort in medicine. It is essential that practitioners of the art of medicine be well-rounded human beings who are interested in people and not just in pathological processes, and who constantly strive to put themselves in the position of the patients they are caring for. Such a quality is indispensable, especially in palliative care.

The Chinese character for 'benevolence' is a combination of the character for 'person' and the character for the number 'two', and indicates two people in a relationship of friendship and trust. It also means 'to be kind and to feel compassion for'.

Recently, however, there has been concern expressed about the deteriorating quality of doctor-patient relationships. Medical school teachers know that this is an increasingly worrying issue. To reverse this trend is a challenge that we all have to courageously take up.

It is therefore with much expectation that I welcome the publication of this book that contains the wisdom derived from the many years of experience of a dedicated palliative care physician who is trying his best to practice humanistic medicine. I sincerely wish this book the great success that it deserves.

Professor Dato' Dr Christopher Boey Chiong Meng
MBBS DCH MRCP FAMM MD PhD FRCPCH FRCP
Deputy Dean (Postgraduate)
Faculty of Medicine
University of Malaya

15th September 2016

Foreword

by Catherine Yee Chiew Huei

I lost both my parents to cancer, one after the other within a span of three years. When my parents were diagnosed -- first my mother, and later, my father -- I experienced a reversal of our parent-child roles. Despite the roller-coaster of emotions we encountered, I learnt to juggle my new responsibilities as caregiver. I was lost, yet, just like any parent who hoped the best for their child, I was hopeful. At first, I hoped that they would recover and continue what they enjoyed doing daily. As time and the disease progressed, my only hope was to take their pain and suffering away. As I write this foreword, my hope is that they are happy wherever they are.

Over the last three years, I learnt that palliative care is not a miracle cure, but a journey filled with hope, love and care. I still remember the first time we were referred to palliative care's Dr SB Tan. It was back in March 2013. "How do I tell my mom she's dying? Do I tell her how long she has left?", I asked Dr Tan. I had so many questions but I couldn't seem to ask or hear anything. "Practitioners will normally help to break the news," he replied, trying to calm me down. Trying to hold back my tears, I said, "I will tell her but you need to teach me how". And that was my introduction to palliative care. From that day onwards, it was "Dr Tan, I will learn but please teach me how." Little did I know, three years later, I would have to relay this unfortunate news again - this time round, to my dad. Honestly, doing it the second time did not make it any easier. It was actually a lot more difficult.

As unfortunate as the circumstances were, both experiences were truly a blessing. Taking care of them, although extremely painful, brought great joy and wonderful discoveries. I learnt a lot about myself and saw how just being human was extraordinary. Beyond the pain of being vulnerable and fragile is the beauty of our own individuality and the wonders of our adaptability.

Each day was unique and every moment was different. My dad wanted to be pain-free so he could just sleep through the ordeal, whereas my mom fought to stay awake just to enjoy her time with us and do what she liked.

Learning from the doctors how to organise the cocktails of medication and their frequencies was overwhelming. There was never a quiet day, and each day brought new challenges. Whilst cleaning my mom one day I found small blisters on her thigh. The oncologist confirmed the blisters were early signs of shingles and gave her some medication. A week later, as the shingles healed, I discovered pressure sores on her body. I ran to the nearest pharmacy for cream and a ripple bed. The pharmacy was like my local grocery store.

Later, when my dad was bedridden, there were episodes where he soiled himself as a result of the laxatives he was on. Once, while cleaning my dad up, I found some blood stains between his thighs. The skin had cracked and was inflamed. It was back to the pharmacy again. And so it went on.

Many a time I was conflicted by what I wanted for them rather than what they actually needed. In the midst of all the worries, frustrations and tiredness, it was so easy to forget what I was actually doing and more importantly, how they were coping. I constantly reminded myself that my actions were in their best interest - it was for THEM and how THEY would like it at THAT moment. The more aware I was of their feelings and the more I listened to what they wanted, the more I learnt about myself. And I'm sure they learnt about me too. Sometimes, I laughed at the assumptions I made of my parents. My only rule of thumb was to keep them happy and at the same time, not beat myself up when I didn't manage to. I told myself that they would know if I was unhappy. They did not knock their head somewhere, they were just ill. When I learnt to embrace that fluidity, I started truly enjoying each passing moment with them and was thankful for what little time we had left together.

There were bouts of mixed emotions and lots of teeth-grinding moments. There were many questions that I didn't know how to answer. "Why won't you just let me die?", "How did I get this?", "Am I going to get well soon?", "Am I going to die?". Over time, I learnt that it was just them being truly human – it was the frustration of being taken care of by their child instead of them taking care of me; the anger of not being able to do what they enjoyed with me; the sadness of having their future taken away; and not being able to watch my kids grow up. Despite their ordeal, they still tried to be as strong as they could, and I was overwhelmed by the realisation. It made me so proud of them, and never had I been more proud being their daughter than I was then.

Two months have gone by since my dad passed away. As I watched him slowly and peacefully slip away, I remembered Dr Tan's words from three years ago. "Dying is a natural and beautiful process. The body will know when it's dying and will slowly shut down. It will be peaceful if we do not struggle with it." I remember the day my mom passed away just as clearly. I held her hand, repeated Dr Tan's words of advice, and wished her a wonderful journey ahead. She smiled as she drew her last breath.

The journey with palliative care has made my life in this boundless universe more beautiful and meaningful.

"When you want something, all the universe conspires in helping you to achieve it" – Paulo Coelho

In memory of my wonderful father and loving mother.

Thank you Dr Tan for sharing your positive energy with us.

- Catherine Yee Chiew Huei, 2016

Preface

My own first exposure to palliative care happened in November 1998 when I did my elective posting at Hualien Tzu Chi Hospital of Taiwan. With my batchmates, we did a project on types of pain control used in the palliative care ward, also called the Heart Lotus Ward. The ward was named so with the conviction that terminally ill patients can bloom beautifully like lotus flowers from the mud of suffering.

I remember we were asked to do a performance at the hospital three days before Christmas. My batchmates sang a song called Using the Malaysian Weather to Say I Love You. I sang The Heart Sutra, a Buddhist scripture of 260 Chinese characters that describes the experience of liberation from suffering of Avalokiteśvara, the Bodhisattva of Compassion. It was a memorable experience.

We met Master Cheng Yen, the founder of the Tzu Chi Foundation, at the corridor beside the canteen. She said, "You are all from Malaysia. One day you will all become great doctors. Use your heart." We felt very blessed. But I didn't understand what was the exact meaning of 'use your heart'.

In 2006, I joined Hospis Malaysia. During that period, I had my first glimpse of the vast amount of suffering people were going through at their end of life. I was completely unprepared to help them despite my 6 years of experience in medicine. What I learnt in medicine was when and how to treat, but not when and how to stop, and how to continue caring after stopping.

During a hospice home visit, I saw a dying patient lying on a mattress on the floor. She couldn't speak to me. She grabbed my right hand. Eyes fixed on me. I could see her suffering. I didn't say anything. She passed on while she was still holding my hand. It was a deep connection. Although I have seen and related well with many patients during my medical years, I have never felt as deep a connection as that time.

After 5 months in Hospis Malaysia, I went to National Cancer Centre, Singapore to learn palliative medicine under Professor Cynthia Goh, who is one of the pioneers of hospice and palliative care development in Singapore. She taught me many things. But what I remember most is her dedication and compassion towards patients. What I have learnt most from the fellowship is the delicate balance between giving and stopping treatment.

In 2008, I came back to Malaysia to work at University of Malaya Medical Centre. My colleague Dr Loh Ee Chin and I were recruited to set up a palliative care unit in the medical centre. I began writing The Little Handbook of Palliative Care to serve as a reference for myself. With time, the little handbook has become not so little as I added more and more details to it.

Since 2008, I started to have more time for myself. I began to invest more and more time in practicing mindfulness. My favourite book of mindfulness is Present Moment Wonderful Moment written by Vietnamese Zen Master Thich Nhat Hanh. The book contains many mindfulness verses that I use to incorporate mindfulness into my day-to-day life.

I also started to meditate after reading The Joy of Living from Yongey Mingyur Rinpoche. I noticed my stress level reduced to zero after months of meditation practices. I still have breakthrough stress once in a while but it quickly returns to zero once I am aware and once I stop sustaining it. I am able to regulate my stress and emotions much better.

Then, I realized that 'use your heart' means mindfulness. Master Cheng Yen planted the seeds of mindfulness in me during the brief encounter. The seeds grew only after more than a decade! It really has become an indispensable asset for me. Mindfulness protects me from being overwhelmed by the intense emotions in palliative care. It gives me a *psychological holiday*. This is why I never take leave due to exhaustion reasons.

The journey of my learning in medicine has been so: first, I learnt when and how to treat in medicine. Second, I learnt when and how to stop, and how to take care of patients after stopping treatment, a skill grossly deficient in most physicians or surgeons. Third, I learnt the delicate balance between giving and stopping treatment. Last but not least, I learnt how to take care of myself.

I have tried my best to summarize what palliative care is in this book. The sequence of the book is as follows, Part I: Introduction to Palliative Care, Part II and III: Symptom Control, Part IV: Management of Death and Dying, Part V: Psychosocial and Spiritual Care and Part VI: Self-Care.

I pray this book will help you in the alleviation of suffering of terminally ill patients and their family members; and introduce you to the wonderful practices of mindfulness in medicine.

Dr Tan Seng Beng
23rd August 2016

You are like a candle. Imagine you are sending light out around you. All your words, thoughts and actions are going in many directions. If you say something kind, your kind words go in many directions, and you yourself go with them.

Thich Nhat Hanh

True Love

Introduction

Love is the foundation of palliative care. Love is to bring happiness. We may be very good in relieving suffering of patients, but that is not enough. We need to be good in bringing happiness to patients too. Thich Nhat Hanh, a Vietnamese Zen Master described true love as following:

Being there

- Love is being there.
- Love is paying one hundred percent attention to our patients when we are with them.
- To be fully there, we may remind ourselves with the following thought: *Dear one, I am here for you.*
- When we are fully present, we feel real. Patients feel real. And life becomes real in the moment.
- This is the greatest gift we can give to our patients.

Recognizing the presence of others

- We can spend a lot of time with our patients, but if we are not recognizing their presence, we cannot bring happiness to them.
- The second thought can be: *Dear one, I know that you are there and it makes me very happy.*

Deep listening

- The next thing we can do is to listen deeply to our patients without judging them.
- As we listen, we do not say anything. We breathe deeply and open our heart to really listen.

- The third thought: *Dear one, I know you are suffering, that is why I am here to listen.*

Loving speech

- After listening to patients and understanding their situations, we speak in such a way that eases suffering and brings comfort.
- The fourth thought: *Dear one, I am aware that how unkind speech brings hurt and loving speech brings comfort. And I will be mindful of my speech.*

Little experiment

When you meet someone today, think to yourself "Dear one, I am here for you." And truly be there for the person.

Do not think that love, in order to be genuine, has to be extraordinary. What we need is to love without getting tired.

Mother Teresa

Dignity and the Essence of Medicine

Introduction

To reinstate kindness, humanity and respect in patient care, Professor Harvey Max Chochinov, a distinguished Professor of Psychiatry, introduced *ABCD of dignity conserving care*.

A=attitude

- Examine our attitude towards patients. Ask ourselves: How would I be feeling in this situation? Am I aware how my attitude may be affecting patients?
- Make a conscious effort in reflecting these questions in each individual patient.
- Discuss this during ward round and teaching. Make this discussion and teaching a culture within the healthcare setting.

B=behaviour

- Modify our behaviour by changing our attitude.
- Treat contact with patients as we would any important clinical intervention, with respect and kindness.

C=compassion

- Get exposed to human life and experiences by listening to patients' stories, reading novels and watching films on life experiences.
- Cultivate ways to show compassion, such as an understanding look, a gentle touch and communication that acknowledges patients' experiences.

D=dialogue

- Acknowledge the personhood beyond the illness.
- Get to know our patient as a person. Ask: What should I know about you as a person to help me take the best care of you that I can?

Little opinion

One of the key components in developing palliative care is education. Teaching medical students about the ABCD of dignity conserving care is as important as teaching them the ABC of resuscitation.

Palliative Care

Introduction

Palliative care comes from the Latin word pallium, which means a cloak. Palliative care can be likened to providing someone with a cloak when he or she is feeling cold.

Little story

I once gave a blanket to a leukemic patient who was feeling cold at the hematology daycare. He was very grateful and he often mentioned my name when he spoke to others. This led me to think that palliative care is a blanket in the modern setting. We are blanket providers.

WHO Definition of palliative care

Palliative care is an approach that

- *Improves quality of life* of patients and their families facing the problem associated with life-limiting illness
- Through the prevention and *relief of suffering* by means of early identification and impeccable assessment and treatment of pain and other problems, physical, psychosocial and spiritual

Explaining the term 'palliative care' to patients

- Palliative care is a specialized medical care provided by a team of specialists to improve quality of life of patients with serious illnesses through reducing pain and suffering.

Communication caution

Exercise caution while using terms like dying, terminal illnesses or life-threatening illnesses to avoid causing unnecessary distress to patients or their families.

Common conditions requiring palliative care

- Cancer
- Organ failure – heart, lung, liver, kidney
- Neurological conditions – motor neuron disease, Parkinson's disease, multiple sclerosis, stroke
- Geriatric conditions – dementia, frailty
- Human immunodeficiency virus infection
- Intensive care unit patients
- Paediatric illnesses

Important concepts of palliative care

- Palliative care is applicable early in the course of illness, in conjunction with other life-prolonging therapies.
- Palliative care is about helping patients to live.

You matter because you are you,
and you matter to the end of your life.
We will do all we can not only to help you die peacefully,
but also to live until you die.

Cicely Saunders

Little story

My colleague and I once brought a terminally ill child to ride LRT (Light Rail Transit). His wish was to ride a train because he used to stay beside a train station but never had a chance to ride one. We took him out for lunch and drove him to take the LRT from one station to another station. He enjoyed the trip a lot. And he passed away not long after the trip.

The Palliative Care Approach

Introduction

The palliative care approach is a vital part of *all clinical practice*, whatever the illness or its stage, informed by knowledge and practice of palliative care principles and supported by specialist palliative care. (NHS Executive 1996)

Palliative care principles

Palliative care principles should be practised by *all health care professionals*:

- Whole person approach
  - Seeing patient as a person
  - Focusing on quality of life
  - Respecting patient autonomy
  - Emphasizing good communication to patients
- Whole family approach
  - Extending care to family
  - Emphasizing good communication to family
- Whole team approach
  - Emphasizing team cooperation
  - Emphasizing caring of the whole team
  - Emphasizing good communication to colleagues
- Whole journey approach
  - Emphasizing care of the entire journey of illness
  - Emphasizing the practice of nonabandonment

Little summary

4 Ws – whole person, whole family, whole team, whole journey

Little reminder

As health care providers, if we are unable to alleviate the suffering of patients, at least we should not contribute to their suffering. Common suffering caused by health care providers are:

- Lack of attention
- Lack of listening
- Lack of empathy
- Lack of communication
- Lack of hope-giving

Remember, never say "There is nothing more can be done" or "There is no more hope".

Palliative Care Referral

Traditional model of palliative care

Curative or life-prolonging treatment	Palliative care

- The traditional practice is to refer palliative care when nothing more can be done to cure or treat the disease.
- This practice often results in increased suffering and late referral (time from referral to death < 2 months).

Integrated model of palliative care

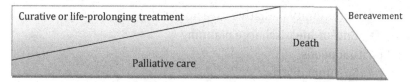

- The integrated model involves palliative care from the start of a life-limiting illness, concurrent with disease-directed care.
- This model is a key to successful patient care. It triggers early referral.
- This model is supported by:
  - World Health Organization (WHO)
  - National Comprehensive Cancer Network (NCCN)
  - American Society of Clinical Oncology (ASCO)
  - European Society for Medical Oncology (ESMO)
- One additional point to decide on referral is whether patient has palliative care needs or not.

Palliative care needs

- Screening question: Is the patient suffering?
- Physical needs
    - Unresolved physical symptoms
    - Complex functional needs
    - Complex nursing needs
- Psychological needs
    - Persistent psychological distress
    - Information needs
    - End-of-life decision-making
    - Advance care planning
- Social needs
    - Caregiver stress
    - Family conflict
    - Staff stress
    - Community palliative care needs
    - End-of-life discharge planning
- Spiritual needs
    - Spiritual distress
    - Existential distress
    - End-of-life discussion
    - End-of-life care
    - Grief and bereavement

Clinical evidence

Temel published a landmark article in New England Journal of Medicine at 2010 reporting improved quality of life and increased median survival of 2.7 months with early palliative care referral in patients with metastatic non-small cell lung cancer.

Palliative Care Assessment

Introduction

A palliative care assessment should focus on finding out the palliative care needs of patients and their family members instead of thinking about our own agenda, such as filling up certain assessment forms.

Physical assessment (symptoms)

- Open-ended questions
    - How are you doing?
    - Are you comfortable?
    - Are there any symptoms that are bothering you?
- Screen for common symptoms
    - Pain
    - Breathlessness
    - Nausea and vomiting
    - Fatigue
    - Constipation
    - Insomnia
- Detailed symptom assessment forms
    - Edmonton Symptom Assessment Scale (ESAS) (10 items) by Eduardo Bruera
    - M.D. Anderson Symptom Inventory (MDASI) (19 items) by Charles Cleeland
    - Memorial Symptom Assessment Scale (MSAS) (32 items) by Russell Portenoy

Physical assessment (functions)

- Open-ended questions
  - What are the things that you do in a day?
  - What are the things that you need help with?
- Screen for problems in performing important activities
  - Bathing
  - Grooming
  - Toileting
  - Ambulating
  - Feeding
  - Shopping
- Assess performance status
  - ECOG score by Oken and Zubrod
  - Barthel index by Mahoney and Barthel
  - Karnofsky Performance Scale by Karnofsky
  - Palliative Performance Scale by Anderson

ECOG (European Cooperative Oncology Group)

- ECOG 0 – asymptomatic
- ECOG 1 – symptomatic but completely ambulatory
- ECOG 2 – symptomatic and <50% in bed during the day
- ECOG 3 – symptomatic and >50% in bed, not bedbound
- ECOG 4 – bedbound
- ECOG 5 – death

Psychological assessment (emotions)

- Open-ended questions
    - How are you feeling today?
    - How are you affected by your emotions?
    - How do you deal with your emotions?
- Screen for distress
    - Distress Thermometer
        - Zero is no distress
        - Ten is extreme distress
- Assess coping mechanisms
    - Problem-focused coping
    - Emotion-focused coping
- Detailed assessment
    - Hospital Anxiety and Depression Scale (HADS) (14 items) by Zigmond and Snaith
    - Mental Adjustment to Cancer Scale (MAC) (40 items) by Watson and Greer
    - Courtauld Emotional Control Scale (CEC) (3 items) by Watson and Greer
    - Cancer Coping Questionnaire (21 items) by Moorey, Frampton and Greer

Psychological assessment (cognitions)

- Open-ended questions to explore ideas, concerns, expectations
    - Are you aware of what is going on?
    - What has the doctor told you about your illness?
    - What are your concerns?
    - What are you hopes?
    - What are your expectations?
- Detailed assessment
    - Cancer Concerns Checklist (14 items)
    - Herth Hope Index (12 items)

- Screen for delirium using Confusion Assessment Method (CAM)
  - Acute onset and fluctuating course
  - Inattention
  - Disorganized thinking
  - Altered level of consciousness

Social assessment (family and friends)

- Open-ended questions
  - Could you tell me about your family?
  - What about your friends?
- Explore
  - Home address for hospice referral
  - Social and cultural background
  - Main caregivers and decision maker
- Draw family tree (genogram)
- Arrange for family meeting
  - Assess family ideas, concerns and expectations
  - Explore caregiver stress and coping
  - Explore family dynamics

Spiritual assessment

- Open-ended questions
  - Could you tell me about your experience of illness?
  - Could you tell me a little about yourself?
  - What is important to you now?
  - How is your quality of life affected by your illness?
  - Could you tell me about your religion?
- Use FICA spiritual history tool
  - F = Tell me about your *faith*
  - I = What *importance* does your faith have in your life?
  - C = Are you part of a spiritual *community*?
  - A = How would you like me to *address* these issues?

- Quality of life assessment forms
  - Short Form 8 (SF-8)
  - Short Form 12 (SF-12)
  - Short Form 36 (SF-36)
  - WHO Quality of Life Assessment Form (WHOQOL)
  - Functional Assessment of Chronic Illness Therapy – Spiritual Well-being (FACIT-Sp-12)
  - European Organization for Research and Treatment of Cancer – Quality of Life Questionnaire (EORTC-QLQ-C30)
- Palliative care specific quality of life assessment forms
  - McGill Quality of Life Questionnaire (MQOL)
  - Health-related Quality of Life for the dying (HRQOL)
  - Missoula-VITAS Quality of Life Index
  - Schedule for the Evaluation of Individual Quality of Life (SEIQOL)

Peeling the onion

Assessing a palliative care patient can be seen like peeling an onion. The first layer is the physical layer. Second is psychological. Third is social. The innermost is the spiritual core. If patients feel that we care, they will be more willing to allow us to peel their deeper layers of difficulties and suffering. If not, we will only see their surfaces.

Little opinion

It is not uncommon for patients to express their frustration when they are being asked too many questions, especially so when they are already very tired. We may have our personal agendas like filling up certain assessment forms or exploration of psychosocial issues, but the most important thing is to find out what are the agendas of patients, not ours.

Pain Terms

Introduction

Pain is defined by IASP (International Association for the Study of Pain) as an unpleasant sensory and emotional experience associated with actual or potential tissue damage. It is a subjective experience. Margo McCaffrey, an American Pain Management Nurse described pain as what the person says it is.

Background pain

- Constant or continuous pain of long duration, $\geq 12h/day$ (Ferrell 1999)
- Also called basal pain, baseline pain or persistent pain
- Treated with around-the-clock (ATC) medication

Breakthrough pain

- A transitory exacerbation of pain experienced by the patient who has relatively stable and adequately controlled baseline pain (Portenoy 2004)
- Also called episodic pain, exacerbation of pain, pain flare, transient pain, transitory pain
- Treated with rescue medication

Types of breakthrough pain (Davis 2005)

- Spontaneous pain (idiopathic pain) – unexpected pain
- Incident pain (precipitated pain) – pain caused by movement
- End-of-dose failure – pain caused by declining analgesic level

Types of incident pain

- Volitional – eating, drinking, swallowing, walking, turning
- Non-volitional – coughing, sneezing, urinating, defecating
- Procedural – investigation (blood taking), therapeutic procedures (intravenous line insertion, wound dressing)

Pain terminology

- Nociceptive pain is pain transmitted through a normal nervous system
- Neuropathic pain is pain transmitted through a damaged nervous system
- Sensitization is increased responsiveness of neurons to their normal input
- Allodynia is pain due to a stimulus that does not normally provoke pain
- Hyperalgesia is increased pain from a stimulus that normally provokes pain
- Hyperpathia is a painful syndrome characterized by an abnormally painful reaction to a stimulus

I coined the term 'total pain,' from my understanding that dying people have physical, spiritual, psychological, and social pain that must be treated.

Cicely Saunders

Types of Pain

Introduction

Making an effort to differentiate nociceptive pain from neuropathic pain is important in pain management.

Types of pain

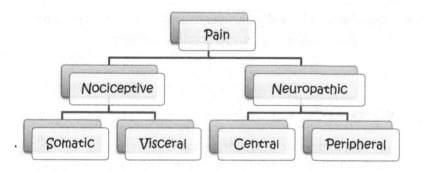

Frequency of cancer pain

- Mixed nociceptive-neuropathic – most common
- Nociceptive – second common
- Neuropathic – third common

Nociceptive pain (superficial somatic pain)

- Pain is usually superficial, sharp and well-localized
- Examples: superficial wound, small pressure sore, cellulitis, abscess, skin metastasis, mucositis and perianal excoriation

Nociceptive pain (deep somatic pain)

- Pain is deep, dull, aching and less well-localized
- Examples: deep wound, huge pressure sore, muscle spasm, chest wall infiltration, psoas infiltration, arthritis, acetabular syndrome, bone metastasis

Nociceptive pain (visceral pain)

- Pain is usually deep, dull and poorly localized
- Associated with referred pain in somatic sites distant from the lesion
- Examples: esophageal pain, liver capsular pain, pancreatic pain, biliary colic, bowel colic, ureteric colic, bladder pain

---

Examples of referred pain

- Left arm, upper interscapular pain (heart)
- Throat and upper abdominal pain (esophagus)
- Epigastric and lower interscapular pain (stomach)
- Back pain (pancreas)
- Right shoulder pain (liver and gallbladder)
- Supraumbilical pain (small bowel)
- Periumbilical pain (appendix)
- Infraumbilical (large bowel)
- Paraumbilical pain (ovary)
- Loin to groin pain (ureter)
- Suprapubic pain (bladder)

Neuropathic pain (central neuropathic pain)

- Pain can be burning, shooting, stabbing, crushing
- Examples: stroke (most common), Parkinson's disease, multiple sclerosis, syringomyelia and cord compression

Neuropathic pain (peripheral neuropathic pain)

- Pain can be burning, shooting, lancinating
- Pain can present as dysesthesia
- Examples: cranial neuropathy, brachial or lumbosacral plexopathy, radiculopathy, peripheral neuropathy (tumour infiltration, chemotherapy like cisplatin, oxaliplatin, vincristine, vinblastine, paclitaxel, thalidomide, post-radiotherapy, post-radical neck dissection, post-mastectomy, post-thoracotomy, post-herpetic neuralgia)

Interesting fact

The brain has no pain receptors. Brain metastasis itself does not cause pain. Headache from brain metastasis is due to pressure on surrounding nerves and blood vessels.

Pain Receptors

Introduction

Pain receptors (nociceptors) transduce noxious stimuli to electrical activities.

Location of nociceptors

- Cutaneous nociceptors are free nerve endings that end at stratum granulosum of epidermis.
- 5 layers of epidermis
    - Stratum corneum
    - Stratum lucidum
    - Stratum granulosum
    - Stratum spinosum
    - Stratum basale

Types of nociceptors (based on conduction)

- $A\delta$ fibers
    - Myelinated fibers
    - Fast conduction at 20m/s
    - Responsible for fast pain or first pain, which is sharp, brief, pricking and well-localized
    - Distributed over body surfaces, muscles and joints
- C fibers
    - Unmyelinated fibers
    - Slow conduction at 2m/s
    - Responsible for slow pain or second pain, which is dull, prolonged, aching, burning and poorly-localized
    - Distributed over most tissues, including visceral tissues, except the brain

Types of nociceptors (based on modalities)

- High threshold mechanoreceptors
    - Aδ fibers
    - Respond to mechanical stimuli only
- Polymodal nociceptors
    - C fibers
    - Respond to multiple modalities
- Silent nociceptors
    - Not respond to any stimuli but may be recruited during tissue injury

Types of nociceptors (based on stimuli)

- Noxious hot stimuli
    - TRPV1-4 (transient receptor potential vanilloid receptor)
- Noxious cold stimuli
    - TRPM8 (transient receptor potential melastatin receptor)
    - TRPA1 (transient receptor potential ankyrin receptor)
- Noxious mechanical stimuli
    - DEG (degenerin receptor)
    - DRASIC (dorsal root acid sensing ion channel receptor)
    - TWIK-1 (tandem pore domain weakly inward-rectifying K channel)
    - TREK-1 (tandem pore domain related K channel)
- Noxious chemical stimuli
    - TRPV1 (transient receptor potential vanilloid receptor)
    - P2X3 (purinoreceptor)
    - ASIC (acid sensing ion channel receptor)
    - DRASIC (dorsal root acid sensing ion channel receptor)

> **Interesting fact:** The spicy sensation of eating chilli is caused by the activation of vanilloid receptors (TRPV1). The pungent sensation of eating wasabi is caused by the activation of ankyrin receptors (TRPA1).

Primary Afferent Neurons

Introduction

Aδ fibers and C fibers are pseudounipolar neurons with cell bodies within dorsal root ganglions. They are primary afferent neurons (first order neurons) which synapse at dorsal horn of spinal cord.

Dorsal horn of spinal cord

- In early 1950s, Bror Rexed identified ten layers of grey matter at the spinal cord.
- They are labelled Rexed laminae I-X.
- The first six laminae are at the dorsal horn.
  - Marginal nucleus (lamina I)
  - Substantia gelatinosa of Rolando (lamina II)
  - Nucleus proprius (lamina III, IV and V)
  - Lamina VI

Synapses of primary afferent neurons

- Aδ fibers
  - Transmit fast pain messages
  - Synapse with second order neuron at lamina I and outer part of lamina II to form neospinothalamic tract
- C fibers
  - Transmit slow pain messages
  - Synapse with interneurons at inner part of lamina II which synapse with second order neurons at lamina V
  - Also synapse with dendrites of second order neurons extending from lamina V
  - Second order neurons form the paleospinothalamic tract

Neurotransmitters

Introduction

Neurotransmitters can be excitatory or inhibitory. The two types of excitatory neurotrasmitters for pain transmission are glutamate and substance P.

Glutamate

- Most common excitatory neurotransmitter
- Major neurotransmitter released from Aδ fibers
- Binds to glutamate receptor:
    - Ionotropic glutamate receptor
        - AMPA receptor
        - NMDA receptor
        - Kainate receptor (role undefined)
    - Metabotropic glutamate receptor

AMPA receptor (AMPAR)

- AMPA: α-amino-3-hydroxy-5-methyl-4-isoxazolepropionic acid
- GluR1, GluR2, GluR3 and GluR4 subunits
- Causes Na^{2+} influx with minimal K^+ efflux
- Generates excitatory post-synaptic potential (EPSP)
- Mediates fast synaptic transmission

NMDA receptor (NMDAR)

- NMDA: N-methyl-D-aspartate
- NR1 and NR2 subunits
- Sufficient depolarization by AMPAR removes Mg^{2+} which blocks the NMDAR
- Causes Na^{2+} and Ca^{2+} influx

- Ca^{2+} influx activates Ca^{2+}/calmodulin-dependent protein kinase II (CaMKII) and protein kinase C (PKC)
- Causes long-term potentiation (LTP) through modifying structure and number of synapses (synaptic plasticity)
- NMDAR also plays a role in glutamate excitotoxicity, where excess Ca^{2+} influx activates calcium-dependent proteases and lipases, degrading proteins and lipids, causing cell death

Metabotropic glutamate receptor

- mGluR1, mGluR2, mGluR3, mGluR4, mGluR5, mGluR6, mGluR7 and mGluR8 subunits
- G-protein-coupled receptor (GPCR)
- Activates phosphoinositol system postsynaptically and increases NMDAR activity or inhibits cyclic AMP system presynaptically and decreases NMDAR activity
- Modulates the activity of NMDAR and regulates neuron vulnerability to glutamate excitotoxicity

Substance P

- Tachykinin neuropeptide
- Major neurotransmitter released from C fibers
- Binds to neurokinin-1 receptor (NK-1), a GPCR which activates the phosphoinositol system
- Integrates pain, stress and anxiety

Little fact

NMDAR plays a crucial role in learning and memory formation.

Ascending Pain Pathways

Introduction

Pain pathway can be ascending or descending. Ascending pain pathways transmit pain impulses to cortex. Descending pain pathways modulate pain transmission.

Projection neurons (Second order neurons)

- Types of projection neurons
    - Nociceptive specific neurons
        - Respond to noxious stimuli only
    - Wide dynamic range neurons (WDR)
        - Respond to all sensory modalities
        - Important in wind-up phenomena
- Cross midline to form lateral and medial pain pathway

Lateral pain pathway (Neospinothalamic tract)

- Fast pain pathway
- Aδ fibers synapse with projection neurons at lamina I (marginal nucleus) and outer part of lamina II of dorsal horn
- Cross at anterior white commissure of spinal cord
- Ascend as lateral spinothalamic tract (LST)
- Synapse with third order neurons at ventral posterior lateral (VPL) and ventral posterior inferior (VPI) nuclei of lateral thalamus
- Third order neurons extend from lateral thalamus to primary somatosensory cortex (SI)
- Responsible for sensory-discriminatory component of pain, like location, intensity and quality

Medial pain pathway (Paleospinothalamic tract)

- Slow pain pathway
- C fibers synapse with interneurons at inner part of lamina II (substantia gelatinosa) of dorsal horn
- Interneurons synapse at lamina V
- Cross at anterior white commissure of spinal cord
- Ascend as anterior spinothalamic tract (AST)
- 1/10 of fibers synapse with third order neurons at intralaminar nuclei (parafascicular and centromedian PF-CM complex) of medial thalamus
- Third order neurons extend from medial thalamus to the whole cortex diffusely, notably secondary somatosensory cortex (SII), anterior cingulate cortex and insular cortex
- Responsible for affective-adversive component of pain, like negative emotions and unpleasantness
- Remaining fibers terminate at:
    - Tectum of midbrain (spinotectal tract): turning eyes, head, trunk toward sources of pain (visuospinal effect)
    - Periaqueductal gray of midbrain (spinomesencephalic tract): descending pain inhibition
    - Reticular formation (spinoreticular tract): arousal effect
        - From reticular formation to hypothalamus (spinohypothalamic tract): autonomic effects
        - From reticular formation to limbic system (spinolimbic tract): fear (amygdala)

Face and head

- Trigeminothalamic tract
    - Sends fast discriminative pain messages to ventral posterior medial nucleus (VPM) of lateral thalamus
    - Sends slow affective pain messages to intralaminar nuclei of medial thalamus and reticular formation

Descending Pain Pathways

Introduction

Descending pain pathways can be excitatory or inhibitory. Only inhibitory pathways or antinociceptive pathways are described here.

Reticular formation

- A polysynaptic network in brainstem
- Filters sensory information
- Antinociceptive neurons in reticular formation:
  - Serotonergic neurons
  - Noradrenergic neurons

Serotonergic pathways

- Periaqueductal gray matter (PAG) in midbrain sends excitatory projection to magnus raphe nucleus (MRN) in medulla.
- MRN descends bilaterally as raphespinal tract within the posterolateral tract of Lissauer to end in substantia gelatinosa at all levels of the spinal cord.
- Releases serotonin to excite inhibitory interneurons in dorsal horn – GABAergic and enkephalinergic
- Inhibitory interneurons inhibit pain transmission from first to second order neurons through inhibiting the transmission of impulse from excitatory interneurons to projection neurons of medial pain pathway, presynaptically or postsynaptically.
- This is called gating, which means the control of synaptic transmission from one set of neurons to the next.
- Inhibit slow pain pathway

GABAergic interneurons

- Release gamma-aminobutyric acid (GABA), which is the chief inhibitory neurotransmitter in CNS
- $GABA_A$ receptors – ionotropic receptors that generate inhibitory post-synaptic potentials by causing Cl^- influx
- $GABA_B$ receptors – metabotropic receptors or GPCRs that cause hyperpolarization indirectly by reducing cyclic AMP and directly by expelling K^+ through G-protein inwardly rectifying K^+ channels (GIRK channels)

Enkephalinergic interneurons

- Also called opiate interneurons
- Enkephalin, like endorphin, endomorphin, dynorphin and nociceptin, is an endogenous opioid. It acts on opioid receptor.
- Opioid receptors are GPCRs:
  - Inhibit neurotransmitter release by inhibiting N-type Ca^{2+} channels presynaptically
  - Inhibit adenylate cyclase presynaptically, causing reduction in cAMP and reduction in neurotransmitter release
  - Open voltage sensitive K^+ channels, causing K^+ efflux and postsynaptic hyperpolarization
- Three main opioid receptors – μ, δ and K
- The endogenous ligands of opioid receptors:
  - Enkephalins act on δ opioid receptors.
  - β-Endorphins act on μ and δ opioid receptors.
  - Endomorphins act on μ opioid receptors.
  - Dynorphins act on K receptors.
  - Nociceptins (Orphanin FQ) act on nociceptin receptors (NOP, ORL-1).

Noradrenergic pathways

- For the noradrenergic pathways, cerulean nucleus or locus ceruleus at the floor of fourth ventricle at upper pons descends bilaterally as ceruleospinal tract to end in dorsal horn to inhibit projection neurons of both medial and lateral pain pathways directly.
- Inhibit both fast and slow pain pathways

Differences between nociception and pain

Nociception refers to the processing and transmission of harmful messages to the brain in the form of electrical activities. Pain refers to the complex sensory, psychological, social and spiritual experiencing of such messages. Pain is often magnified by self-cherishing negative thoughts about 'I'. Examples:

- I feel bad.
- I do not want to feel bad.
- I am suffering.
- I do not want to live.

If we are able to remove these thoughts, pain may be reduced to pure nociception. Then we can say, "Nociception is inevitable. Pain is optional."

Miscellaneous Antinociceptive Pathways

Introduction

Apart from the descending pain pathways, pain can also be suppressed by the following pathways.

Tactile-induced analgesia

- Pain relief with rubbing the painful area and TENS
- Aβ fibers give off collaterals to GABA interneurons to inhibit excitatory interneurons which pass pain messages from C fibers to projection neurons

Diffuse noxious inhibitory controls

- Pain relief with acupuncture and pain elsewhere
- Pain elsewhere activates MRN via spinoreticular or trigeminoreticular tract, which in turn inhibits pain

Stress-induced analgesia

- Absence of pain awareness during fight and flight response
- Stress causes hypothalamus to release β-endorphins which disinhibit the inhibitory interneurons of PAG, activating the serotonergic pathways

Thalamic gating

- Serotonergic and noadrenergic afferents send projections to ventral and intralaminar nuclei of thalamus, gating pain transmission in thalamus

Interesting facts

In a study by Zeidan in 2011, practicing mindfulness meditation 20 minutes daily for 4 days reduced pain sensitivity.

fMRI findings:

- Deactivation of primary somatosensory cortex (SI) – sensory discrimination of pain
- Deactivation of thalamus – thalamic gate control of pain
- Activation of anterior cingulate cortex (ACC) – cognitive regulation of pain processing
- Activation of right anterior insula (AI) – interoceptive awareness
- Activation of bilateral orbitofrontal cortex (OFC) – emotional regulation of pain processing

Greatest activation of right AI and bilateral ACC correlates with greatest reduction in pain intensity. Greatest activation of bilateral OFC plus greatest deactivation of thalamus correlate with greatest reduction in pain unpleasantness.

Peripheral Sensitization

Introduction

Repetitive pain transmission can cause structural and functional changes in the neural system, sensitizing the pain pathways and making pain worse.

Pathophysiology

- Peripheral sensitization is caused by sensitization of nociceptors by inflammatory mediators released from damaged tissues and activated immune and inflammatory cells.
- Characterized by spontaneous pain, hyperalgesia and allodynia
- Spontaneous pain is caused by direct activation of specific receptors on nociceptor terminals by inflammatory mediators
- Hyperalgesia and allodynia are caused by:
    - Early post-translational changes of nociceptors
    - Later transcriptional-dependent changes in effector genes

Post-translational changes of nociceptors

- Inflammatory mediators activate intracellular signaling pathways
    - Protein kinase A (PKA)
    - Protein kinase C (PKC)
- Protein kinases phosphorylate membrane receptors
    - TRPV1 receptors
    - Tetrodotoxin-resistant sodium channels (TTXr)

Transcriptional-dependent changes of nociceptors

- Nerve growth factors (NGFs) play a key role
- NGFs bind tyrosine kinase A receptors (TrkA)
- NGF-TrkA complexes are internalized and transported from peripheral terminals to cell bodies of dorsal root ganglion
- Activate transcriptional factors
    - cAMP-responsive element-binding protein (CREB)
        - Also activated by CaMK via calcium influx
    - Mitogen-activated protein kinases (MAPK)
        - Extracellular signal-regulated kinases (ERK)
        - C-Jun N-terminal kinases (JNK)
        - P38 enzymes
- Increase TRPV1 and TTXr at peripheries
- Increase substance P, calcitonin gene-related peptide (CGRP) and brain-derived neurotrophic factor (BDNF) at synapses

---

Interesting facts

Tetrodotoxin is a potent sodium channel blocker produced by pufferfish. Ingestion causes paraesthesia of lips and tongue within 30 minutes, then face and extremities, followed by paralysis of voluntary muscles, including diaphragm, and even death.

Inflammatory Mediators

Introduction

The cardinal features of inflammation described by Aulus Cornelius Celcus, a Roman encyclopaedist, are pain (dolor), redness (rubor), heat (calor) and swelling (tumor). Various plasma-derived and cell-derived inflammatory mediators are involved in peripheral sensitization.

Plasma-derived mediators

- Kinin system (Bradykinin is involved in pain)
- Coagulation system (Thrombin is involved in pain)
- Fibrinolysis system
- Complement system

Cell-derived mediators

- Preformed mediators in secretory granules
  - Histamine
  - Serotonin
- Newly synthesized mediators
  - Eicosanoids
  - Cytokines
  - Nitric oxide

Miscellaneous mediators

- Protons
- Adenosine
- Glutamate
- Substance P
- Nerve growth factor

Bradykinin

- Produced by proteolytic cleavage of kininogen
- Activation of B1 receptors releases prostaglandins
- Activation of B2 receptors sensitizes TRPV1 via PKC

Thrombin

- Produced by proteolytic cleavage of prothrombin
- Activation of PAR1 (proteinase-activated receptors) releases histamine, substance P, calcitonin gene-related peptide (CGRP), cytokines

Histamine

- Released from mast cell by substance P, IL-1, CGRP and NGF
- Produces itch at low concentration
- Produces pain at high concentration
- Activation of H1 receptors increases Ca^{2+} influx and evokes release of neuropeptides and eicosanoids

Serotonin

- Released from platelets by platelet activating factor
- Activation of 5-HT1 receptors decreases K^+ permeability
- Activation of 5-HT2 receptors decreases K^+ permeability
- Activation of 5-HT3 receptors increases Na^+ influx
- Activation of 5-HT4 receptors sensitizes TTXr via PKA

Eicosanoids

- Step 1: Liberation of arachidonic acid from cell membranes by phospholipase A2 (inhibited by steroids)
- Step 2: Metabolism of arachidonic acid to prostaglandin by cyclooxygenase or to leukotriene by 5-lipooxygenase
- Activation of prostaglandin receptors (EP1) by prostaglandin E2 (PGE2) sensitizes TRPV1 via PKC

- Activation of prostaglandin receptors (IP) by prostacyclin (PGI2) sensitizes TTXr via PKA
- Activation of leukotriene B4 receptors (BLTR) by leukotriene B4 releases 8R, 15SdiHETE from leucocytes to sensitize nociceptors

Cytokines

- Polypeptides produced by lymphocytes and macrophages
- TNF-α, IL-1β and IL-6
- Release eicosanoids
- Increase expression of bradykinin and NGF receptors

Nitric oxide (Endothelium-derived relaxing factor EDRF)

- Released from endothelium
- Sensitizes TRPV1 and TRPA1 through S-nitrosylation

Protons

- Released from inflamed tissue
- Low pH sensitizes DRASIC/ASIC-3
- Low pH sensitizes TRPV1

Adenosine and ATP

- Released from inflamed tissue
- Activation of adenosine A2 receptors by adenosine decreases K^+ permeability
- Activation of purinergic receptors (P2X3) by ATP sensitizes nociceptors

Glutamate

- Presence of peripheral glutamate receptors (iGlu and mGlu)
- Role in peripheral sensitization

Substance P

- Released from C fibers
- Activation of NK1 increases prostaglandins

Nerve growth factor

- Produced by fibroblasts and mast cells
- Binds tyrosine kinase A receptor (TrkA)
- Sensitizes TRPV1
- Enhances release of substance P and CGRP
- Increases expression of TRPV1 and TTXr at peripheries
- Increases expression of substance P, CGRP, BDNF at synapses

---

Little story

I used to aspire to be a neurologist because I love to memorize facts and make difficult diagnoses. But I changed my mind to subspecialize in Palliative Medicine after joining Hospis Malaysia. I noticed the difference between being competent and being caring. The former emphasized knowledge, skills and efficiency (brain). The latter involved love, compassion and spending more time to comfort patients (heart). Both sets of values are important, but I was so moved by my experiences that I chose the latter. I followed my heart.

Intracellular Signaling Pathways

Introduction

Extracellular messages from inflammatory mediators (first messengers) may be propagated intracellularly by second messengers via various intracellular signaling pathways. These pathways include the cAMP pathway, the phosphoinositol pathway, the MAPK pathway and the JAK/STAT pathway.

The cAMP pathway

- Activation of GPCR by first messenger
- Release of G_α subunit to link with GTP
- Conversion of ATP to cAMP with adenylate cyclase
- cAMP is a second messenger
- Activation of protein kinase A (PKA) by cAMP
  - Phosphorylates ion channel
  - Phosphorylates protein
  - Activates transcription factor CREB

The phosphoinositol pathway

- Activation of GPCR by first messenger
- Release of G_α subunit to link with phospholipase C (PLC)
- PLC splits phosphatidylinositol 4, 5-biphosphate (PIP2), a membrane phospholipid, into diacylglycerol (DAG) and inositol 1, 4, 5-triphosphate (IP3)
- DAG and IP3 are second messengers
- Activation of protein kinase C by DAG
  - Phosphorylates ion channel
  - Phosphorylates protein
  - Activates transcription factor via MAPK

- IP3
  - Opens calcium channel
  - Releases Ca^{2+} from smooth endoplasmic reticulum
  - Binds calmodulin
  - Activates Ca^{2+}/calmodulin-dependent protein kinase
  - Activates transcription factor CREB

The MAPK pathway

- Activation of tyrosine kinase receptor by growth factor
- Activation of GTP-binding protein Ras
- Ras-GTP is a second messenger
- Interaction with Raf protein kinase (MAP kinase kinase kinase)
- Raf phosphorylates MEK (MAP kinase kinase)
- MEK phosphorylates ERK (MAP kinase)
- ERK phosphorylates transcription factors
  - C-Myc
  - Elk-1
  - C-Fos
  - C-Jun
- ERK also phosphorylates transcription factor CREB via Rsk2 activation

The JAK/STAT pathway

- Activation of cytokine receptor by cytokine
- Activation of Janus kinase (JAK)
- Activation of signal transducer and activator of transcription (STAT) proteins
- Translocation to nucleus
- Stimulation of transcription of target genes
- No second messenger

Central Sensitization

Introduction

Peripheral sensitization mediates pain hypersensitivity at the injured site (primary hyperalgesia). It continues as long as the peripheral pathology is present. Central sensitization mediates pain hypersensitivity at the uninjured site surrounding the injury (secondary hyperalgesia). It continues even if the peripheral pathology is no longer present.

Pathophysiology

- Central sensitization is caused by sensitization of spinal neurons by neurotransmitters released from C fibers
- Characterized by secondary hyperalgesia and allodynia
- Secondary hyperalgesia and allodynia are caused by:
  - Early post-translational changes of spinal neurons
  - Later transcriptional-dependent changes of spinal neurons

Post-translational changes of spinal neurons

- Repetitive activation of C fibers causes temporal summation of second pain (TSSP), resulting in wind-up phenomena
  - TTSP: each 'second pain' of C fibers becomes stronger and spreads outside the area of injury
  - Wind-up phenomena: like tightening the spring
- Release of neurotransmitters from C fibers
  - Glutamate binds AMPAR – depolarization, Na^+ influx
  - Glutamate binds group I mGluR – activates PKC
  - Substance P binds NK1 – activates PKA and PKC
  - CGRP binds CGRP1 – activates PKA and PKC

- Brain-derived neurotrophic factor (BDNF) binds tyrosine kinase B receptor (TrkB) – activates PKC
- Activation of NMDAR
  - Key step in central sensitization
  - NMDAR is blocked by Mg^{2+} under normal condition
  - Sustained release of glutamate and neuropeptides leads to sufficient depolarization that removes Mg^{2+} block, activating NMDAR
  - Na^+ and Ca^{2+} influx
- Increase in intracellular Ca^{2+}
  - Caused by:
    - Ca^{2+} influx through NMDARs (predominant)
    - Ca^{2+} influx through calcium-permeable AMPARs
    - Ca^{2+} influx through voltage-gated calcium channels
    - Ca^{2+} release from endoplasmic reticulum in response to mGluR-NMDAR coupling (IP3-mediated)
  - Activates protein kinases
    - Calcium/calmodulin-dependent protein kinase II (CaMKII)
    - Protein kinase C (PKC)
    - Mitogen-activated protein kinase/extracellular-signal-regulated kinase (MAPK/ERK) via PKC
- Activated protein kinases
  - Phosphorylate membrane AMPARs and NMDARs
    - PKA (via neuropeptides)
    - PKC
    - CaMKII
    - MAPK
  - Recruit AMPARs to membrane
    - PKA (via neuropeptides)
    - CaMKII
    - MAPK

- Result in increased neuronal excitability

Transcriptional-dependent changes of spinal neurons

- Activated protein kinase MAPK
    - Phosphorylates transcription factors
        - cAMP response element binding (CREB)
        - ELK-1
    - Causes genes transcription
        - Immediate-early genes (IEG)
            - c-Fos
            - Cox-2 – produces prostaglandin for neural and glial cell plasticity (apoptosis, axonal sprouting, new afferent connections)
        - Late-response genes
            - NK1
            - TrkB
            - Dynorphin – increases neuronal excitability
    - Results in increased protein production
        - Synaptic plasticity
            - Modification of structure of synapses
            - Modification of number of synapses
        - Sustained neuronal excitability

Interesting theory

Hebbian theory: Cells that fire together, wire together. Cells that fire out of sync, lose their link.

Pain Assessment

Introduction

A comprehensive pain assessment involves taking a detailed history, performing a targeted examination and ordering relevant investigations.

History taking

- Open-ended question: Could you tell me about your pain?
- Mnemonic: SOCRATES
  - S = Site
  - O = Onset
  - C = Character
  - R = Radiation
  - A = Associated symptoms
  - T = Time
  - E = Exacerbating and relieving factors
  - S = Severity

Determining the type of pain

- Nociceptive pain (superficial somatic pain)
  - Described as superficial, sharp, burning, cutting, pricking, tingling and stabbing pain
  - Well-localized around injured tissues
- Nociceptive pain (deep somatic pain)
  - Described as deep, dull, cramping, aching, throbbing, boring, and crushing pain
  - Less well-localized around injured tissues

- Nociceptive pain (visceral pain)
  - Described as vague, dull, aching, cramping, squeezing, gnawing and pressure pain
  - Poorly-localized in relation to affected organ
  - Presence of referred pain remote from the location of the affected organ
  - Presence of visceral hyperalgesia with pain during normal functioning of affected organ
- Neuropathic pain
  - Described as constant, burning, tingling and numbing in dysesthetic pain
  - Described as episodic, electric-like, shooting, stabbing, lancinating and jabbing in lancinating pain
  - Localized to area innervated by damaged nerves
  - Presence of central sensitization with persistent pain, hyperalgesia and allodynia
  - Presence of neurological symptoms like anaesthesia, paraesthesia, dysesthesia and paralysis

Determining the cause of pain

- Cancer-related pain
  - Bone pain syndromes (most common)
    - Head: skull metastases
    - Chest: rib metastases
    - Back: vertebral metastases
    - Pelvis: acetabular metastases
    - Limbs: pathological fracture
  - Visceral pain syndromes (second common)
    - Head: brain metastases
    - Chest: mediastinal metastases
    - Abdomen: liver metastases, peritoneal metastases, bowel obstruction, ureteric obstruction

- Back: pancreatic cancer, retroperitoneal infiltration
- Pelvis: gynaecological cancer, bladder spasm, rectal spasm, perineal pain
- Neuropathic pain syndromes (third common)
  - Head: leptomeningeal metastases, cranial neuralgias
  - Chest: brachial plexopathy, intercostal neuropathy
  - Abdomen: celiac plexopathy
  - Back: spinal cord compression, radiculopathy
  - Pelvis: lumbosacral plexopathy
  - Limbs: peripheral neuropathy
- Treatment-related pain
  - Chemotherapy-related pain
    - Chemotherapy-induced headache
      - Intrathecal methotrexate meningitic syndrome
      - L-asparaginase-related dural sinus thrombosis
      - Trans-retinoic acid headache
    - Chemotherapy mucositis
    - 5-Fluorouracil-induced angina
    - Post-chemotherapy gynaecomastia
    - Hormonal therapy pain flare
    - Interferon-induced pain
    - Diffuse bone pain from trans-retinoic acid or colony stimulating factor
    - Steroid pseudorheumatism
    - Intravenous steroid-induced perineal discomfort
    - Peripheral neuropathy
    - Intravenous infusion pain
    - Hand-foot syndrome
  - Radiotherapy-related pain
    - Radiation mucositis
    - Radiation brachial plexopathy
    - Radiation enteritis

- Radiation myelopathy
- Radiation cystitis
- Radiation proctitis
- Avascular necrosis
- Surgery-related pain
  - Post-radical neck dissection pain
  - Post-mastectomy pain
  - Post-thoracotomy pain
  - Phantom pain
    - Phantom breast pain
    - Phantom bladder pain
    - Phantom anus pain
    - Phantom limb pain

Determining the pattern of pain

- Background and breaktrough pain
- Fluctuation in location, severity and quality
- Frequency of breakthrough pain
- Aggravating and relieving factors
- Analgesic history, including pain score pre and post-analgesia

Determining the impact of pain

- Activities of daily living
- Instrumental activities
- Leisure activities

Determining the perception of pain

- Ideas, concerns and expectations regarding pain
- Ideas, concerns and expectations regarding analgesia
- Ideas, concerns and expectations of family members
- Associated emotions
- Pain and suffering

Bone Pain Syndromes

Introduction

Cancer-induced bone pain has a nociceptive component caused by skeletal remodelling and inflammatory mediators; and a neuropathic component caused by damage to sensory and sympathetic nerves together with pathological sprouting. Bone pain syndromes caused by skull metastases, rib metastases, vertebral metastases and acetabular metastases will be discussed.

Skull metastases

- Orbital syndrome
    - Metastasis to bony orbit
    - Unilateral supraorbital pain
    - Dull, continuous and progressive
    - Associated features (ipsilateral)
        - Proptosis, chemosis, papilloedema
        - Complete ophthalmoplegia (III, IV, VI)
        - Reduced sensation of V1
- Parasellar syndrome
    - Also called sphenocavernous syndrome
    - Metastasis to petrous apex or sella turcica with secondary extension to cavernous sinus
    - Unilateral frontal pain
    - Dull, continuous and progressive
    - Associated features (ipsilateral)
        - Proptosis, chemosis, papilloedema
        - Hemianopia or quadrantanopia
        - Complete ophthalmoplegia (III, IV, VI)
        - Reduced sensation of V1 and V2

- Middle fossa syndrome
  - Also called Gasserion ganglion syndrome
  - Metastasis to middle fossa
  - Unilateral facial pain
  - Dull, continuous and progressive
  - May have lancinating facial pain (trigeminal neuralgia)
  - Associated features (ipsilateral)
    - Reduced sensation of V2 and V3
    - Weakness of pterygoids and masseters muscles
- Jugular foramen syndrome
  - Metastasis to jugular foramen
  - Unilateral occipital or postauricular headache
  - Exacerbated by movement
  - May have lancinating throat pain (glossopharyngeal neuralgia)
  - Associated features (ipsilateral)
    - Horner's syndrome
    - Hoarseness and dysphagia (IX, X)
    - Neck weakness (XI)
    - Syncope
- Occipital condyle syndrome
  - Metastasis to occipital condyle
  - Unilateral occipital headache or neck pain
  - Exacerbated by neck flexion and rotation
  - Severe, continuous and progressive
  - Associated features (ipsilateral)
    - Neck stiffness
    - Dysarthria and dysphagia due to tongue paresis (XII)
- Clivus syndrome
  - Metastasis to clivus (front of foramen magnum)
  - Vertex headache
  - Exacerbated by neck flexion

- Associated features (ipsilateral, then bilateral)
    - Diplopia (VI)
    - Facial weakness (VII)
    - Hoarseness, dysarthria and dysphagia (IX, X)
    - Neck weakness (XI)
    - Tongue weakness (XII)
- Sphenoid sinus syndrome
    - Metastasis to sphenoid sinus
    - Bifrontal headache and retroorbital pain
    - Radiating to temporal regions
    - Associated features
        - Nasal stuffiness
        - Diplopia (unilateral or bilateral VI)

Rib metastases

- Rib metastasis – no pain or mild pain
- Rib fracture – transient severe chest pain triggered by:
    - Trunk movement (bending, lateral bending and twisting) due to attachment of abdominal muscles to lower ribs
    - Deep breathing
    - Coughing
    - Laughing

Vertebral body syndromes

- Odontoid process syndrome
    - Severe neck pain
    - Radiating to occiput and vertex
    - Exacerbated by neck flexion
    - Progressive sensory and motor involvement beginning in upper limbs

- C7-T1 syndrome
  - Dull lower neck pain
  - Radiating to shoulders and interscapular area
  - May have C7-T1 radicular pain
  - May have C7-T1 percussion tenderness
  - Associated with Horner's syndrome
- T12-L1 syndrome
  - Dull midback pain
  - Radiating anteriorly causing a girdle-like band or to both paraspinal and lumbosacral areas
  - Exacerbated by lying or sitting but relieved by standing
  - May have referred pain to sacroiliac joint and iliac crest
  - May have T12-L1 radicular pain
- Sacral syndrome
  - Localized severe low back pain or coccygeal pain
  - Radiating to buttocks, perineum or posterior thigh
  - Exacerbated by lying or sitting but relieved by walking
  - Lateral extension causes incident hip pain
  - Perianal sensory loss ± bladder and bowel dysfunction
  - May cause impotence

Acetabular or head of femur metastases

- Also called hip joint syndrome
- Localized hip pain
- Radiation to medial thigh or knee
- Exacerbated by hip movement and weight bearing
- May have lumbosacral plexopathic pain from medial extension

Visceral Pain Syndromes

Introduction

Visceral afferents from thoracic and abdominal organs utilize autonomic pathways to reach the central nervous system.

Visceral pain pathways

- Vagal pathway
    - Vagal afferents with cell bodies in nodose ganglion
    - Project to nucleus tractus solitarius
    - Project to thalamus, hypothalamus and limbic system
- Spinal pathway
    - Spinal afferents with cell bodies in dorsal root ganglion
    - Travel alongside:
        - Sympathetic efferents
            - Thoracic splanchnic nerves
                - Greater splanchnic nerve
                - Lesser splanchnic nerve
                - Least splanchnic nerve
            - Lumbar splanchnic nerves
            - Sacral splanchnic nerves
        - Parasympathetic efferents
            - Pelvic splanchnic nerves
    - Terminate in dorsal horn
    - Project to higher centers through:
        - Dorsal column pathways
        - Spinothalamic tracts
        - Spinoparabrachial tracts

Liver metastases

- Innervation of liver capsule (Glisson's capsule)
    - Lower intercostal nerves
    - Phrenicoabdominal branches of phrenic nerve
- Innervation of liver parenchyma
    - Hepatic plexus
        - Sympathetic nerves (from celiac plexus)
        - Parasympathetic nerves (from vagus nerve)
- Liver capsular pain
    - Dull, continuous, aching right hypochondrial pain
    - Exacerbated by movement, pressure and deep inspiration
    - Associated with nausea and anorexia
    - Caused by:
        - Stretching of liver capsule
        - Intrahepatic bleeding
            - Rapidly increasing pain
        - Traction of coronary and falciform ligaments
            - Standing pain
            - Walking pain
        - Distension and compression of biliary tract vessles
        - Diaphragmatic irritation
            - Referred pain to right shoulder, neck, scapula
- Other causes of pain
    - Outward pressure on rib cage
        - Bilateral lower rib cage pain
    - Pinching parietal peritoneum against rib cage
        - Intermittent sharp right hypochondrial pain
    - Pinching abdominal wall
        - Abdominal pain
    - Straining of lumbar spine
        - Back pain

Pancreatic cancer

- Innervation of pancreas
    - Sympathetic (Celiac plexus)
        - Greater splanchnic nerves
    - Parasympathetic (Vagus nerves)
- Pancreatic pain
    - Dull, continuous aching epigastric pain
    - Exacerbated by lying down
    - Eased by bending forward
    - Worse at night
    - Localization of pain
        - Head of pancreas
            - Pain at right of epigastrium
            - Mediated by right splanchnic nerves
            - Associated with jaundice
            - Associated with small bowel obstruction
                - Pain after eating
            - Tumour compression of portal vessels
                - Acute right hypochondrial pain
        - Body of pancreas
            - Pain at mid epigastrium
            - Mediated by bilateral splanchnic nerves
        - Tail of pancreas
            - Pain at left of epigastrium and left upper back
            - Mediated by left splanchnic nerves
    - Radiation of pain to the back
        - Invasion of celiac plexus
        - Similar to midline retroperitoneal syndrome
        - Positive retroperitoneal stretch compared to pain from spinal cord compression

Peritoneal metastases

- Innervation of parietal peritoneum
  - Somatic nerves
  - Anterior abdominal wall
    - Lower six thoracic nerves
    - First lumbar nerves
  - Diaphragmatic peritoneum
    - Lower six thoracic nerves – peripheral
    - Phrenic nerves – central
  - Pelvic peritoneum
    - Obturator nerves (branch of lumbar plexus)
- Innervation of visceral peritoneum
  - Same visceral nerve as the viscera it invests
- Peritoneal pain
  - Pathology of parietal peritoneum
    - Somatic pain
    - Well-localized
    - Lateralized
  - Pathology of visceral peritoneum
    - Visceral pain
    - Poorly localized
    - Midline
    - Associated with referred pain
      - Foregut – epigastrium
      - Midgut – umbilicus
      - Hindgut – suprapubic
- Other causes of pain
  - Ascites – stretching pain
  - Malignant adhesion – colicky pain
  - Malignant bowel obstruction – colicky pain
  - Mesenteric tethering – diffuse abdominal pain or low back pain

Malignant bowel obstruction

- Innervation of gut
  - Foregut (esophagus to duodenum)
    - Sympathetic (Celiac plexus)
      - Greater splanchnic nerves
    - Parasympathetic (Vagus nerves)
  - Midgut (duodenum to proximal 2/3 transverse colon)
    - Sympathetic (Superior mesenteric plexus)
      - Lesser splanchnic nerves
      - Least splanchnic nerves
    - Parasympathetic (Vagus nerves)
  - Hindgut (distal 1/3 transverse colon to anus)
    - Sympathetic (Inferior mesenteric plexus)
      - Lumbar splanchnic nerves
    - Parasympathetic (Pelvic splanchnic nerves)
- Constant pain
  - Abdominal distension
  - Bowel compression by tumour
  - Bowel wall ischemia
  - Mesenteric tension
- Colicky pain
  - Bowel contractions
    - Small bowel obstruction
      - Early onset
      - Periumbilical
      - Intense
      - Short intervals
    - Large bowel obstruction
      - Late
      - Peripheral
      - Less intense
      - Longer intervals

Malignant ureteral obstruction

- Innervation of ureters
    - Ureteric plexus
        - Renal plexus – upper part
        - Superior hypogastric plexus – middle part
        - Inferior hypogastric plexus – lower part
- Usually asymptomatic and detected on imaging
- May present with ureteric colic
    - Unilateral loin pain
    - Radiating to the groin
    - Exacerbated by standing
    - Partially relieved by sitting
    - Colicky breakthrough pain may be induced by:
        - Urination
        - Defecation

Pelvic cancers

- Innervation of pelvic organs
    - Branches of inferior hypogastric plexus
        - Uterus (Uterovaginal plexus)
        - Bladder (Vesical plexus)
        - Prostate (Prostatic plexus)
        - Rectum (Rectal plexus)
    - Inferior hypogastric plexus
        - Sympathetic (Superior hypogastric plexus)
            - Thoracic splanchnic nerves
            - Lumbar splanchnic nerves
        - Sympathetic (Sacral splanchnic nerves)
        - Parasympathetic (Pelvic splanchnic nerves)
- Causes of pain
    - Ovarian mass
        - Paraumbilical pain

- Bladder or uterine mass
  - Suprapubic pain
- Rectal mass
  - Pain on sitting
  - Mild pressure or severe pain till cannot sit down
- Deeper rectal mass with myofascial infiltration
  - No pain on sitting
  - Increasingly severe dragging pain on standing for a few minutes or walking 50-100m
- Lateral pelvic wall invasion
  - Obturator internus muscle infiltration
    - Unilateral iliac fossa pain
  - Iliopsoas muscle infiltration
    - Painful fixed flexion of the hip
    - Exacerbation of pain by passive hip extension (positive psoas test)
    - Pain exacerbated by walking
    - May be bedridden because of pain on walking
- Posterior pelvic wall invasion (presacral mass)
  - Piriformis and coccygeus muscles infiltration
    - Unilateral buttock pain
    - Radiating to posterior thigh (sciatic nerve)
  - Lumbosacral plexopathy
  - Sacral plexopathy
  - T12-L1 syndrome
  - Sacral syndrome

Malignant perineal pain

- Anatomical boundaries of perineum
  - Superior – pelvic diaphragm
  - Anterior – pubic symphysis
  - Posterior – coccyx

- Lateral – inferior pubic rami, inferior ischial rami
- Contents of perineum
  - Urogenital triangle – distal urethra, external genitalia
  - Anal triangle – distal rectum, anus
- Innervation of perineum
  - Visceral nerves (Follow parasympathetic nerves)
    - Sacral nerves (S2, S3, S4)
    - Travel with pelvic splanchnic nerves to inferior hypogastric plexus
    - Supply rectum and upper 2/3 anal canal
  - Visceral nerves (Follow sympathetic nerves)
    - Ganglion impar
    - Supply distal urethra, vagina and rectum; vulva, anus, coccyx and perineum
  - Somatic nerves (Pudendal nerves)
    - Inferior rectal nerve
      - External anal sphincter
      - Lower 1/3 anal canal
    - Perineal nerve
      - Urogenital diaphragm
      - External urethral sphincter
      - External genitalia
    - Dorsal nerve of penis or clitoris
      - Penis (male)
      - Clitoris (female)
- Vague, poorly localized, constant aching pain
- Exacerbated by sitting and standing
- Associated with bladder or rectal tenesmus

Neuropathic Pain Syndromes

Introduction

Neuropathic pain is pain caused by damage to the nervous system. It is mediated by a combination of peripheral and central mechanisms.

Mechanisms of neuropathic pain

- Peripheral sensitization
  - Abnormal ion channel expression
    - Increase in TTXs Na expression
      - Type III TTXs Na channel – NGF-dependent
    - Decrease in TTXr Na expression
      - SNS TTXr Na channel – NGF-dependent
      - NaN TTXr Na channel – GDNF-dependent
    - Translocation of SNS from cell body to neuroma
    - Altered N-type Ca channel expression
    - Decrease in K channel expression
  - Upregulation of nociceptors
    - TRPV1
    - P2X3
  - Neuronal hyperexcitability
    - From abnormal ion channel expression
    - Causes ectopic discharges – spontaneous firing
    - Causes ephaptic conduction – cross-excitation
  - Sprouting of primary afferents into skin – NGF-dependent
  - Coupling between sympathetic and sensory nerves
    - Peripheral sensitization from sympathetic nerves
    - Cross-excitation from sympathetic nerves
    - Sympathetic sprouting into DRG – NGF-dependent

- Central sensitization
  - Spinal cord hyperexcitability
    - Activation of NMDAR
      - Removal of Mg^{2+} block
      - NMDAR phoshorylation
    - Spinal cord reorganization
      - Aβ fibers sprouting into lamina II – NGF-dependent
    - Cortical reorganization
    - Changes in inhibitory pathways

Leptomeningeal metastases

- Meningeal irritation
  - Severe, intractable headache
  - Associated with:
    - Photophobia
    - Nuchal rigidity
    - Nausea and vomiting
- Cerebral involvement
  - Headache
  - Confusion
  - Memory loss
  - Lethargy
  - Behavioural changes
  - Gait disturbances
  - Incontinence
  - Seizures
- Cranial nerve involvement
  - Diplopia – III, IV, VI
  - Facial pain (resembling cluster headache), numbness – V
  - Facial weakness – VII
  - Hearing loss and vertigo – VIII
  - Glossopharyngeal neuralgia – IX

- Spinal nerve root involvement
    - Nuchal rigidity
    - Neck pain
    - Back and radicular pain
    - Weakness and paraesthesia of lower extremities
    - Bowel and bladder dysfunction

Tumour infiltration of cervical plexus

- Cervical plexus
    - Formed from ventral rami of C1-C4
- Severe, deep, constant, boring pain localized to the neck
    - Anterior neck pain – transverse cervical nerves
    - Periauricular pain – great auricular nerve
    - Occipital scalp pain – lesser occipital nerve
    - Shoulder pain – supraclavicular nerve
- May referred to throat, shoulder, face and head
    - Overlap of innervations from cranial nerve V, VII, IX, X
- May have intermittent sharp component or causalgic features
- Exacerbated by neck movement, swallowing, coughing
- Associated with:
    - Horner's syndrome – superior cervical ganglion
    - Dyspnoea – paralyzed hemidiaphragm (phrenic nerve)
    - Shoulder weakness – spinal accessory nerve
    - Head tilt – sternocleidomastoid
- Complication
    - Sharp, severe pain on neck movement
        - Cervical spine involvement
        - Impending epidural extension

Tumour infiltration of brachial plexus

- Brachial plexus
    - Formed from ventral rami of C5-T1
- Lower brachial plexopathy (C8-T1)
    - Tumour infiltrates plexus from below due to anatomy
        - Pancoast syndrome
        - Breast cancer
    - Dull, aching shoulder pain
        - Axillary pain
            - T2 involvement
            - Intercostobrachial nerve
            - Not part of brachial plexus
            - May be the first nerve affected
            - Axilla, anterior chest, medial upper arm pain
        - Pain over medial aspects of arm, elbow and forearm
            - T1 involvement
            - Freezing sensation and hypersensitivity along medial aspect of arm
            - Lancinating pain over elbow
            - Cramp-like, crushing pain over forearm
        - Burning, dysesthetic pain of 4th and 5th fingers
            - C8 involvement
    - Associated with weakness:
        - Small muscles of hand (T1)
        - Finger gripping (C6, C7, C8)
        - Wrist flexion (C6, C7)
        - Wrist extension (C7, C8)
        - Elbow extension (C7, C8)
    - Complication
        - Suspect epidural extension
            - Horner's syndrome
            - Weakness of serratus anterior or rhomboid

- Upper brachial plexopathy (C5-C6)
  - Primary brachial plexus tumour
    - Neurofibromas
    - Schwannomas
  - Breast cancer with supraclavicular node
  - Dull, aching shoulder pain
    - Pain over lateral aspects of arm, elbow and forearm
      - C5 involvement
    - Pain over tips of thumb and 2nd finger
      - C6 involvement
  - Associated with weakness:
    - Shoulder abduction (C5)
    - Elbow flexion (C5, C6)
    - Wrist flexion (C6, C7)
    - Finger gripping (C6, C7, C8)
  - Presence of myokimia on EMG suggests radiation fibrosis rather than tumour infiltration
- Pan brachial plexopathy (C5-T1)
  - Progression from lower plexus infiltration
  - Pain can progress to complex regional pain syndrome
  - Neurological dysfunction can spread from lower to upper plexus, leading to paralysis of entire upper limb
  - Associated with lymphoedema in late stage

Tumour infiltration of lumbosacral plexus

- Lumbosacral plexus
  - Lumbar plexus
    - Formed from ventral rami of L1-L4
    - Received T12 contribution
  - Sacral plexus
    - Formed from ventral rami of S1-S4
    - Received L4-L5 contribution via lumbosacral trunk

- Lower lumbosacral plexopathy (L4-S1)
    - Dull, aching back pain near iliac crest
    - Radiating to buttock and posterior thigh and leg
    - Causes footdrop
    - Associated with weakness:
        - Ankle dorsiflexion (L4, L5), plantar flexion (S1, S2)
        - Knee flexion: hamstrings (L5, S1)
        - Hip abduction (L5, S1), adduction (L3, L4)
    - Associated with:
        - Positive straight leg raising test
        - Absent ankle jerk
        - Sensory loss over posterior thigh and sole
        - Rectal mass
        - Sphincter weakness
- Upper lumbosacral plexopathy (L1-L4)
    - Dull, aching back pain near costovertebral angle
    - Radiating to groin and anteromedial thigh
    - Causes difficulty in climbing stairs
    - Associated with weakness:
        - Hip flexion: iliopsoas (L2, L3, L4)
        - Knee extension: quadriceps (L2, L3, L4)
        - Hip adduction (L3, L4)
    - Associated with:
        - Positive psoas test
        - Absent knee jerk
        - Sensory loss over anterior thigh
- Pan lumbosacral plexopathy (L1-S3)
    - Dull aching back pain
    - Radiating to anterior and posterior thigh and leg
    - Exacerbated by sudden movement or lying supine
    - Relieved by standing and walking (compared to pelvic metastases)

Painful peripheral neuropathies

- Mononeuropathy
    - Nerve compression from bone metastases
        - Ulnar nerve – elbow
        - Radial nerve – humerus
        - Intercostal nerve – ribs
        - Obturator nerve – obturator canal
        - Sciatic nerve – pelvis
        - Peroneal nerve – fibula
    - Entrapment neuropathy from lymphedema
        - Carpal tunnel syndrome
    - Rarely nerve metastasis from breast cancer or melanoma
    - Pain, then sensory and motor loss over distribution of involved nerve
    - Palpable mass compressing the nerve
    - Radiating paraesthesia when nerve is percussed near site of involvement
- Polyneuropathy
    - Chemotherapy-induced polyneuropathies
    - Paraneoplastic polyneuropathies
        - Sensory neuropathy from dorsal root ganglionitis
        - Sensorimotor neuropathy
        - Guillain-Barré syndrome (Rarely)
    - Direct invasion of multiple nerves
        - Lymphomas
        - Leukemias
    - Burning paraesthesias
    - Tingling sensation in the extremities
    - Occasional lancinating and lightning pain
    - May associated with:
        - Sensory ataxia
        - Distal weakness

Pain from Spinal Cord Compression

Introduction

Pain from spinal cord compression could be somatic, visceral or neuropathic.

Somatic pain

- Deep somatic pain from mechanical instability
    - Causes: damaged ligaments or bone fractures
    - Bilateral non-radicular back pain
    - With or without radiation
    - Radiation to buttocks, upper thighs, inguinal, abductors
    - Radiation not below the knees
    - Exacerbated by movement: catch sensation on movement
    - When pain is extreme, patient remains absolutely still
    - Not exacerbated by coughing and straining
    - Full range of spine movement
    - Absence of root tension signs
- Deep somatic pain from muscle spasm
    - Causes: hyperactive stretch reflexes and cutaneomuscular reflexes in spastic muscle groups
    - Triggers: stretching a muscle or stimulating the body below the level of injury
    - Sometimes putting on trousers is enough to produce spasm of the hip and knee flexors
    - Relieved by daily range of motion exercise and treatment of muscle spasm
    - Associated with autonomic effects: sweating, increased blood pressure and urinary incontinence

- Deep somatic pain from secondary overuse syndrome
  - Cause: repetitive microtraumatic injuries
  - Onset: months or years after injury
  - Affects proximal muscles of joints
  - Exacerbated by the use of affected muscles or joints
  - Relieved by proper posture and rest
  - Example: rotator cuff tendinitis in shoulder pain

Visceral pain

- Cause: intact visceral pain pathway post-injury
- Pathology: no obvious visceral pathology
- Onset: delayed after spinal cord injury
- Constantly fluctuating burning or cramping abdominal pain
- Other causes: dysreflexic headache, renal calculus, bowel problems, sphincteric dysfunction

Neuropathic pain

- Complex regional pain syndrome
  - Above-level neuropathic pain – above the level of injury
  - Unilateral throbbing, burning or shooting upper limb pain
  - Presence of hyperalgesia and allodynia
  - Exacerbated by limb movement, dependent position and temperature changes
  - Autonomic dysfunction: skin temperature asymmetries, skin colour changes, oedema, hyper/hypohidrosis
  - Motor dysfunction: weakness, limited movement, tremor, dystonia (rare and late)
  - Trophic changes: disturbed nail and hair growth, palmar or plantar fibrosis, hyperkeratosis, distal osteoporosis

- Compressive mononeuropathy
    - Above-level neuropathic pain
    - Example: carpal tunnel syndrome
- Radicular pain from nerve root compression
    - At-level neuropathic pain
    - Cause: nerve root entrapment
    - Burning, lancinating or stabbing pain
    - Extent: single dermatome unilaterally or bilaterally
    - Exacerbated by spinal movement, coughing and straining
    - Relieved by decompression
- Segmental deafferentation pain
    - At-level neuropathic pain
    - Terms: girdle pain, border pain or transitional zone pain
    - Cause: spinal cord damage at dorsal horn
    - Spontaneous burning or tingling pain
    - Onset: 1st few months post-injury
    - Location: border of normal sensation and anaesthetic skin
    - Extent: 2-4 dermatomes unilaterally or bilaterally
    - Description: half belt or full belt
    - Presence of segmental hyperalgesia and allodynia
    - Stimulus independent
- Syringomyelia
    - At-level neuropathic pain
    - Onset: years post-injury
    - Radicular pain in a cape-like distribution, interscapular pain or central cord pain
    - Dysesthetic pain: burning sensations, pins and needles, stretching of skin
    - Trophic changes: hyperhidrosis, glossy skin, coldness, paleness

- Cauda equina syndrome
  - At-level neuropathic pain
  - Burning pain
  - Location: legs, feet, perineum, genitals and rectum
  - Associated with saddle-shaped loss of sensation and loss of bladder and bowel control
- Deafferentation pain
  - Below-level neuropathic pain
  - Terms: spinal cord injury pain, dysesthetic pain, central dysesthesia syndrome
  - Diffuse, constant, burning, aching or throbbing pain in anaesthetic regions below the level of injury
  - Asscociated with numbness and tingling
  - Exacerbated by infection
  - Not affected by movement or position
  - Usually not relieved by opioids

Pain Assessment Tools

Introduction

Various pain assessment tools can be used to rate the intensity of pain and to document response to pain management.

Numerical rating scale (NRS)

- Pain is rated from 0 to 10
- Ask patient to score his or her pain from 0 to 10
- 0= no pain, 10= worst possible pain
- Clinically significant pain reduction = 2
- Easier to complete than visual analogue scale
- No need to carry the pain ruler

Visual analogue scale (VAS)

- Pain is rated from a 10cm line on a pain ruler
- Ask patient to mark a point that best describes his or her pain
- 0= no pain, 10=worst possible pain
- Clinically significant pain reduction = 2

Categorical rating scale (CRS)

- Pain is rated as mild, moderate or severe
- Ask patient to rate his or her pain as mild, moderate or severe
- Useful in elderly

Wong-Baker faces pain rating scale

- Pain is rated from faces on a Wong-Baker ruler
- Ask patient to point to the face that best matches the type of pain he or she is feeling
- Left end= smiling face, right end= crying face

FLACC scale

- Pain is rated from observing the behaviour of patient
- Originally designed to assess pain in children and babies
- Useful in non-communicative adult patients

Criteria	0	1	2
Face	Normal	Grimace	Clenched jaw
Legs	Normal	Restless	Kicking
Activity	Normal	Squirming	Arched
Cry	Normal	Moaning	Screaming
Consolability	Normal	Reassurable	Nonreassurable

Little story

Once I received a present and a thank you card from a family member of a patient that I could not remember. My boss was a little upset for my forgetfulness. After some effort, I remembered I saw a patient in the haematological ward who was referred to me to find out whether he was in pain. Patient was semi-comatose. I observed him and started him on morphine infusion because he was exhibiting behaviour suggestive of pain. I told his son, "He is in pain. I need to start him on morphine infusion to make him comfortable. Then I asked his son, "How are you?" It was a short encounter. In the thank you card he wrote, "Although I have brought my father to see so many doctors, but I have never come across a doctor who is so kind." The encounter was short. Maybe I was the first doctor who asked about him.

Principle of Pain Management

Introduction

WHO analgesic ladder is a useful guide in cancer pain management. It is 90% effective in pain control.

Step 3
Severe pain (7-10)
Non-opioid
+ strong opioid
± adjuvants

Step 2
Moderate pain (4-6)
Non-opioid
+ weak opioid
± adjuvants

Step 1
Mild pain (1-3)
Non-opioid
± adjuvants

Principles

- By the mouth – give orally
- By the clock – give regularly
- By the ladder – give according to ladder
- For the individual – give according to individual
- Attention to details – give with attention to details

Non-opioids

- Paracetamol
- NSAIDs

Weak opioids

- Codeine
- Dihydrocodeine
- Tramadol

Paracetamol + weak opioid

- Panadeine (Paracetamol 500mg + codeine 8mg)
- Panadeine Extra (Paracetamol 500mg + codeine 15mg)
- Panadeine Forte (Paracetamol 500mg + codeine 30mg)
- Ultracet (Paracetamol 325mg + tramadol 37.5mg)

Strong opioids

- Morphine
- Oxycodone
- Hydromorphone
- Fentanyl
- Buprenorphine
- Methadone

Adjuvants

- Steroids
- Antidepressants
- Anticonvulsants
- NMDA receptor blockers
- Muscle relaxants
- Bisphosphonates

Paracetamol

Introduction

Paracetamol is a non-opioid that has been used in the management of mild pain and fever for more than 50 years.

Mechanisms of action

- The exact mechanism is still undefined
- Proposed mechanisms
  - Central COX inhibition (predominantly COX-2)
    - Inhibits PGE2 production from arachidonic acid
      - Activates serotonergic pathway to reduce pain
      - Lowers hypothalamic set point to reduce fever
  - Anandamide uptake inhibition by paracetamol metabolite (N-arachidomoylphenolamine or AM404)
    - Increases endogenous cannabinoids
      - Activates serotonergic pathway
      - Lowers body temperature
  - Direct NMDAR inhibition
  - Inhibition of substance P-dependent synthesis of NO through the L-arginine-nitric oxide pathway

Recommendations

- Typical dose in palliative care: PO Paracetamol 1g tds-qid
  - Timing for qid: 8am, 12pm, 4pm, 8pm
    - Especially if patient is on syrup morphine q4h
  - Timing for qid: 8am, 12pm, 6pm, 10pm
    - Especially if patient is not on syrup morphine q4h
  - Timing for qid: 6am, 12pm, 6pm, 12am
    - 12am dose may affect sleep

- Timing for qid: morning, afternoon, evening, bedtime
  - Especially at home
- PO Paracetamol 1g q4h with morphine q4h (Stockler 2004)
  - Timing: 8am, 12pm, 4pm, 8pm, 12am, 4am
  - Exceeds maximum recommended daily dose of 4g/day
  - Palliative care input recommended
- Syrup Paracetamol
  - Concentration = 125mg/5ml, 250mg/5ml
  - Not suitable for patients who cannot drink ≥20ml
- PR Paracetamol 1g tds-qid
  - 1 paracetamol suppository = 500mg
- IV Paracetamol 1g q6h if >50kg
  - 1 vial = 500mg/50ml
  - Infusion over 15min
  - Maximum 4g/day
- IV Paracetamol 15mg/kg q6h if <50kg
  - Maximum 60mg/kg/day

Additional information

- PO Paracetamol 1g qid is preferred to tds for maximal benefit
- If definite benefit not seen within 2 days after adding paracetamol to strong opioid, discontinue it (Axelsson and Christensen 2003)
- Use of paracetamol ≤4g/day is not contraindicated in stable chronic liver disease (Benson 1983)
- Limit paracetamol use to single dose 1g prn in decompensated chronic liver disease
- Use of paracetamol ≤4g/day is not contraindicated in severe renal impairment with CC<30ml/min
- 5HT3-receptor antagonists may block the analgesic effect of paracetamol completely (Pickering 2006)

Little experience

A patient once complained to me that he was aroused during midnight to take paracetamol. He was unhappy because he felt that it didn't make sense to wake him up for the sole reason of taking paracetamol.

NSAIDs

Introduction

Use an NSAID if it provides better pain relief than paracetamol.

Mechanisms of action

- Peripheral COX inhibition
  - Reduces prostaglandin production from arachidonic acid
    - COX-1 inhibition
      - Reduced cytoprotective prostaglandins
        - Gastrointestinal toxicity
    - COX-2 inhibition
      - Reduced inflammatory prostaglandins
        - Analgesia
      - Reduced renoprotective prostaglandins
        - Renal toxicity
- Central COX inhibition

NNTs from single dose studies (≥50% pain relief)

- Etoricoxib 120mg = 1.6
- Ibuprofen 800mg = 1.6
- Ketorolac 20mg = 1.8
- Diclofenac 100mg = 1.9
- Lumiracoxib 400mg = 2.1
- Diclofenac 50mg = 2.3
- Naproxen 440mg = 2.3
- Ibuprofen 400mg = 2.4
- Celecoxib 400mg = 2.6
- Topical NSAIDs = 3.1
- Celecoxib 200mg = 4.2

Risk of GI bleeding (RR compared to ibuprofen)

- Ibuprofen = 1.0 (lowest risk among nonselective NSAIDs)
- Diclofenac = 1.8
- Naproxen = 2.2
- Indomethacin = 2.4
- Piroxicam = 3.8
- Ketoprofen = 4.2

Risk of UGI bleeding with NSAID ≥ 2 months (Tramer 2000)

- Risk of endoscopic ulcer   1 in 5
- Risk of symptomatic ulcer   1 in 70
- Risk of bleeding ulcer   1 in 150
- Risk of death from bleeding ulcer   1 in 1,300

COX-2 selectivity ratio

- Etoricoxib = 106
- Celecoxib = 7.6
- Diclofenac = 3.0
- Meloxicam = 2.0
- Indomethacin = 0.4
- Ibuprofen = 0.2
- Piroxicam = 0.08

Low gastrointestinal toxicity of ibuprofen

- R(-)-ibuprofen enantiomer is metabolized to active S(+) isomer
- Active S-ibuprofen inhibits prostaglandin synthesis
- Inactive R-ibuprofen masks interaction of S-ibuprofen with COX-1, reducing inhibition of gastric prostaglandin production

Risk factors for GI toxicity

- Age >65 years
- Peptic ulcer disease

- Long term use of NSAIDs
- Serious comorbidity
  - Cancer
  - Diabetes mellitus
  - Hypertension
  - Cardiovascular disease
  - Hepatic impairment
  - Renal impairment
- Concurrent use of steroids, aspirin or anticoagulant
- Concurrent use of SSRI
- Platelet $<50 \times 10^9/L$

Choices of NSAID in palliative care

- PO Ibuprofen 400-800mg tds-qid + GI prophylaxis
- PO Diclofenac 50-100mg tds-qid + GI prophylaxis
- PO Diclofenac SR 75-150mg bd + GI prophylaxis
- PO Naproxen 550-1100mg bd + GI prophylaxis
- PO Etoricoxib 60-120mg daily + GI prophylaxis
- PO Celecoxib 200-400mg bd + GI prophylaxis
- CSCI Diclofenac 75-150mg/24h + GI prophylaxis (PCT advice)
- CSCI Ketorolac 60-90mg/24h + GI prophylaxis (PCT advice)

PCT = palliative care team

GI prophylaxis

- PO Omeprazole 20mg om
- PO Pantoprazole 20mg om
- PO Lansoprazole 30mg om
- PO Ranitidine 300mg bd
- PO Misoprostol 400mcg bd (Rostom 2002)

Additional information

- Limit NSAID use for ≤ 2 months if possible
- For long term NSAIDs, seek palliative care input
- Use of NSAID should be avoided in renal disease unless preservation of renal function is no longer wanted
- Since risk of GI toxicity in palliative care patients is high, consider GI prophylaxis for all palliative care patients
- Consider single dose NSAID for highly selected patients with relative contraindications to NSAID
- Omeprazole and lansoprazole can be given as orodispersible tablets or granules from opening the capsules
- SC Omeprazole 40mg in 100ml normal saline over 3 hours can be used in the symptomatic treatment of GI toxicity when intravenous access is a burden (PCT advice)

Weak Opioids

Introduction

Weak opioids are often used to manage moderate pain in step 2 WHO analgesic ladder. However, step 2 can be skipped. A direct move to third step with small doses of morphine improves pain control compared to traditional three-step strategies (Maltoni 2005). Step 2 is reserved for patients who are not ready to use strong opioids.

Mechanisms of action

- Tramadol: $\mu > \kappa > \delta$
- Codeine and dihydrocodeine: $\mu > \delta > \kappa$
- Additional mechanisms of tramadol
    - Stimulates neuronal release of serotonin
    - Inhibits re-uptake of serotonin and noradrenaline (SNRI)

Pharmacology

- Onset of action
    - Tramadol: 30min
    - Codeine: 30min
    - Dihydrocodeine: 30min
- Duration of action
    - Tramadol: 4h
    - Codeine: 4h
    - Dihydrocodeine: 4h
- Metabolism in liver
    - Tramadol: converted to O-desmethyltramadol (active)
    - Codeine: converted to morphine (active)
    - Dihydrocodeine: converted to dihydromorphine (active)

- Potency
    - Tramadol: 5 times weaker than oral morphine
    - Codeine: 8 times weaker than oral morphine
    - Dihydrocodeine: 10 times weaker than oral morphine
    - Tramadol injection: 2 times weaker than oral tramadol

Doses

- PO Tramadol 50-100mg tds-qid
- PO Codeine 30-60mg tds-qid
- PO Dihydrocodeine 30-60mg tds-qid
- SC Tramadol 50-100mg tds-qid
- CSCI Tramadol 100-600mg/24h (PCT advice)
- CSCI Dihydrocodeine 100-350mg/24h (PCT advice)

Combinations

- Ultracet (Paracetamol 325mg + tramadol 37.5mg)
- Panadeine (Paracetamol 500mg + codeine 8mg)
- Panadeine Extra (Paracetamol 500mg + codeine 15mg)
- Panadeine Forte (Paracetamol 500mg + codeine 30mg)

Combination doses

- PO Ultracet 1-2 tablets tds-qid
- PO Panadeine 1-2 tablets tds-qid
- PO Panadeine Extra 1-2 tablets tds-qid
- PO Panadeine Forte 1-2 tablets tds-qid

Recommendations

- Consider prophylactic antiemetic for first 3-5 days
- Consider regular laxatives
- Consider switching to strong opioid rapidly if pain is uncontrolled or breakthrough analgesia is required

Little experience

Once my boss started a patient on tramadol. After the first dose she went up to the ward to review the patient for pain control and side effects. The patient was so touched that her eyes brimmed with tears. It was not about the tramadol. It was the care and concern that my boss had towards her.

Five Principles of Using Syrup Morphine

Introduction

The five principles of using syrup morphine can serve as an initial guide to manage moderate to severe pain in palliative care.

The five principles

- Prescribe syrup morphine q4h for background pain
- Prescribe syrup morphine prn/q1h for breakthrough pain
- Prescribe regular antiemetic for the first 5 days
- Prescribe regular laxatives
- Provide opioid education

Background pain

- Common error: prescribing syrup morphine prn, on, q6h or q8h for background pain
- Rationale: increasing the interval results in end-of-dose pain because the duration of action of syrup morphine is four hours
- Exception: severe renal failure with CC<30ml/min or severe liver impairment with prolonged prothrombin time

Breakthrough pain

- Common error: not prescribing syrup morphine prn/q1h for breakthrough pain
- Rationale: breakthrough pain needs additional analgesia
- Some centers practice prescribing syrup morphine prn/q2h or prn/q4h for breakthrough pain
- Increasing the interval may result in poorly controlled breakthrough pain

Opioid-induced emesis

- Common error: not prescribing regular antiemetic
- Rationale: some patients refuse to take morphine again once they have vomited even though the chance of vomiting is 25%
- Recommendation: PO Metoclopramide 10mg tds x 5/7 or PO Haloperidol 1.5mg bd x 5/7
- Exception: patients with recent history of using morphine without nausea or vomiting

Opioid-induced constipation

- Common error: not prescribing regular laxatives
- Rationale: opioid-induced constipation is common
- Recommendation: PO Senna 15mg bd ± PO Lactulose 10ml bd
- Exception: patients with diarrhoea or with iliostomy

Opioid education

- Common error: prescribing morphine without explaning about side effects and without addressing fear of morphine
- Rationale: some patients refuse to take morphine due to their fear, some relatives refuse to give patient morphine due to their fear and misconception about morphine
- Recommendation: educate patients and relatives about the common side effects of morphine and address their fear of morphine

---

Opioid teaching

The 5 principles of using syrup morphine is a preliminary guide that we can share with our medical and surgical colleagues on how to start morphine.

Opioid Education

Introduction

The successful use of syrup morphine depends largely on opioid education. The proper amount of information should be communicated to patients and their relatives to improve compliance.

Three common side effects

- Drowsiness
- Nausea and vomiting
- Constipation

Three common fears

- Fear of addiction
- Fear of tolerance
- Fear of using morphine when one is not dying

Opioid-induced drowsiness

- Mild to moderate drowsiness for the first 24 hours of using morphine and during dose increase (Pasero 2011)
- Should be easily arousable to talk and eat as usual
- Drowsiness usually disappears within 3-5 days
- Severe drowsiness needs dose reduction

Opioid-induced emesis

- 1 in 4 will experience nausea or vomiting
- Usually disappears within 3-5 days
- Can be prevented by taking anti-vomiting drug for 3-5 days

Opioid-induced constipation

- Morphine can cause constipation
- Need regular laxatives to assist in bowel opening

Fear of addiction

- Misconception: I don't want to get addicted to morphine
- Explanation: Addiction is extremely uncommon if you are taking morphine to control pain or other symptoms like cough and breathlessness.

Fear of tolerance

- Misconception: If my pain gets worse, there will be nothing left for me to control my pain.
- Explanation: When the pain gets worse, usually it can be controlled by increasing the dose. Besides, there are many alternatives which are stronger than morphine if morphine does not work well for you.

Fear of using morphine when one is not dying

- Misconception: I am not dying yet. Morphine is for the dying.
- Explanation: Morphine is not meant for the dying, but is used when there is a need, even early in the disease. When the pain is controlled, you can continue your daily activities in life.

Little secret

Majority of patients who refuse morphine given by the primary team are willing to take morphine prescribed by the palliative care team after proper information is given to them. The secret is communication.

Opioid Side Effects

Introduction

Opioid can cause a range of side effects. Effective opioid management requires active prevention of common side effects and regular assessment of opioid toxicity.

Drowsiness

- Mild to moderate drowsiness is not a sign of opioid toxicity
- Tolerance develops within first few days
- Persistent drowsiness can be treated with psychostimulants
  - PO Methylphenidate 5-10mg at 8am ± 12pm
  - PO Dextroamphetamine 10-30mg at 8am ± 12pm
  - PO Modafinil 200-400mg at 8am ± 12pm
  - PO Donepezil 2.5-5mg at 8am ± 12pm
- Excessive drowsiness is an early sign of opioid toxicity
  - Causes of excessive drowsiness
    - Opioid naïve
    - Frailty
    - Mild pain
    - Nerve block
    - Acute kidney injury
    - CNS depression
      - CNS depressants
      - Infection
      - Metabolic disturbances
      - Brain metastases
  - Management of excessive drowsiness
    - Opioid dose reduction
    - Opioid rotation

Nausea and vomiting

- Nausea and vomiting occur in 25% of patients
- Tolerance develops within first few days
- High risk group
  - Age < 65 years
  - Female
  - Breast cancer
  - Stomach cancer
  - Gynaecological cancer
- Prescribe prophylactic antiemetic for all patients
  - PO Metoclopramide 10mg tds for 5 days or
  - PO Haloperidol 1.5mg bd for 5 days
- Opioid-induced nausea and vomiting (OINV)
  - Delayed gastric emptying
    - IV/SC Metoclopramide 10mg tds
  - Direct chemoreceptor trigger zone (CTZ) stimulation
    - IV/SC Haloperidol 1.5mg bd for CTZ stimulation
  - Increased vestibular sensitivity
    - IV Promethazine 12.5-25mg tds
    - Scopolamine patch 1.5mg q72h to mastoid
  - Persistent nausea and vomiting
    - IV/SC Dexamethasone 8mg at 8am and 12pm
  - Refractory nausea and vomiting (PCT advice)
    - IV/SC Metoclopramide 10-20mg q4h
    - CIVI/CSCI Metoclopramide 60-120mg/24h

Constipation

- Opioid-induced constipation occurs in 90% of patients
- Tolerance does not develop
- Prescribe prophylactic laxative for all patients unless diarrhoea
  - PO Senna 15mg bd or
  - PO Docusate 100mg bd

- Opioid-induced constipation (OIC)
  - PO Senna 15mg bd + Syrup Lactulose 15ml bd or
  - PO Bisacodyl 10mg bd + Syrup Lactulose 15ml bd or
  - PO Co-danthrusate (Dantron + Docusate) 1-3 cap on-bd
  - PO Co-danthramer (Dantron + Poloxamer) 1-3 cap on-bd
- Education of laxative titration
  - Hard stool: double the dose of stool softener
    - Maximum docusate 400mg qid (4 tablets qid)
    - Maximum lactulose 30ml qid
  - No stool: double the dose of stool pusher
    - Maximum senna 30mg qid (4 tablets qid)
    - Maximum bisacodyl 20mg qid (4 tablets qid)
  - Diarrhoea: stop 3/7, then restart with half the usual dose
- Rectal measures required in 1/3 patients
  - PR Glycerin enema II/II prn if NBO for 3/7 or
  - PR Bisacodyl 10-20mg prn if NBO for 3/7
  - PR Fleet enema I/I prn if still NBO
- Alternative options for OIC
  - PAMORA
    - Peripherally acting μ-opioid receptor antagonists
    - SC Methylnaltrexone 8mg EOD if 40-60kg
    - SC Methylnaltrexone 12mg EOD if 60-120kg
    - PO Naloxegol 25mg om
  - Locally acting chloride channel activator
    - PO Lubiprostone 24mcg bd
- Avoid bulk laxatives for OIC
  - Increase impaction
    - Opioid reduces water in lumen
    - Bulk laxatives draw fluid into lumen

Little knowledge

Drowsiness, nausea and vomiting are side effects that occur during rising serum opioid levels. They tend to resolve as steady state is achieved. Constipation persists despite steady state opioid levels.

Opioid Toxicity

Introduction

Opioid-induced neurotoxicity is a syndrome that includes some or all of the following features: severe drowsiness, respiratory depression, delirium, hallucination, hyperalgesia, allodynia, myoclonus and seizures. The clue to prevent opioid toxicity is frequent review.

Risk factors of opioid toxicity

- Frail patients
- Excessive dose initiation or increment
- Dehydration and renal failure
- Infection
- Pain acutely relieved by procedure like nerve block

Clinical features of opioid toxicity

- Central nervous system depression (inhibitory neurotoxicity)
    - Excessive drowsiness
    - Hypoactive delirium
    - Coma
    - Respiratory depression: respiratory rate <8-10/min
- Central nervous system stimulation (excitatory neurotoxicity)
    - Agitation
    - Hyperalgesia and allodynia
    - Hyperactive delirium
    - Hallucinations and delusions
    - Myoclonus and seizures
    - Coma
    - Respiratory arrest

Excessive drowsiness

- Mild to moderate drowsiness is not a sign of opioid toxicity
- Excessive drowsiness is an early sign of opioid toxicity
- Excessive drowsiness is characterized by poor arousability
- Screen for hypoactive delirium
- Review CNS depressants
- Treat contributory factors
    - Dehydration
    - Infection
    - Hypercalcemia
- Opioid dose reduction
- Opioid rotation

Delirium

- Stable opioid dose does not impair cognition (Bruera 1989)
- Cognitive function improves with pain control
- Median precipitating factors = 3 per episode in palliative care
- Treat precipitating factors
    - Pain
    - Fecal impaction
    - Urinary retention
    - Dehydration
    - Renal failure
    - Infection
    - Hypercalcemia
    - Hypoxia
    - Metabolic encephalopathy
- Rehydration to reduce opioid metabolites
- Opioid dose reduction
- Opioid rotation

- Treat hypoactive delirium with unpleasant hallucinations
  - PO Haloperidol 0.75mg on-bd
  - IV/SC Haloperidol 0.5mg on-bd
- Treat all hyperactive delirium
  - Mild agitation: PO/IV/SC Haloperidol 1.5mg on-bd
  - Moderate agitation: PO/IV/SC Haloperidol 2.5mg on-bd
  - Severe agitation: PO/IV/SC Haloperidol 5mg on-bd

Respiratory depression

- Uncommon in cancer patients with chronic pain
- Does not occur with proper opioid titration (Sykes 2007)
- Risk factors
  - Advanced age
  - Multiple comorbidities
  - Renal failure
  - Morbid obesity
  - Sleep apnoea
  - Nerve block
  - Opioid rotation to methadone
- Naloxone in palliative care (American Pain Society 1992)
  - RR ≥8/min + easily arousable
    - Wait and see
    - Consider opioid dose reduction or omission
  - RR <8/min + poorly arousable
    - Dilute 400mcg (1 ampoule) to 10ml with NS
    - Give 20mcg (0.5ml) q2min IV or q5min SC till RR ≥8/min
    - Further boluses prn if RR<8/min
    - Duration of action of naloxone is 0.5-1.5h
    - Aim for partial reversal, not complete reversal
    - Restart opioid with a lower dose after sustained improvement in consciousness

- Use of naloxone may precipitate a withdrawal syndrome, arrhythmias, seizures and severe pain (Manfredi 1996)

Opioid-induced hyperalgesia (OIH)

- Mechanisms
  - Excitatory opioid metabolites, such as:
    - Morphine-3-glucuronide (M3G)
    - Hydromorphone-3-glucuronide (H3G)
  - Activation of NMDAR
  - Activation of glial cells
  - Alteration in G protein coupling of opioid receptors
    - With G_s rather than G_i or G_o
- Characteristics
  - Worsening pain despite opioid dose escalation
  - Presence of hyperalgesia and allodynia
  - Pain becomes more diffuse, extending beyond area of pre-existing pain
  - Pain of lesser quality and harder to pinpoint
- Management
  - Rehydration to reduce opioid metabolites
  - Rapid opioid dose reduction to 25% of peak dose
  - Switch to an opioid with less risk of OIH
    - Fentanyl (highest risk) > morphine > methadone > buprenorphine (lowest risk)
  - Add paractemol or NSAID
  - Consider neuropathic adjuvant: gabapentin
  - Consider ketamine
  - Consider spinal or epidural opioid
  - Correct hypomagnesemia
  - Consider ultralow doses of opioid antagonist
  - Prescribe benzodiazepine for seizures or distressing myoclonus

Little caution

High index of suspicion is needed to detect opioid excitatory neurotoxicity because these patients may be fully alert. Be cautious when patients are requesting higher and higher doses of opioid without much pain control.

Opioid Concerns

Introduction

It is common for laypeople or healthcare staff to express concerns in using opioids due to various misunderstandings. These misunderstandings can result in undertreatment of pain.

Addiction

- Concern: I don't want to become a drug addict
- Physical dependence
    - Not addiction
    - Patients depend on morphine to reduce pain
- Withdrawal symptoms
    - Not addiction
    - Occur when morphine is stopped abruptly
    - Prevented by reducing morpine gradually
- Psychological dependence
    - Is addiction
    - Presence of mental craving and drug-seeking behaviour in the absence of pain
    - Rare in patient without history of drug abuse: 4 in 12,000 patients (Porter 1980)

Tolerance

- Concern: If the pain gets worse, I will have nothing to use
- Tolerance
    - Requiring higher and higher doses to achieve analgesia
    - Need of increasing dose is due to increasing pain from disease progression, not tolerance
    - Significant tolerance is uncommon

- Broad therapeutic range of morphine allows dose escalation when pain gets worse
- Availability of other strong opioids when morphine fails

Dying

- Concern: I am not dying yet
- Morphine is not used exclusively in dying patients
- Morphine can be used to treat pain in early stages of disease
- Patients can resume their activities when pain is under control

Allergy

- Concern: I am allergic to morphine
- True allergy is rare
- Nausea and vomiting are often mistaken as allergy
- Nausea and vomiting are preventable side effects

Respiratory depression and hastening of death

- Concern of healthcare staff: morphine hastens death
- Proper titration of morphine does not cause clinically significant respiratory depression
- Proper titration of morphine does not hasten death
- Lethal dose of morphine is ≥200mg for opioid naïve patients

---

Little opinion

Misperceptions about opioid are mistaken first impressions about opioid. Misconceptions about opioid are mistaken beliefs about opioid after substantial thinking. The former is easier to rectify than the latter.

Morphine

Introduction

Morphine is named after the Greek God of Dream, Morpheus, because of its sedative effect. It is derived from opium poppy (Papaver somniferum).

Mechanisms of action

- μ opioid receptor agonist
- Presynaptic inhibition of neurotransmitter release at dorsal horn (predominant mechanism)
  - Activation of G_i protein coupled receptors
    - Increased K^+ efflux
      - Hyperpolarization
      - Reduced neurotransmitter release
    - Decreased Ca^{2+} conductance
      - Reduced Ca^{2+} influx
      - Reduced depolarization
      - Reduced neurotransmitter release
    - Inhibition of adenylate cyclase
      - Reduced cAMP dependent cellular processes
      - Reduced neurotransmitter release
- Postsynaptic inhibition of neuron firing at dorsal horn
- Activation of descending pain pathways
  - GABA disinhibition – suppression of GABAergic inputs onto descending pain pathways

Pharmacology

- Metabolites: morphine-6-glucuronide (M6G), morphine-3-glucuronide (M3G)

- Morphine-6-glucuronide (M6G)
    - 10-15%
    - Active metabolite
    - 100x more potent than morphine
    - Less abundant in CNS due to poor penetration of blood brain barrier
    - Activation of opioid receptor: can cause nausea, vomiting, sedation, respiratory depression
- Morphine-3-glucuronide (M3G)
    - 80%
    - Inactive metabolite
    - Indirect activation of NMDAR: excitatory neurotoxicity
- Immediate release oral morphine
    - Bioavailability: 35%
    - Onset of action: 30-45min
    - Plasma half-life: 2-4h
    - Duration of action: 4h

Titration of oral morphine

- Use immediate release oral morphine for titration because the dose can be adjusted up or down rapidly in view of the short half-life
- Starting dose
    - Syrup morphine 2.5mg q4h for moderate pain
    - Syrup morphine 5mg q4h for severe pain
    - Syrup morphine 10mg q4h if on maximum weak opioid
- Breakthrough dose
    - Use 1/6 of oral morphine daily dose (Hanks 2001)
    - Given as frequent as required up to hourly
- Examples of prescription
    - Syrup morphine 5mg q4h
    - Syrup morphine 5mg prn/q1h for breakthrough pain

- Timing of baseline morphine
  - Syrup morphine at 8am, 12pm, 4pm, 8pm, 12am, 4am
- Alternative timing
  - Syrup morphine at 8am, 12pm, 4pm, 8pm
  - Double dose at 12am to avoid waking up for 4am dose
- Titration based on breakthrough doses
  - Titrate the baseline dose if ≥ 3 breakthough doses per day
  - Add the total breakthrough doses to the baseline dose
  - Example
    - Baseline: syrup morphine 5mg q4h
    - Breakthrough: syrup morphine 5mg x 6 doses/day
    - Titration = (5mg x 6) + (5mg x 6) = 60mg/day
    - New baseline: syrup morphine 10mg q4h
    - New breakthrough: syrup morphine 10mg prn/q1h
  - Do not increase the dose <25% (no significant change)
  - Do not increase the dose >100% (higher risk of toxicity)
- Alternative titration based on pain severity
  - Mild pain: increase dose by 25%
  - Moderate pain: increase dose by 50%
  - Severe pain: increase dose by 100%
- Alternative titration based on stepwise increment
  - Increase q4h dose every 24-48h till pain is controlled
  - 5–10–15–20–30–40–60–80–100–130
- Frequency of titration
  - Depends on half-life ($T_{1/2}$)of oral morphine ≈ 2-4h
    - Time to 50% concentration = $1T_{1/2}$
    - Time to 75% concentration = $2T_{1/2}$
    - Time to 90% concentration = $3.3T_{1/2}$
    - Time to steady state ≈ $4T_{1/2}$
  - Time to steady state = 8-16h
- Comparison of plasma half-life of different opioids
  - Immediate release oral morphine: 2-4h

- Immediate release oral oxycodone: 3.5h
- Immediate release oral hydromorphone: 2.5h
- Intravenous morphine: 1.5h
- Fentanyl patch: 0.5-1 day
- Oral transmucosal fentanyl citrate: 6h
- Intravenous fentanyl: 3.5h
- Intravenous sufentanil: 2.5h
- Intravenous alfentanil: 1.5h
- Buprenorphine patch (BuTrans): 0.5-1.5days
- Buprenorphine patch (Transtec): 1-1.5 days
- Sublingual buprenorphine: 1-3 days
- Intravenous buprenorphine: 3-16h
- Oral methadone: 8 hours to 3 days
- Recommended frequency of titration for different opioids
  - Immediate release morphine: q24h
  - Immediate release oxycodone: q24h
  - Immediate release hydromorphone: q24h
  - Sustained release morphine: q48h
  - Sustained release oxycodone: q48h
  - Sustained release hydromorphone: q48h
  - Fentanyl patch: q72h
  - Buprenorphine patch (BuTrans): q72h
  - Buprenorphine patch (Transtec): q72h
  - Methadone: weekly

Preparations of syrup morphine

- Common preparations
  - 1mg/ml
  - 2mg/ml
  - 10mg/ml
- Check with pharmacist regarding available concentration
- Prescribe in mg, not in ml

Sustained Release Morphine Tablets (MST)

Introduction

Convert immediate release oral morphine to sustained release morphine tablets (MST) once the pain is adequately controlled for 2-3 days.

Pharmacology

- Onset of action: 2h
- Half-life: 4h
- Duration of action: 12h

Conversion

- Conversion ratio = 1:1
- Examples of conversion
    - Syrup morphine 5mg q4h ≈ MST 20mg q12h
    - Syrup morphine 10mg q4h = MST 30mg q12h
- Examples of prescription
    - MST 30mg q12h at 8am and 8pm
    - Syrup morphine 10mg prn/q1h for breakthrough pain

Instructions for prescribing MST

- Avoid prescribing 8 hourly dosing (higher risk of toxicity)
- Instruct patient not to chew or crush tablets
- For nasogastric or PEG feeding:
    - Use sustained release morphine granules if available or
    - Change back to immediate release oral morphine or
    - Consider using fentanyl patch

Starting dose for opioid-naïve patients

- Standard opioid titration begins with titration of syrup morphine, then convert to MST once pain is stable
- Consider seeking advice from the palliative care team if you intend to start MST without titrating with syrup morphine
- MST 10mg q12h for breathlessness or moderate pain
    - Syrup morphine 2.5mg prn/q1h for breakthrough pain
- MST 20mg q12h for severe pain
    - Syrup morphine 5mg prn/q1h for breakthrough pain
- MST 30mg q12h if on maximal weak opioid
    - Syrup morphine 10mg prn/q1h for breakthrough pain
- Use 1/6 of oral morphine daily dose as breakthrough doses

Titration of MST

- Mild to moderate pain
    - Titrate MST if ≥ 3 breakthrough doses per day
    - Add total breakthrough doses to baseline dose
    - Frequency of titration is at least 48h
    - Maximal titration: 100%
- Severe pain
    - Retitrate by adding syrup morphine q4h or
    - Retitrate by converting back to syrup morphine q4h

Preparations for q12h dosing (MS Contin)

- MST 10mg = pink
- MST 30mg = purple
- MST 60mg = orange

Preparations for q24h dosing (Kadian, Avinca)

- Kadian 10mg, 20mg, 30mg, 50mg, 60mg, 80mg, 100mg, 200mg
- Avinza 30mg, 60mg, 90mg, 120mg

Fentanyl Patch

Introduction

Fentanyl is an alternative strong opioid. It is a strong μ-opioid receptor agonist. It is highly lipophilic.

Pharmacology

- Onset of action: 12h
- Half-life: 0.5-1 day
- Duration of action: 72h

Indications

- Consider converting immediate release oral morphine to fentanyl patch once the pain is adequately controlled for 2-3 days, in the following conditions:
  - Head and neck cancer
  - Swallowing problem
  - Persistent nausea and vomiting
  - Short bowel syndrome
  - Malignant bowel obstruction
  - PEG feeding

Conversion

- Fentanyl is 100x more potent than oral morphine
- To convert oral morphine mg/day to fentanyl patch mcg/h, divide oral morphine daily dose by 3
- Example of conversion
  - Syrup morphine 5mg q4h = 30mg/day
  - $30 \div 3 = 10 \approx 12$
  - Syrup morphine 5mg q4h = fentanyl patch 12mcg/h/72h

- Example of conversion in details
  - Syrup morphine 5mg q4h = 30mg/day
  - Based on conversion ratio = 1: 100
  - $30 \div 100$ mg/day = $30 \div 100$ x 1000 mcg/day

$$= 30 \div 100 \times 1000 \div 24 \text{ mcg/h}$$
$$= 30 \div 2.4 \text{ mcg/h}$$
$$\approx 30 \div 3 \text{ mcg/h}$$
$$= 10\text{mcg/h}$$
$$\approx 12\text{mcg/h}$$

Rapid conversion

- Syrup morphine 5mg q4h = fentanyl patch 12mcg/h/72h
- Syrup morphine 10mg q4h = fentanyl patch 25mcg/h/72h
- Syrup morphine 20mg q4h = fentanyl patch 50mcg/h/72h
- Syrup morphine 30mg q4h = fentanyl patch 75mcg/h/72h
- Syrup morphine 40mg q4h = fentanyl patch 100mcg/h/72h

Starting dose for opioid-naïve patients

- Standard opioid titration begins with titration of syrup morphine, then convert to fentanyl patch once pain is stable
- Consider seeking advice from the palliative care team to start fentanyl patch without titrating with syrup morphine
- Fentanyl patch 12mcg/h/72h for moderate to severe pain
  - Syrup morphine 5mg prn/q1h for breakthrough pain
- Fentanyl patch 25mcg/h/72h if on maximal weak opioid
  - Syrup morphine 10mg prn/q1h for breakthrough pain

Titration of fentanyl patch

- Mild to moderate pain
  - Titrate fentanyl patch if ≥ 3 breakthrough doses per day
  - Add total breakthrough doses to baseline dose
  - Frequency of titration is at least 72h

- Maximal titration: 100%
- Examples of titration: 12–25–37–50–62–75–100
- Severe pain
  - Retitrate by adding syrup morphine q4h or
  - Retitrate by converting back to syrup morphine q4h after 12h of patch removal or
  - Retitrate by adding fentanyl infusion or
  - Retitrate by converting to fentanyl infusion after 8h of patch removal

Preexisting analgesia

- Continue pre-existing baseline analgesia for 12 hours because onset of action for fentanyl patch is 12 hours
  - Continue 3 more q4h doses for syrup morphine
  - Continue 1 more q12h dose for MST
  - Continue 8h for morphine infusion

Additional information

- Apply over chest, abdomen and sometimes limbs
- Do not apply at the back
- Do not apply at pain site
- Do not shave body hair, cut it
- Do not cut the patch
- Do not plaster half
- Cover with a transparent plaster like Tegaderm or Opsite
- Label date and time of change with permanent marker pen
- Do not shower hot water over it
- Change the patch every 72 hours
- Dispose by folding it into half with adhesive side inwards and discarding in a sharps container (hospital) or dustbin (home)

Preparations

- Fentanyl patch 12mcg/h/72h
- Fentanyl patch 25mcg/h/72h
- Fentanyl patch 50mcg/h/72h
- Fentanyl patch 100mcg/h/72h

Opioid Review

Introduction

Regular assessment is important during opioid titration. Patients should be assessed for pain control, side effects and opioid toxicity.

	Peak	Steady state
PO Morphine:	15-60min	8-16h
PO Oxycodone:	60-90min	14h
PO Hydromorphone:	60min	10h
PO Methadone:	4h	1.5-12days
PO MST:	1-6h	16h
PO Oxycontin:	3h	18h
SC Morphine:	10-20min	6h
Fentanyl patch:	1-3days	2-4days
OTFC:	20-40min	1day
IV Fentanyl:	4.5min	14h
IV Alfentanil:	1.5min	6h
IV Sufentanil:	2.5min	10h
Buprenorphine patch (BuTrans):	3days	2-6days
Buprenorphine patch (Transtec):	2.5days	4-6days
Sublingual buprenorphine:	1-2h	4-12days

Principles of opioid review

- Risk of opioid toxicity is highest during rising opioid level from onset to peak to steady state
- Risk of opioid toxicity during steady state if:
  - Acute kidney injury
  - Pain is acutely relieved by a procedure like nerve block

Recommended initial review during opioid titration

- Within 12h (Same day)
  - SC/IV Morphine
  - SC/IV Fentanyl
  - SC/IV Alfentanil
  - SC/IV Sufentanil
- Within 24h (Next day)
  - PO Morphine
  - PO Oxycodone
  - PO Hydromorphone
  - PO MST
  - PO Oxycontin
- Within 24h (Next day) and twice-weekly for one week
  - Fentanyl patch
  - Buprenorphine patch
- Within 24h (Next day) and twice-weekly for two weeks
  - PO Methadone

Additional information

- Educate patients and their families regarding opioid toxicity
  - Mild to moderate drowsiness + easy arousability: observe
  - Excessive drowsiness: seek medical advice
  - Poor arousability: seek medical advice

Opioid Switching

Introduction

For opioid switching, first calculate the oral MEDD (morphine equivalent daily dose) of the existing opioid, then convert to the new opioid and consider dose reduction.

Indications for opioid switching

- Uncontrolled pain with dose escalation
- Unacceptable side effects
- Opioid neurotoxicity

Potency of weak opioids

- PO Hydrocodone is 1.5x weaker than PO Morphine
- PO Tramadol is 5x weaker than PO Morphine
- PO Codeine is 8x weaker than PO Morphine
- PO Dihydrocodeine is 10x weaker than PO Morphine
- PO Dextropropoxyphene is 10x weaker than PO Morphine

Switching weak opioid in mg/day to oral MEDD in mg/day

- PO Hydrocodone ÷ 1.5 = oral MEDD
- PO Tramadol ÷ 5 = oral MEDD
- PO Codeine ÷ 8 = oral MEDD
- PO Dihydrocodeine ÷ 10 = oral MEDD
- PO Dextropropoxyphene ÷ 10 = oral MEDD

Potency of strong opioids

- PO Oxycodone is 2x stronger than PO Morphine
- PO Hydromorphone is 5x stronger than PO Morphine
- Fentanyl patch is 100x stronger than PO Morphine

- Buprenorphine patch is 100x stronger than PO Morphine
- SL Buprenorphine is 100x stronger than PO Morphine

Switching oral MEDD in mg/day to other strong opioid

- Oral MEDD ÷ 2 = PO Oxycodone in mg/day
- Oral MEDD ÷ 5 = PO Hydromorphone in mg/day
- Oral MEDD ÷ 3 = Fentanyl patch in mcg/h/72h
- Oral MEDD ÷ 3 = Buprenorphine patch in mcg/h/72h
- Oral MEDD ÷ 100 = SL Buprenorphine in mg/day

Switching to oral hydromorphone

- Syrup morphine 10mg q4h = 60mg/day
- PO Hydromorphone = 60 ÷ 5 = 12mg/day
- Syrup morphine 10mg q4h ≈ PO Hydromorphone 1.3mg q4h

Switching to sublingual buprenorphine

- Syrup morphine 10mg q4h = 60mg/day
- SL Buprenorphine = 60 ÷ 100 = 0.6mg/day
- Syrup morphine 10mg q4h = SL Buprenorphine 0.2mg q8h

Potency of parenteral opioids

- IV/SC Tramadol is 2x weaker than PO Tramadol
- IV/SC Morphine is 2-3x stronger than PO Morphine
- IV/SC Oxycodone is 2x stronger than PO Oxycodone
- IV/SC Hydromorphone is 2x stronger than PO Hydromorphone
- IV/SC Methadone is 2x stronger than PO Methadone
- IV/SC Buprenorphine is 2x stronger than SL Buprenorphine

Switching to parenteral opioid in mg/day

- PO Tramadol x 2 = IV/SC Tramadol
- PO Morphine ÷ 3 = IV/SC Morphine
- PO Oxycodone ÷ 2 = IV/SC Oxycodone

- PO Hydromorphone ÷ 2 = IV/SC Hydromorphone
- PO Methadone ÷ 2 = IV/SC Methadone
- SL Buprenorphine ÷ 2 = IV/SC Buprenorphine

Potency of parenteral fentanyl and fentanyl analogues

- IV/SC Fentanyl is similar potent as fentanyl patch
- IV/SC Fentanyl is 4x stronger than IV/SC Alfentanil
- IV/SC Fentanyl is 10x weaker than IV/SC Sufentanil
- IV/SC Fentanyl is 10x weaker than IV/SC Remifentanil

Switching of parenteral fentanyl

- IV/SC Fentanyl in mcg/h = Fentanyl patch in mcg/h/72h
- IV/SC Fentanyl in mcg/h x 4 = IV/SC Alfentanil in mcg/h
- IV/SC Fentanyl in mcg/h ÷ 10 = IV/SC Sufentanil in mcg/h
- IV/SC Fentanyl in mcg/h ÷ 10 = IV/SC Remifentanil in mcg/h

Switching from parenteral MEDD in mg/day

- Parenteral MEDD = IV/SC Oxycodone in mg/day
- Parenteral MEDD = IV/SC Fentanyl in mcg/h
- Parenteral MEDD ÷ 1.5 = IV/SC Diamorphine in mg/day
- Parenteral MEDD ÷ 5 = IV/SC Hydromorphone in mg/day
- Parenteral MEDD ÷ 15 = IV/SC Alfentanil in mg/day
- Parenteral MEDD ÷ 40 = IV/SC Buprenorphine in mg/day

Switching from parenteral MEDD in mg/day

- Parenteral MEDD ÷ 10 = Epidural morphine
- Parenteral MEDD ÷ 100 = Intrathecal morphine
- Parenteral MEDD ÷ 1000 = Intraventricular morphine

Dose reduction after switching opioid

- Consider palliative care referral for opioid switching unless adequate pharmacological knowledge and clinical experience in using the alternative opioid are available
- Consider dose reduction for incomplete cross tolerance after opioid switching
    - No dose reduction
        - Switching to fentanyl patch
        - Switching for severe uncontrolled pain
    - 30% dose reduction
        - Switching to any opioid except fentanyl/methadone
    - 50% dose reduction
        - Switching to methadone
        - Elderly
        - Severe renal impairment with CC<30ml/min
        - Severe liver impairment with prolonged PT
        - Severe cardiopulmonary disease
    - 75% dose reduction
        - Oral MEDD >2g/day

Alternative Opioids

Introduction

Oral morphine is the first choice opioid in moderate to severe cancer pain. For opioid switching to alternative opioids, referral to palliative care team is *strongly recommended*.

Oxycodone

- Semisynthetic opioid synthesized from thebaine
- Thebaine is an opioid alkaloid found in Persian poppy
- Receptors
    - μ-opioid receptors (less strong than morphine)
    - κ-opioid receptors (animal studies)
- Pharmacology
    - Bioavailability: 75% (morphine: 35%)
    - Onse of action: 20-30min
    - Half-life: 3.5h, 4.5h in renal failure
    - Duration of action: 4h
    - Metabolites: 90% noroxycodone, 10% oxymorphone
- Potency
    - PO Oxycodone is 2x stronger than PO Morphine
    - IV/SC Oxycodone is similar potent to IV/SC Morphine
- Starting dose for opioid-naïve patients
    - Immediate release: PO Oxycodone (Oxynorm) 5mg q4h
    - Modified release: PO Oxycodone (Oxycontin) 10mg q12h
- Starting dose for mild liver impairment or mild to moderate renal impairment
    - Immediate release: Syrup Oxynorm 2.5mg q4h
    - Modified release: PO Oxycontin 5mg q12h

- Starting dose of CSCI for opioid-naïve patients
    - CSCI Oxycodone 5mg/24h (0.2mg/h): breathlessness
    - CSCI Oxycodone 7.5mg/24h (0.3mg/h): moderate pain
    - CSCI Oxycodone 10mg/24h (0.5mg/h): severe pain
    - Review q12h during initial titration
    - Increase 25-50% if pain is uncontrolled
    - Breakthrough dose = 1/6 SC Oxycodone daily dose
    - Breakthrough dose = 4x SC Oxycodone hourly dose
- Example of CSCI prescription
    - CSCI Oxycodone 0.5mg/h
    - SC Oxycodone 2mg prn/q1h for breakthrough pain
- Preparations
    - Immediate release
        - Capsule Oxynorm
            - 5mg: orange/beige
            - 10mg: white/beige
            - 20mg: pink/beige
        - Syrup Oxynorm 1mg/ml
    - Modified release
        - Tablet Oxycontin
            - 5mg: blue round
            - 10mg: white round
            - 20mg: pink round
            - 40mg: yellow round
            - 80mg: green round
        - Tablet Targin (Oxycontin/Naloxone)
            - 5mg/2.5mg: blue oblong
            - 10mg/5mg: white oblong
            - 20mg/10mg: pink oblong
            - 40mg/20mg: yellow oblong
    - Injection
        - 10mg/ml, 1ml amp, 2ml amp

Fentanyl

- Semisynthetic opioid
- Highly lipophilic (morphine: hydrophilic)
    - Suitable for transdermal route
    - Suitable for transmucosal route
    - Less opioid molecules outside CNS
        - Less constipation
        - Less nausea and vomiting
- Sequestrated in body fats
- Strong μ-opioid receptor agonist
- Pharmacology
    - Fentanyl patch
        - Onset of action: 12h
        - Half-life: 0.5-1day
        - Duration of action: 72h
    - Oral transmucosal fentanyl citrate (OTFC)
        - Bioavailability: 50%
        - Onset of action: 5min
        - Half-life: 6h
        - Duration of action: 2h
    - Intravenous fentanyl
        - Onset of action: 1.5min
        - Half-life: 3.5h
        - Duration of action: 1h
    - Metabolites: norfentanyl
- Potency
    - 100x more potent than oral morphine
- Safe in severe renal failure
- Starting dose of fentanyl patch for opioid-naïve patients
    - Fentanyl patch 12mcg/h/72h
      = syrup morphine 5mg q4h
      = syrup oxycodone 2.5mg q4h

- Starting dose of CSCI for opioid-naïve patients
  - CSCI Fentanyl 10mcg/h
  - Review q12h during initial titration
  - Increase 25-50% if pain is uncontrolled
  - Breakthrough dose = 1/24 – 1/12 SC Fentanyl daily dose
  - Breakthrough dose = 1-2x SC Fentanyl hourly dose
- Example of CSCI prescription
  - CSCI Fentanyl 10mcg/h
  - SC Fentanyl 10mcg prn/q1h for breakthrough pain
- OTFC titration for breakthrough pain
  - OTFC 200mcg prn (background oral MEDD ≥ 60mg/day)
  - Rub OTFC around inside of mouth
  - Remove OTFC if patient feels drowsy, nauseated or giddy
  - Repeat OTFC 200mcg after 15min if pain is uncontrolled
  - Increase OTFC to next dose level if pain is uncontrolled with 2 similar doses of OTFC
  - Maximum 4 doses of OTFC per day
  - Dissolve half-used OTFC under hot tap before disposing
- Sublingual fentanyl titration for breakthrough pain
  - For opioid-tolerant patients only
  - Background oral MEDD ≥ 60mg/day
  - Parenteral formulation of fentanyl 50mcg/ml
  - Start with SL Fentanyl 25mcg (0.5ml of 50mcg/ml)
  - Titrate to 50mcg (1ml), then 100mcg (2ml) if necessary
  - Avoid doses >100mcg (>2ml) to ensure absorption
- Preparations
  - Fentanyl patch in mcg/h/72h
    - 12, 25, 50, 100
  - OTFC (Actiq) in mcg
    - 200, 400, 600, 800, 1200, 1600
  - Fentanyl sublingual tablets (Abstral) in mcg
    - 100, 200, 300, 400, 600, 800

- Fentanyl sublingual spray (Subsys) in mcg
    - 100, 200, 400, 600, 800
- Fentanyl buccal tablets (Fentora) in mcg
    - 100, 200, 400, 600, 800
- Fentanyl nasal spray (Lazanda) in mcg
    - 100, 400
- Fentanyl nasal spray (Instanyl) in mcg
    - 50, 100, 200
- Fentanyl injection
    - 50mcg/ml, 2ml amp, 10ml amp

Alfentanil

- Synthetic derivative of fentanyl
- Useful as alternative to fentanyl when volume is a problem
    - Using syringe driver
    - Sublingual administration
- Pharmacology
    - Onset of action: 0.75min
    - Half-life: 1.5h
    - Duration of action: 0.5h
- Potency
    - 4x less potent than fentanyl
- Starting dose for opioid-naïve patients
    - CSCI Alfentanil 0.5-1mg/24h = CSCI Fentanyl 5-10mcg/h
    - Review q12h during initial titration
    - Increase 25-50% if pain is uncontrolled
    - Breakthrough dose = 1/6 SC Alfentanil daily dose
    - Fentanyl breakthrough = 1/40 SC Alfentanil daily dose
- Example of CSCI prescription
    - CSCI Alfentanil 1mg/24h
    - SC Alfentanil 150mcg prn/q1h for breakthrough pain or
    - SC Fentanyl 25mcg prn/q1h for breakthrough pain

- SC Fentanyl is preferred for breakthrough pain because of longer duration of action
- Preparations
  - Injection: 500mcg/ml, 2ml amp, 10ml amp

Sufentanil

- Synthetic derivative of fentanyl
- Useful as alternative to fentanyl when volume is a problem
  - Using syringe driver
  - Sublingual administration
- Pharmacology
  - Onset of action: 1min
  - Half-life: 2.5h
  - Duration of action: 1h
- Potency
  - 10x more potent than fentanyl
- Starting dose for opioid-naïve patients
  - CSCI Sufentanil 15-25mcg/24h = CSCI Fentanyl 5-10mcg/h
  - Review q12h during initial titration
  - Increase 25-50% if pain is uncontrolled
  - Breakthrough dose = 1/24 – 1/12 SC Sufentanil daily dose
- Example of CSCI prescription
  - CSCI Sufentanil 25mcg/24h
  - SC Sufentanil 1mcg prn/q1h for breakthrough pain
- Preparations
  - Injection: 50mcg/ml, 1ml amp, 2ml amp, 5ml amp

Hydromorphone

- Semisynthetic opioid
- Strong μ-opioid receptor agonist
- Useful when patient needs high doses of subcutaneous opioid

- Pharmacology
  - Bioavailability: 30%
  - Onse of action: 30min
  - Half-life: 2.5h
  - Duration of action: 4h
  - Metabolites: hydromorphone-3-glucuronide (H3G)
- Potency
  - 5x more potent than oral morphine
- Starting dose for opioid-naïve patients
  - Immediate release: PO Hydromorphone 1.3mg q4h = syrup morphine 10mg q4h
  - Modified release: PO Hydromorphone SR 2mg q12h = MST 10mg q12h
- Starting dose of CSCI for opioid-naïve patients
  - CSCI Hydromorphone 2mg/24h = CSCI Morphine 10mg/24h
  - Review q12h during initial titration
  - Increase 25-50% if pain is uncontrolled
  - Breakthrough dose = 1/6 SC Hydromorphone daily dose
- Preparations
  - Immediate release: 1.3mg, 2.6mg
  - Modified release: 2mg, 4mg, 8mg, 16mg, 24mg
  - Injection: 10mg/ml, 1ml amp

Buprenorphine

- Semisynthetic derivative of thebaine
- Highly lipophilic
- Receptors
  - μ-receptor partial agnonist
  - κ-receptor antagonist
  - δ-receptor antagonist
  - Nociceptin receptor partial agonist

- Pharmacology
  - Sublingual buprenorphine
    - Onset of action: 15-45min
    - Half-life: 1-3days
    - Duration of action: 8h
  - Buprenorphine patch (BuTrans)
    - Onset of action: 0.5-1day
    - Half-life: 0.5-1.5days
    - Duration of action: 7 days
  - Buprenorphine patch (Transtec)
    - Onset of action: 0.5-1day
    - Half-life: 1-1.5days
    - Duration of action: 4days
  - Intravenous buprenorphine
    - Onset of action: 5-15min
    - Half-life: 3-16h
    - Duration of action: 8h
  - Metabolites: norbuprenorphine
- Potency
  - 100x more potent than oral morphine
- Starting dose for opioid-naïve patients
  - SL Buprenorphine 0.2mg q8h
    = syrup morphine 10mg q4h
- Doses of buprenorphine patch (BuTrans)
  - Buprenorphine patch (BuTrans) 5mcg/h
    = syrup morphine 2.5mg q4h
  - Buprenorphine patch (BuTrans) 10mcg/h
    = syrup morphine 5mg q4h
  - Buprenorphine patch (BuTrans) 20mcg/h
    = syrup morphine 10mg q4h
- Buprenorphine patch (BuTrans)
  - Change patch every 7th day

- Titrate q72h if pain is uncontrolled
- Rest skin site for 3weeks after using
- Doses of buprenorphine patch (Transtec)
  - Buprenorphine patch (Transtec) 35mcg/h
    = SL Buprenorphine 0.2mg q8h
    = syrup morphine 10mg q4h
  - Buprenorphine patch (Transtec) 52.5mcg/h
    = SL Buprenorphine 0.4mg q8h
    = syrup morphine 15mg q4h
  - Buprenorphine patch (Transtec) 70mcg/h
    = SL Buprenorphine 0.4mg q6h
    = syrup morphine 20mg q4h
  - Buprenorphine patch (Transtec) 140mcg/h
    = SL Buprenorphine 0.8mg q4h
    = syrup morphine 40mg q4h
- Buprenorphine patch (Transtec)
  - Change patch every 3rd day
  - Titrate q72h if pain is uncontrolled
  - Allow 12-24h for maximum effect
  - Allow 12-24h post patch removal for effect to wear off
- Opioid switching to SL Buprenorphine/Naloxone (Suboxone)
  - Useful for opioid-tolerant patients with opioid-induced hyperalgesia (OIH)
  - Background oral MEDD ≥ 60mg/day
  - Stop all opioids
  - SL Suboxone 2mg prn/q6h for breakthrough pain or withdrawal symptoms
  - Maximum dose: 8mg q6h
- Preparations
  - BuTrans: 5mcg/h, 10mcg/h, 20mcg/h
  - Transtec: 35mcg/h, 52.5mcg/h, 70mcg/h
  - Sublingual tablets (Subutex): 0.4mg, 2mg, 8mg

- Sublingual tablets (Temgesic): 0.2mg, 0.4mg
- Sublingual buprenorphine/naloxone (Suboxone) tablets
  - 2/0.5mg (hexagonal orange tablets)
  - 8/2mg (hexagonal orange tablets)
- Sublingual buprenorphine/naloxone (Suboxone) films
  - 2/0.5mg (green box)
  - 4/1mg (purple box)
  - 8/2mg (blue box)
  - 12/3mg (orange box)
- Injection: 0.3mg/ml, 1ml
- Instructions to use suboxone film
  - Not to eat immediately before dosing
  - Take sip of water to moisten mouth
  - Dry hands
  - Hold film by its edge
  - Place under tongue one at a time
  - For multiple films, place two under tongue on either side of frenulum, place the rest onto inside of cheeks
  - Do not move the film after placement
  - Do not chew or swallow
  - Wait until it dissolves in 2-5min
  - Recommended supervision time: <1min because film adheres to mucous membranes within seconds

Methadone

- Synthetic strong opioid
- Lipophilic
- Receptors
  - μ-opioid receptor agonist
  - δ-opioid receptor agonist
  - NMDA receptor blocker
  - Serotonin re-uptake presynaptic blocker

- Pharmacology
  - Bioavailability: 80%
  - Onset of action: < 30min
  - Half-life: 8 hours to 3 days
  - Duration of action: 8-12h with repeated doses
- Potency
  - 10x more potent than oral morphine when oral MEDD <1000mg/day
  - 20x more potent than oral morphine when oral MEDD 1000-2000mg/day
  - 30x more potent than oral morphine when oral MEDD >2000mg/day
- Starting dose for opioid-naïve patients
  - Syrup methadone 5mg q12h and prn/q3h
  - Syrup methadone 2.5mg q12h and prn/q3h for elderly
  - Titrate weekly if necessary
  - Keep the same breakthrough doses
  - If syrup methadone ≥30mg q12h, increase breakthrough dose to 1/10 – 1/6 of the daily dose

Opioid switching to syrup methadone

- Morley-Makin method
  - Stop previous opioid
  - Start syrup methadone as 1/10 of oral MEDD prn/q3h
  - Maximum starting dose 30mg prn/q3h
  - Day 6 (steady state): use average total methadone daily dose used on day 4 and 5 as divided dose q12h
  - Breakthrough: 1/6 of total methadone daily dose prn/q3h
- Modified Morley-Makin method
  - Stop previous opioid
  - Give stat dose of syrup methadone 1/10 of oral MEDD
  - Then start syrup methadone 1/30 of oral MEDD prn/q3h

- Maximum starting dose 30mg prn/q3h
- Day 6 (steady state): use average total methadone daily dose used on day 4 and 5 as divided dose q12h
- Breakthrough: 1/6 of total methadone daily dose prn/q3h
- Titrate weekly if ≥ 2 doses of prn per day
- Reduce dose 30-50% if excessively drowsy
- Give prn/q1h of previous opioid to control withdrawal symptoms or moderate to severe pain < 3h
- Give paracetamol to control mild pain < 3h
- Example for modified Morley-Makin method
  - Stop syrup morphine 50mg q4h (300mg/day)
  - Give stat dose of syrup methadone 30mg
  - Then start syrup methadone 10mg prn/q3h
  - Day 6: if total methadone dose on day 4 and 5 is 60mg, then prescribe syrup methadone 30mg/day = 15mg q12h
  - Breakthrough = 5mg prn/q3h
- Friedman method
  - Oral MEDD (<1000mg/day + age<65) ÷ 10
  - Oral MEDD (<1000mg/day + age>65) ÷ 20
  - Oral MEDD (1000-2000mg/day + any age) ÷ 20
  - Oral MEDD (>2000mg/day + any age) ÷ 30
- Ripamonti method
  - Oral MEDD (30-90mg/day) ÷ 4
  - Oral MEDD (90-300mg/day) ÷ 6
  - Oral MEDD (>300mg/day) ÷ 8
- Mercadante method
  - Oral MEDD (30-90mg/day) ÷ 4
  - Oral MEDD (90-300mg/day) ÷ 8
  - Oral MEDD (>300mg/day) ÷ 12
- Ayonrinde method
  - Oral MEDD (<100mg/day) ÷ 3
  - Oral MEDD (100-300mg/day) ÷ 5

- Oral MEDD (300-600mg/day) ÷ 10
- Oral MEDD (600-800mg/day) ÷ 12
- Oral MEDD (800-1000mg/day) ÷ 15
- Oral MEDD (>1000mg/day) ÷ 20

Rapid switch versus 3-day switch to methadone

- Rapid switch
  - Stop previous opioid and start equianalgesic methadone in 3 daily divided doses
  - Success 77%
  - Side effects 7%
    - Sedation 4%
    - Respiratory depression 0.4%
- Ad libitum switch
  - Morley-Makin or modified Morley-Makin
  - Success 93%
  - Side effects 2%
- 3-day switch
  - Day 1: replace 30% previous opioid with equianalgesic dose of methadone in 3 daily divided doses
  - Day 2: replace 60% previous opioid with equianalgesic dose of methadone in 3 daily divided doses
  - Day 3: replace 100% previous opioid with equianalgesic dose of methadone in 3 daily divided doses
  - Success 93%
  - Less side effects compared to rapid switch

Recommended switch

- Outpatient switch
  - Use modified Morley-Makin method
  - Dose reduce 50% for incomplete cross tolerance

- Review after one week instead of D6 to get the average total methadone daily dose based on previous 2 days
- Breakthrough: 1/6 total daily methadone dose prn/q3h
- Inpatient switch
  - Use Friedman method
  - Dose reduce 50% for incomplete cross tolerance
  - Use 3-day switch
  - Breakthrough options
    - Use previous short-acting opioid prn/q1h
    - Use alternative equianalgesic short-acting opioid prn/q1h if neurotoxic with previous opioid
    - Use 1/6 total daily methadone dose prn/q3h

Tapendatol

- Centrally acting opioid of benzenoid class
- Receptors
  - μ-receptor agonist
  - Noradrenaline reuptake inhibitor
- Pharmacology
  - Bioavailability: 30%
  - Onset of action: 30min
  - Half-life: 4h
  - Duration of action: 4-6h
  - No active metabolites
- Potency
  - 2x more potent than oral tramadol
  - 2.5x less potent than oral morphine
- Conversion
  - Oral Tramadol ÷ 2 = Oral Tapendatol
  - Oral Morphine x 2.5 = Oral Tapendatol
- Dosage
  - Immediate release: 50-100mg q4-6h

- Modified release: 50-250mg q12h
- Preparations
  - Immediate release
    - Nucynta 50mg , 75mg, 100mg
  - Modified release
    - Nucynta ER 50mg, 100mg, 150mg, 200mg, 250mg

Pethidine

- Avoid using pethidine in cancer pain
- Disadvantages of pethidine
  - Excitatory neurotoxicity with chronic use
  - Due to accumulation of toxic metabolite: norpethidine
    - Tremors
    - Multifocal myoclonus
    - Agitation
    - Seizures
  - Ceiling effect due to neurotoxicity
  - Short duration of action 2-3h
  - More emetogenic
  - Contraindicated in renal failure
  - Usually prescribed as intramuscular injection which is painful

Pain Control in Renal Failure

Introduction

The presence of renal failure affects the pharmacokinetics and pharmacodynamics of many drugs. Special precautions are needed before initiating analgesics in renal failure.

Not recommended in renal failure

- Codeine
    - Do not use in renal failure
    - Cumulation of C6G, M6G, M3G
    - Reports of serious side effects
- Dihydrocodeine
    - Do not use in renal failure
    - Cumulation of DHC6G, DHM6G, DHM3G
- Morphine
    - Do not use in renal failure
    - Cumulation of M6G (inhibitory), M3G (excitatory)
    - Opioid toxicity can occur even with small doses
    - Use temporarily only if no other strong opioid available
        - Use immediate release
        - Do not use modified release
        - Do not use infusion
        - Breakthrough: prn/q6h

Dosage reduction recommended by Bunn and Ashley 1999

Morphine	% normal dose	Dose (mg)	Interval
CC20-50	75	5	q6h
CC10-20	50	2.5	q8h
CC<10	25	2.5	q12h

Use cautiously in renal failure

- Tramadol
  - First line weak opioid in renal failure
  - Use with dose reduction in severe renal failure
  - Metabolites: O-desmethyltramadol
  - Use immediate release
  - CC<10: PO Tramadol 50mg tds (on dialysis)
  - CC<10: PO Tramadol 50mg bd (not on dialysis)

Tramadol	% normal dose	Dose (mg)	Interval
CC20-50	100	50-100	q6h
CC10-20	50	50-100	q8h
CC<10	50	50	q12h

- Oxycodone
  - Use with dose reduction and careful monitoring
  - Metabolites: noroxycodone, oxymorphone
  - Case report of CNS-depressant effect in renal failure
  - Use temporarily only if hydromorphone is unavailable
    - Use immediate release in the form of syrup
    - Use in low doses only
    - Do not use modified release
    - Do not use infusion
    - Breakthrough: prn/q6h

Oxycodone	% normal dose	Dose (mg)	Interval
CC20-50	50	2.5-5	q6h
CC10-20	25-50	2.5-5	q8h
CC<10	25-50	2.5-5	q12h

- Hydromorphone
  - First line oral strong opioid in renal failure
  - Use with careful monitoring

- Metabolites: H3G (excitatory)
- Use if oral strong opioid is needed in renal failure
  - Use immediate release
  - Do not use modified release
  - Do not use infusion
- Dose: PO Hydromorphone 1.3mg q4h and prn/q4h
- Keep the total daily dose low by using fentanyl patch when >12mg/day

Fentanyl patch (mcg/h/72h)	PO Hydromorphone prn/q4h (mg)
12	No data
25	1.3
50	2.6
75	5.2
100	7.8
125	9.1

Generally safe with close monitoring in renal failure

- Fentanyl
  - First line strong opioid in renal failure
  - Metabolites: norfentanyl (inactive)
  - Titrate with oral hydromorphone or fentanyl infusion
  - Then convert to fentanyl patch once pain is stable
  - Dose
    - CSCI Fentanyl 5mcg/h for breathlessness
    - CSCI Fentanyl 10mcg/h for moderate/severe pain
    - Breakthrough: 1-2x the hourly dose prn/q1h
- Alfentanil
  - Drug of choice for use in syringe driver
  - Metabolites: noralfentanil (inactive)
  - Use when CSCI Fentanyl > 25mcg/h or 600mcg/24h
  - Not recommended for titration due to short duration of action: 30min

- Dose
  - CSCI Alfentanil 0.5mg/24h for breathlessness
  - CSCI Alfentanil 1mg/24h for moderate/severe pain
  - Breakthrough: 1/10 – 1/6 total daily dose prn/q1h
- Sufentanil
  - Safe with close monitoring
  - Metabolites: N-desalkylsufentanil, O-desmethylsufentanil
  - Dose
    - CSCI Sufentanil 15mcg/24h for breathlessness
    - CSCI Sufentanil 25mcg/24h for pain
    - Breakthrough: 1/24 – 1/12 total daily dose prn/q1h
- Remifentanil
  - Safe with close monitoring
  - Metabolized by esterases
  - Metabolites: remifentanil acid (inactive)
- Buprenorphine
  - Safe with close monitoring
  - Metabolites: norbuprenorphine
    - Does not cross blood-brain barrier
    - Little central effect
- Methadone
  - Safe with close monitoring
  - Metabolites: methadone pyrrolidine (inactive)
  - Pyrrolidine is excreted in feces
  - Some recommend 50% dose reduction when CC<10

Pain Control in Liver Impairment

Introduction

Most opioids are metabolized by liver through phase 1 reactions by cytochrome P450 enzymes 2D6 and 3A4. Some are through phase 2 glucuronidation. Liver impairment may lead to increased risk of opioid toxicity because the parent drug is not adequately converted to metabolites for elimination.

- CYP2D6: O-demethylation
- CYP3A4: N-demethylation

Not recommended in severe liver impairment

- Codeine
    - Do not use in severe liver impairment
    - Not converted to active metabolite morphine
- Dihydrocodeine
    - Do not use in severe liver impairment
    - Not converted to active metabolite dihydromorphine
- Methadone
    - Do not use in severe liver impairment
    - Methadone is highly protein-bound: 80-90%
    - Increased free-drug level due to reduced albumin and α-1-acid glycoprotein production in liver impairment
- Buprenorphine
    - Do not use in severe liver impairment
    - Buprenorphine is highly protein-bound: 96%
    - Increased free-drug level due to reduced albumin and α-1-acid glycoprotein production in liver impairment

Dose adjustment in severe liver impairment (prolonged PT)

- Tramadol
    - PO Tramadol 50mg bd (maximum dose)
    - Use immediate release
    - Do not use modified release
- Morphine, oxycodone, hydromorphone
    - Parent drug may not be converted to metabolites
    - Use oral
    - Use immediate release
    - Do not use modified release
    - Reduce dose 50%
        - PO Morphine 2.5-5mg q8h
        - PO Oxynorm 5mg q8h
        - PO Hydromorphone 1.3mg q8h
- Alfentanil
    - Accumulate in severe liver impairment
    - Reduce dose 50%

Generally safe with close monitoring in severe liver disease

- Fentanyl, sufentanil and remifentanil
    - First line strong opioids in severe liver impairment
    - Pharmacokinetics unaffected by severe liver impairment
    - Fentanyl is affected by reduced hepatic blood flow
    - No dosage adjustment needed
    - Close monitoring for precipitation or aggravation of hepatic encephalopathy

Pain Crisis

Introduction

Pain crisis is a palliative care emergency. Patient needs to be attended immediately.

Definition

- Pain score ≥7
- Patient is in acute distress because of the pain

Rapid parenteral opioid titration

Definitions

- Opioid-tolerant
  - Patients who are taking oral morphine ≥ 60mg/day or an equianalgesic dose of another opioid for a week or longer

- Opioid-naïve
  - Patient who are not taking any opioid
  - Patients who do not meet the definition of opioid-tolerant

Opioid-naïve patients with normal renal function

- Give IV/SC Metoclopramide 10mg stat
- Titrate with IV Morphine 2mg q5min or
- Titrate with SC Morphine 2mg q10min if no IV access
- Check respiratory rate (RR) before each titration
- Titrate till patient is in less distress or pain score <4
- Calculate the total morphine dose given during titration
- Divide the total dose by 4 to get the hourly infusion dose
- Breakthrough: 1-4x hourly dose prn/q1h
- Example:
  - Total IV Morphine given = 10mg
  - CIVI/CSCI Morphine = 10/4 = 2.5mg/h
  - Breakthrough dose = 2.5-10mg prn/q1h
- Preparation: 10mg/ml amp
- Dilution: 50mg morphine into total 50ml saline = 1mg/ml
- Half-life of intravenous morphine = 1.5h
- Time to steady state is 4 x 1.5h = 6h
- Do not increase the continuous infusion dose > 2x/day
- Convert to oral morphine once pain is stable for 2-3 days

Opioid-naïve patients with renal failure

- Give IV/SC Metoclopramide stat
- Titrate with IV Fentanyl 10mcg prn q5min or
- Titrate with SC Fentanyl 10mcg prn q10min if no IV access
- Check respiratory rate (RR) before each titration
- Titrate till patient is in less distress or pain score <4
- Calculate the total fentanyl dose given during titration
- Divide the total dose by 2 to get the hourly infusion dose

- Breakthrough: 1-2x hourly dose prn/q1h
- Example:
  - Total IV Fentanyl given = 50mcg
  - CIVI/CSCI Fentanyl = 50/2 = 25mcg/h
  - Breakthrough dose = 25-50mcg prn/q1h
- Preparation: 100mcg/2ml amp
- Dilution: 500mcg into total 50ml saline = 10mcg/ml
- Half-life of intravenous fentanyl = 3.5h
- Time to steady state is 4 x 3.5h = 14h
- Do not increase the continuous infusion dose > 2x/day
- Convert to fentanyl patch once pain is stable for 2-3 days

"1 + 1" titration method for hydromorphone

- IV Hydromorphone 1mg stat, then 1mg prn 15min later
- Adequate analgesia within 1h in 96% (Chang 2009)

Opioid-tolerant patients

- Refer palliative care team for advice
- Use the breakthrough dose as bolus for rapid titration
- Example:
  - Syrup morphine 30mg q4h
  - Oral morphine breakthrough dose = 30mg
  - Parenteral morphine breakthrough dose = 10mg
  - IV Morphine 10mg q5min or SC Morphine 10mg q10min

Patient controlled analgesia (PCA)

- Opioid-naïve patients
  - PCA IV Morphine
    - Strength: 1mg/ml
    - Dose: 1-3mg
    - Lockout: 10min
    - Total dose over 4h ÷ 4 = infusion rate in mg/h

- New PCA dose = 50% hourly infusion rate
- Max PCA doses/hour = 3-5x estimated required dose
  - PCA IV Hydromorphone
    - Strength: 0.2mg/ml
    - Dose: 0.2-0.4mg
    - Lockout: 10min
  - PCA IV Fentanyl
    - Strength: 10mcg/ml
    - Dose: 10-20mcg
    - Lockout: 10min
- Opioid-tolerant patients
  - PCA IV Morphine
    - Continuous infusion rate in mg/h
    - PCA dose = 50% hourly infusion rate

Dosage increase and opioid toxicity

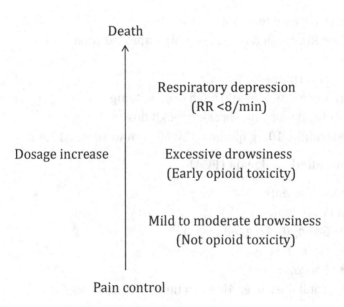

Monitoring in the hospital

- Pain control
    - Numerical pain score q4h
    - End point
        - Patient is less distressed by the pain or
        - Pain score <4
        - Do not reduce pain to 0 during rapid titration to minimize the risk of opioid toxicity
    - Give breakthrough dose if pain score ≥4
- Drowsiness
    - Pasero Opioid-induced Sedation Scale (POSS) q4h
        - S = Sleep, easily arousable
        - 1 = Awake and alert
        - 2 = Slightly drowsy, easily arousable
        - 3 = Frequently drowsy, arousable, drifts off to sleep during conversation
        - 4 = Somnolent, minimal or no response to verbal and physical stimulation
    - S, 1, 2: increase opioid dose if pain is uncontrolled
    - 3: decrease 25-50% opioid dose
    - 4: decrease 50% opioid dose if RR≥8/min; give naloxone 20mcg prn q2min IV or q5min SC if RR<8/min
- Respiratory depression
    - Check RR q1h for first 24h, then q4h
    - Count 1min
    - Give naloxone if RR<8/min
        - Dilute 400mcg (1 ampoule) to 10ml with NS
        - Give 20mcg (0.5ml) q2min IV or q5min SC till RR ≥8/min

Neuropathic Pain Management

Introduction

Neuropathic pain is pain caused by damage to the somatosensory system. The damage is associated with somatosensory signs and symptoms that can be picked up using various neuropathic pain screening tools.

Neuropathic pain screening tools

- LANSS (Leeds Assessment of Neuropathic Symptoms and Signs)
- DN4 (Douleur Neuropathique 4)
- NPQ (Neuropathic Pain Questionnaire)
- PainDETECT
- ID Pain

LANSS (Bennett 2001)

- Does your pain feel like strange, unpleasant sensations in your skin? Words like pricking, tingling, pin and needles might describe these sensations. (5 marks) *Dysesthetic pain*
- Does your pain make the skin in the painful area look different from normal? Words like mottled, looking more red or pink might describe the appearance. (5 marks) *Skin appearance*
- Does your pain make the affected skin abnormally sensitive to touch? Getting unpleasant sensations when lightly stroking the skin, or getting pain when wearing tight clothes might describe the abnormal sensitivity. (3 marks) *Allodynia*
- Does your pain come on suddenly and in bursts for no apparent reason when you are still? Words like electric shocks, jumping and bursting describe these sensations. (2 marks) *Lancinating pain*

- Does your pain feel as if the skin temperature in the painful area has changed abnormally? Words like hot and burning describe these sensations. (1 mark) *Skin temperature*
- Unpleasant sensations like tingling and nausea while lightly stroking cotton wool across painful area. (5 marks) *Allodynia*
- No sensation, reduced sensation or very painful sensation during pinprick examination on painful area. (3 marks) *Anaesthesia, hypoesthesia or hyperalgesia*
    - Score <12: neuropathic mechanisms are unlikely
    - Score ≥12: neuropathic mechanisms are likely
    - Sensitivity 80%, specificity 85%

NNTs of neuropathic agents (Finnerup 2005, 2007)

Antidepressants	NNT

Tricyclic antidepressants (TCAs)
- Balanced SNRIs
   - Amitriptyline
   - Imipramine
   - Clomipramine
	2-3
	2.1

- Predominantly NRIs
   - Nortriptyline
   - Desipramine
   - Maprotiline
	2.5

Serotonin-noradrenaline reuptake inhibitors (SNRIs) - Duloxetine - Venlafaxine	5.1
Dopamine-noradrenaline reuptake inhibitors (DNRIs) - Bupropion	1.6
Selective serotonin reuptake inhibitors (SSRIs) - Paroxetine - Citalopram - Fluoxetine	7

Anticonvulsants	NNT
Gabapentin (all doses)	5.1
Gabapentin 800mg tds	3.8
Pregabalin 150-300mg bd	3.7
Sodium valproate 400mg tds	2.5
Phenytoin	2.1
Carbamazepine	2.0
Lamotrigine 400mg dly	4.9
Topiramate	7.4

NNTs of opioids

- Morphine   2.5
- Oxycodone   2.6
- Tramadol   3.9

NNTs of miscellaneous agents

- Topical lignocaine   4.4
- Topical capsaicin   6.7

Choices of neuropathic medications in palliative care

- Step 1: strong opioid ± NSAID/steroid
- Step 2: tricyclic antidepressant or anticonvulsant
- Step 3: tricyclic antidepressant and anticonvulsant
- Step 4: ketamine
- Step 5: spinal opioid

Tricyclic antidepressant titration

- Standard titration
  - Day 1: PO Amitriptyline 25mg on
  - Day 3: PO Amitriptyline 50mg on
  - Week 2: PO Amitriptyline 75mg on

- Week 2: PO Amitriptyline 100mg on
- Week 3: PO Amitriptyline 150mg on (often unnecessary)
- Frail elderly
  - Day 1: PO Amitriptyline 10mg on
  - Day 3: PO Amitriptyline 25mg on
  - Week 2: PO Amitriptyline 50mg on
  - Week 4: PO Amitriptyline 75mg on
  - Week 6: PO Amitriptyline 100mg on
  - Week 8: PO Amitriptyline 150mg on (often unnecessary)
- Amitriptyline
  - Mechanism: serotonin-noradrenaline reuptake inhibitor
  - Analgesic effect: after 3-7 days
  - Antidepressant effect: after 2-4 weeks
  - Contraindicated in significant heart disease
  - Taken at night
  - Taken 2h pre-bed if early morning drowsiness
  - Significant blood level indicated by dry mouth
  - Stop if <50% pain reduction despite reasonable doses
  - Length of trial: 4-6 weeks
  - Stop gradually over 2-3 weeks
  - When switching from one antidepressant class to another, overlap the gradual stopping of old antidepressant with the gradual introduction of new antidepressant over 2-3 weeks

Other antidepressants

- Second generation TCAs
  - Secondary amines
  - First line antidepressant for neuropathic pain
  - Recommended by NeuPSIG of IASP
  - NeuPSIG: Neuropathic Pain Special Interest Group
  - Less adverse effect than first generation TCAs

- - - PO Nortriptyline 25-150mg on
    - PO Desipramine 25-150mg on
  - First generation TCAs
    - Tertiary amines
    - First line antidepressant for neuropathic pain
    - Recommended if secondary amines are not available
    - More analgesic property than second generation TCAs
      - PO Amitriptyline 25-150mg on
      - PO Imipramine 25-150mg on
- PO Duloxetine (Cymbalta)
  - Second line antidepressant for neuropathic pain
  - Mechanism: serotonin-noradrenaline reuptake inhibitor
  - Week 1: 30mg on
  - Week 2: 60mg on (more nausea if initiate at 60mg dly)
  - Week 2: 60mg bd (more analgesia and more side effects)
  - Optimal dose: 60mg on
  - Contraindicated if CC<30ml/min
  - Stop if no benefit despite maximum dose
  - Length of trial: 4 weeks
  - Stop gradually over 2-3 weeks
- PO Venlafaxine (Effexor)
  - Second line antidepressant for neuropathic pain
  - Mechanism: serotonin-noradrenaline reuptake inhibitor
  - Week 1: 37.5mg dly
  - Week 2: 37.5mg bd
  - Week 4: 75mg bd
  - Optimal dose: 75mg bd
  - May increase systolic BP ≥10mm with 75mg bd
  - Contraindicated if CC <10ml/min or PT>18s
  - Stop if no benefit despite maximum dose
  - Length of trial: 4-6 weeks
  - Stop gradually over 2-3 weeks

- PO Venlafaxine MR (Effexor XL)
  - Week 1: 37.5mg dly
  - Week 2: 75mg dly
  - Week 4: 150mg dly
- PO Bupropion (Wellbutrin)
  - Mechanism: serotonin-noradrenaline reuptake inhibitor, dopamine reuptake inhibitor
  - Psychostimulant properties
  - Starting dose: 75mg bd
  - Average dose: 100-150mg bd
  - Maximum dose: 300mg bd (risk of seizure)
- PO Citalopram (Celexa)
  - Mechanism: selective serotonin reuptake inhibitor
  - Starting dose: 10mg om
  - Average dose: 20-40mg om
  - Maximum dose: 60mg om
  - Taper gradually
- PO Paroxetine (Paxil)
  - Mechanism: selective serotonin reuptake inhibitor
  - Starting dose: 10mg on
  - Average dose: 20-40mg on
  - Maximum dose: 60mg on
  - Taper gradually

Gabapentin titration in normal renal function

- Rapid titration
  - Day 1: PO Gabapentin 300mg on
  - Day 2: PO Gabapentin 300mg bd
  - Day 3: PO Gabapentin 300mg tds
  - Day 6: PO Gabapentin 600mg tds
  - Day 9: PO Gabapentin 800-900mg tds
  - Day 12: PO Gabapentin 1200mg tds (often unnecessary)

- Slow titration in frail elderly
    - Week 1: PO Gabapentin 300mg on
    - Week 2: PO Gabapentin 300mg tds
    - Week 3: PO Gabapentin 600mg tds
    - Week 4: PO Gabapentin 800-900mg tds
    - Week 5: PO Gabapentin 1200mg tds (often unnecessary)

Gabapentin titration in renal impairment

CC in ml/min	Starting dose	Maximum dose
>80	300mg tds	800mg tds
50-80	200mg tds	400mg tds
30-50	300mg on	300mg bd
15-30	300mg EOD	300mg on
<15	300mg EOD	300mg EOD
After 4h HD	200-300mg stat	

- Gabapentin (Neurontin)
    - First line anticonvulsant in neuropathic pain
    - Mechanism: $\alpha2\delta$ subunit calcium channel blocker
    - GABA analogue but no activity at GABA receptor
    - Analgesic effect: from immediate to 1-2 weeks
    - Maximum analgesic effect: 2 months
    - Synergism: Gabapentin 600mg tds+nortriptyline 50mg on
        - More effective than either drug alone at high doses
        - Without significant side effects
    - Drowsiness in 50%: resolves in 7-10 days
    - Capsule can be opened
    - Contents can be mixed with water or fruit juice
    - Stop if no benefit despite ≥800mg tds
    - Length of trial: 8 weeks
    - Stop gradually over 1-2 weeks

Pregabalin titration in normal renal function

- Standard titration
  - Day 1: PO Pregabalin 75mg bd
  - After 3-7 days: PO Pregabalin 150mg bd
  - After 3-7 days: PO Pregabalin 225mg bd
  - After 3-7 days: PO Pregabalin 300mg bd
- Slow titration in frail elderly
  - Day 1: PO Pregabalin 75mg on
  - Increase cautiously every week if necessary

Pregabalin titration in renal impairment

CC in ml/min	Starting dose	Maximum dose
>60	75mg bd	300mg bd
31-60	25mg tds	150mg bd
15-30	25-50mg on	150mg on
<15	25mg on	75mg on
After 4h HD	25mg stat	150mg stat

- Pregabalin (Lyrica)
  - First line anticonvulsant in neuropathic pain
  - Mechanism: $\alpha2\delta$ subunit calcium channel blocker
  - GABA analogue but no activity at GABA receptor
  - Analgesic effect: <24h
  - Maximum analgesic effect: 2 weeks
  - Compared to gabapentin
    - More rapid onset of pain relief
    - Linear pharmacokinetics: less individual variability
    - Less dose-related side effects: faster titration
    - Twice daily dosing
    - Maximum benefit at 2 weeks (gabapentin 2 months)

- Stop if no benefit despite 300mg bd
- Length of trial: 8 weeks
- Stop gradually over 1-2 weeks

Other anticonvulsants

- PO Sodium valproate (Epilim)
  - Mechanism: GABA reuptake inhibitor, GABA transaminase inhibitor, sodium channel blocker
  - Week 1: 200mg tds
  - Week 2: 400mg tds
  - Week 3: 600mg bd
- PO Phenytoin (Dilantin)
  - Mechanism: sodium channel blocker
  - 100mg tds
- PO Carbamazepine (Tegretol)
  - Mechanism: sodium channel blocker
  - Starting dose: 100-200mg bd
  - Titration: 200mg increment every 1-2 weeks
  - Maximum dose: 600mg bd
- PO Lamotrigine (Lamictal)
  - Mechanism: sodium channel blocker
  - Starting dose: 25-50mg on
  - Titration: 50mg increment every 2 weeks
  - Maximum dose: 400mg on
- PO Topiramate (Topamax)
  - Mechanism: sodium channel blocker, GABA potentiation
  - Starting dose: 50mg on
  - Titration: 50mg increment every 2 weeks
  - Maximum dose: 200mg bd
- PO Levetiracetam (Keppra)
  - Mechanism: calcium channel blocker
  - Starting dose: 500mg bd

- Titration: 1000mg increment every 2 weeks
- Maximum dose: 1500mg bd
- PO Zonisamide (Zonegran)
  - Mechanism: sodium channel blocker, calcium channel blocker, GABA release
  - Starting dose: 100mg dly for 2 weeks
  - Titration: 200mg increment every week
  - Maximum dose: 200mg bd

Miscellaneous neuropathic agents

- PO/SC/IV Dexamethasone
  - Dexamethasone 4-8mg om for plexus or root compression
  - Dexamethasone 12-16mg om for spinal cord compression
  - Trial of 5-7 days
- PO Ketamine
  - Mechanism: NMDAR blocker
  - Day 1: 10mg tds-qid
  - Day 2: 20mg tds-qid
  - Day 3: 40mg tds-qid
  - Day 4: 60mg tds-qid
  - Day 5: 80mg tds-qid
  - Day 6: 100mg tds-qid
  - Consider the following:
    - 30-50% opioid dose reduction at the beginning
    - Further opioid dose reduction during titration
    - PRN/tds ketamine equivalent to regular dose
    - Q4h dosing for end-of-dose pain
    - Smaller doses and q4h dosing for neuropsychiatric side effects or drowsiness despite opioid reduction
    - Prevention of neuropsychiatric side effects
      - PO Haloperidol 1.5-3mg on
      - PO Diazepam 2.5-5mg on

- Lignocaine patch 5% (Lidoderm)
  - Useful in localized neuropathic pain
  - 1-3 patches daily
  - 12h on, 12h off: to avoid tachyphylaxis (acute tolerance)
  - Applied to intact skin to cover the most painful area
- Capsaicin patch 8% (Qutenza)
  - Useful in localized neuropathic pain
  - 1-4 patches every three months
  - Application techniques
    - Wear gloves
    - Mark painful area
    - Wash the area with mild soap and water
    - Dry thoroughly
    - Anaesthetize skin with topical LA
    - Wash and dry the area
    - Cut patch to fit area
    - Leave patch in place
      - 30min for feet
      - 60min for other locations
    - Remove patch by gently rolling it inward
    - Apply cleansing gel to area for 1 minute
    - Wash the area with mild soap and water
    - Dry thoroughly
  - Side effects in 5%: redness, pain, itching, papules
- Capsaicin cream 0.075%
  - Useful in localized neuropathic pain
  - Applied to painful area tds-qid
  - Causes severe burning sensation
  - Stop if no benefit after 1 week
- EMLA cream
  - Useful in localized neuropathic pain
  - Eutectic mixture of LA: prilocaine and lignocaine

Neuropathic pain crisis

- Step 1: rapid parenteral morphine titration or IV PCA opioid
- Step 2: parenteral opioid switching
- Step 3: parenteral lignocaine or ketamine
- Step 4: spinal opioid

Parenteral lignocaine

- Mechanism: sodium channel blocker
- Standard dose: IV Lignocaine 5mg/kg over 30-60min
    - <250mg: dilute with 100ml D5
    - ≥250mg: dilute with 500ml D5
    - Maximum dose: 900mg
- Low dose: IV Lignocaine 1mg/kg over 30min
- Syringe driver dose
    - CSCI Lignocaine 1-2mg/kg/h or
    - CSCI Lignocaine 500-1000mg/24h
    - Useful for patients who require frequent IV Lignocaine

Parenteral ketamine

- Mechanism: NMDAR blocker
- Standard titration of subcutaneous ketamine infusion
    - Day 1: CSCI Ketamine 50mg/24h (2mg/h)
    - Day 2: CSCI Ketamine 100mg/24h (4mg/h)
    - Day 3: CSCI Ketamine 200mg/24h (8mg/h)
    - Day 4: CSCI Ketamine 300mg/24h (12mg/h)
    - Day 5: CSCI Ketamine 400mg/24h (16mg/h)
    - Day 6: CSCI Ketamine 500mg/24h (20mg/h)
    - Day 7: CSCI Ketamine 600mg/24h (25mg/h)
    - Consider the following:
        - Starting at 25mg/24h (1mg/h) for frail elderly
        - Loading dose of 10mg in 1ml NS
        - 50-100% q8h titration in severe uncontrolled pain

- 30-50% opioid dose reduction at the beginning
- Further opioid dose reduction during titration
- Prevention of neuropsychiatric side effects
  - CSCI Haloperidol 1.5-3mg/24h
  - CSCI Midazolam 5-10mg/24h
- Burst ketamine
  - Day 1: CSCI Ketamine 100mg/24h
    - Effective: continue for 3 days, then stop
    - Ineffective: titrate
  - Day 2: CSCI Ketamine 300mg/24h
    - Effective: continue for 3 days, then stop
    - Ineffective: titrate
  - Day 3: CSCI Ketamine 500mg/24h
    - Effective: continue for 3 days, then stop
    - Ineffective: stop
- Preparation: 50mg/ml in 10ml vial
- Conversion to oral ketamine
  - Oral ketamine is metabolized by CYP3A4 to norketamine
  - Norketamine
    - 1/3 as potent as parenteral ketamine as anaesthetic
    - Equipotent to parenteral ketamine as analgesia
  - Switch to oral ketamine q6h with 1:1 conversion

Miscellaneous parenteral neuropathic agents

- IV Dexmedetomidine 0.2-0.6mcg/kg/h over 50min
- IV Phenytoin 600mg over 24h
- IV Phenytoin 15mg/kg over 2h
- IV Sodium valproate 200-400mg tds
- IV Ondansetron 8mg once
- IV Magnesium sulfate 30mg/kg over 30min

Bone Pain Management

Introduction

Optimal management of bone metastases needs integration of opioid and non-opioid analgesia, bone-targeted agents, cancer-directed treatment and sometimes orthopaedic surgery.

Clinical features of bone pain

- Dull and constant pain
- Increases gradually with time
- May be aggravated by movement or weight-bearing
- Progresses to spontaneous pain with time
- Spontaneous pain can be acute, severe and unpredictable

Mechanisms of cancer-induced bone pain

- Nociceptive component
  - Inflammatory mediators
  - Skeletal remodelling
- Neuropathic component
  - Damage to sensory and sympathetic nerves
  - Pathological sprouting

Analgesia

- Use WHO analgesic ladder
  - Paracetamol
  - NSAIDs: reduce inflammatory mediators
  - Steroids: reduce inflammatory mediators
  - Opioid
  - Neuropathic agents: target neuropathic component

Bone-targeted agents

- Biphosphonates
    - Osteoclast inhibitor
    - Target skeletal remodelling
    - Benefits
        - Reduce frequency of skeletal-related events (SREs)
        - Reduce bone pain
        - Reduce hypercalcemia
    - Onset of analgesia: 2 weeks
    - NNT for pain control: 11 at 4 weeks, 7 at 12 weeks
    - Long term use ≥6 months reduces new SREs in breast cancer, prostate cancer and myeloma
    - Non-nitrogen containing bisphosphonates
        - Clodronate and etidronate
        - Converted intracellularly into methylene-containing ATP analogue
        - Accumulate in macrophages and osteoclasts
        - Cause direct apoptosis
    - Nitrogen containing bisphosphonates
        - Pamidronate, zoledronate, ibandronate
        - Also inhibit farnesyl diphosphate synthase (rate-limiting enzyme of mevalonate pathway)
            - Prevent protein prenylation of small GTPase (Ras, Rho, Rab): important signalling proteins that regulate osteoclast survival
    - Indications
        - Breast cancer with symptomatic bone mets
        - Hormone-resistant prostate cancer with bone mets
        - Myeloma requiring chemotherapy ± bone mets
    - Dosages
        - IV Pamidronate (Aredia) 90mg over 4h monthly
        - IV Zoledronate (Zometa) 4mg over 15min monthly

- Avoid in renal failure
- Side effect: osteonecrosis of the jaw
  - Long term pamidronate 4%
  - Long term zoledronate 10%
- Stop if declining performance status
- Denosumab
  - RANK-L antibody
  - Osteoclast inhibitor
  - Superior over zoledronate in preventing SREs
  - Dosage: SC Denosumab (XGEVA) 120mg monthly
  - No need dose adjustment in renal failure

External beam radiotherapy

- For localized bone metastases
- Pain relief within 4-6 weeks
  - 60%: partial pain relief
  - 30%: complete pain relief
  - 10%: pain flare during first few days
- Single fraction 8Gy as efficacious as 5 fractions 20Gy
- Single fraction: re-treatment rate 2.5x higher

Radiopharmaceuticals

- For widespread painful bone metastases
- Response rate: 40-95%
- Strontium-89 or samarium-153
- Side effect: bone marrow suppression (mild, reversible)

Spinal cord compression

- Combined surgery and radiotherapy for fit patients
  - Superior to radiotherapy alone in functional outcome
- Radiotherapy alone
  - For unfit patients with poor prognosis

Miscellaneous treatment

- Radiofrequency ablation (RFA)
- High intensity focused ultrasound (HIFU)
- Vertebroplasty
- Surgical fixation of pathological fracture or impending pathological fracture

---

Interesting facts

Chronic pain can be unlearned through 6 weeks of visualization based on neuroplasticity because neurons that fire together wire together, neurons that fire apart wire apart. The techniques are summarized in the acronym MIRROR (Moskowitz 2013).

- **M**otivation: Stay motivated to change the brain even without immediate success.
- **I**ntention: Focus on changing the brain to stop persistent pain.
- **R**elentlessness: Counter-stimulate every pain intrusion using thoughts, images, sensations, memories, soothing emotions, movement and beliefs.
- **R**eliability: Count on the brain to make positive change.
- **O**pportunity: Use pain intrusions as an opportunity to practice neuroplastic treatment approaches to stop pain.
- **R**estoration: Disconnect expanded pain map to its important role of sounding and alarm about danger.

Incident Pain Management

Introduction

Incident pain is pain caused by a specific event like movement.

Types of breakthrough pain (BTP)

- Spontaneous pain
- Incident pain
    - Volitional: movement, sitting, eating, drinking
    - Non-volitional: cough, micturition, defecation
    - Procedural: wound dressing
- End-of-dose failure

Simple measures

- Movement-related pain
    - Make use of a draw sheet correctly
    - Turn patient gently
    - Pay attention to facial expression or vocalization of pain
- Cough-related pain
    - Give cough suppressant
    - Advise to reduce smoking if appropriate
    - Advise to reduce food or drink which aggravates cough
- Meal-related pain
    - Treat oral candidiasis
    - Use lignocaine viscous or coating agent for mucositis
    - Consider alternative feeding route like NG feeding
- Micturition-related pain
    - Rapid response to request for help
    - Urinary catheter for urinary retention
    - Rapid diaper change for perianal excoriation

- Defecation-related pain
  - Rapid response to request for help
  - Laxatives for constipation
  - Local anaesthetic for haemorrhoids
  - Rapid diaper change for perianal excoriation
- Procedure-related pain
  - Explanation about the procedure
  - Distract patient by talking if appropriate
  - Stop immediately if requested
  - Local anaesthetic before procedure

Analgesics and onset of analgesia

- Onset of analgesia ≤5min
  - IV Alfentanil: 0.75min
  - IV Sufentanil: 1min
  - IV Fentanyl: 1.5min
  - IV Morphine: 5min
- Onset of analgesia ≤10min
  - SL Sufentanil: 4-6min
  - SL Alfentanil: 5-10min
  - SL Fentanyl: 5-10min
  - IN Fentanyl: 5-10min
  - OTFC: 5-10min
  - SC Morphine: 10min
  - IN Ketamine: 10min
- Onset of analgesia ≤30min
  - Neb Fentanyl: 15min
  - SL Buprenorphine: 15-30min
  - SC Ketamine: 15-30min
  - Syrup Morphine: 20-30min
  - PO Methadone: 30min
  - PO Ketamine: 30min

Sedatives and onset of sedation

- Nitrous oxide: <1min
- IV Midazolam: 2-3min
- SC Midazolam: 5-10min
- SL Lorazepam: 5min
- PO Lorazepam: 10-15min
- Buccal Midazolam: 15min

Characteristics of BTP

- Rapid onset BTP (ROBTP)
    - Peaks within 5min
    - Fades within 15min
- Gradual onset BTP (GOBTP)
    - Peaks within 15-30min
    - Fades within 1h

	ROBTP	Syrup morphine	OTFC
Onset	Immediate	20-30min	5-10min
Peak	5min	40-60min	20min
Duration	15min	4h	1-2h

Management of GOBTP and ROBTP

- Triple opioid therapy (TOT)
    - Baseline pain: long acting opioid
    - GOBTP: short acting opioid
    - ROBTP: rapid onset opioid
- Rapid onset opioids
    - OTFC
    - SL Fentanyl
    - IN Fentanyl
    - SL Alfentanil
    - SL Sufentanil

Management of non-volitional incident pain

- Step 1: SL Fentanyl 25mcg
- Step 2: SL Fentanyl 50mcg
- Step 3: SL Sufentanil 12.5mcg or SL Alfentanil 0.5mg
- Step 4: SL Sufentanil 25mcg or SL Alfentanil 1mg
- Step 5: SL Sufentanil 50mcg or SL Alfentanil 2mg

Management of volitional incident pain and procedural pain

- Step 1: PO Analgesia ± PO Sedative
  - PO Analgesia 60min before incidence/procedure
    - PO Diclofenac 50-100mg or
    - PO Dihydrocodeine 30-60mg or
    - PO Tramadol 50-100mg or
    - Syrup morphine 1/6 total oral daily dose
  - PO Sedative 60min before incidence/procedure
    - PO Lorazepam 0.5-1mg or
    - PO Diazepam 5mg
- Step 2: SL/SC Analgesia ± SL/SC Sedative
  - SL/SC Analgesia 30min before incidence/procedure
    - OTFC (Actiq) 200mcg or
    - Fentanyl buccal tablet (Effentora) 100mcg or
    - Fentanyl sublingual tablet (Abstral) 100mcg or
    - Fentanyl intranasal spray (Lazanda) 100mcg or
    - Fentanyl sublingual solution 50-100mcg or
    - Alfentanil sublingual solution 250-500mcg or
    - Sufentanil sublingual solution 12.5-25mcg or
    - SC Morphine 1/6 total SC daily dose
  - SL/SC Sedative 30min before incidence/procedure
    - SL Lorazepam 0.5-1mg
    - SL Alprazolam 0.25-0.5mg
    - SC Midazolam 2.5-5mg
    - Buccal Midazolam 2.5-5mg

- Step3: IV Analgesia ± IV Sedative
  - IV Analgesia 5min before incidence/procedure
    - IV Morphine 1/6 total IV daily dose
    - IV Fentanyl 1/12 total IV daily dose
    - IV Ketamine 25-50mg
      - Give 5mg q1min till sedation
  - IV Sedative 5min before incidence/procedure
    - IV Midazolam 2.5-5mg
      - Give 0.5mg q1min till sedation

Cautions

- Health care providers must be competent in:
  - Opioid and sedative titration
  - Airway management
  - Reversal of analgesia and sedation
    - Benzodiazepine reversal
      - IV Flumazenil 0.2mg prn/q1min
      - Maximum 4 doses
      - Repeat after 20min if re-sedation
      - Benzodiazepine tolerance
        - Aim: partial reversal
        - Endpoint: RR≥8/min
    - Opioid reversal
      - IV Naloxone 20mcg prn/q2min
      - Opioid tolerance
        - Aim: partial reversal
        - Endpoint: RR≥8/min

Anaesthetic Procedure in Pain Control

Introduction

Interventional pain management is considered 'step 4' in WHO analgesic ladder. (Miguel 2000)

Neuraxial infusions

- Indications
    - Unacceptable side effects with systemic opioids
    - Poor pain control with systemic opioids
    - Unsuccessful opioid switching
- Epidural opioid infusion
    - Short term use ≤ 3 weeks
    - Higher rate of catheter migration and occlusion
    - Divide parenteral morphine daily dose by 10 to get the epidural morphine daily dose
- Intrathecal opioid infusion
    - Long term use 3 weeks to 3 months
    - Lower rate of catheter migration and occlusion
    - Divide parenteral morphine daily dose by 100 to get the intrathecal morphine daily dose
    - Consider an implantable pump system if:
        - Long term use ≥ 3 months
        - Able to afford the implant pump
        - Diffuse pain from widespread metastases
        - Access to pump refill/reprogramming capabilities
        - Favourable response to intrathecal trial with >50% pain relief

- Absence of severe incident pain requiring frequent patient-controlled doses
- Absence of the need for an epidural infusion which requires a higher volume
- Implantable pump system
  - Fixed rate pump
    - 0.5ml/day or 1ml/day
    - Titration based on changing concentration
    - Refillable drug reservoir up to 60ml
  - Programmable rate pump
    - Titration based on programming the pump
    - Refillable drug reservoir 20-40ml

Intrathecal analgesia

- Step 1: morphine/hydromorphone
- Step 2: morphine/hydromorphone + bupivacaine
- Step 3: morphine/hydromorphone + bupivacaine + clonidine
- Switch to fentanyl/sufentanil if side effects or lack of analgesia

Equianalgesic opioid switching in mg

Opioid	Parenteral	Epidural	Intrathecal
Morphine	100	10	1
Hydromorphone	20	2	0.25
Fentanyl	1	0.01	0.001

Maximum long term IT drug concentrations and doses

- Proposed to minimize risk of catheter tip granuloma

Drug	Max concentration (mg/ml)	Maximum daily dose (mg)
Morphine	20	15
Hydromorphone	10	4
Bupivacaine	40	30
Clonidine	2	1

Spinal drugs

- Morphine and hydromorphone
    - First line spinal opioids
    - Hydrophilic
    - Penetrate spine effectively
    - Slow redistribution
- Fentanyl and sufentanil
    - Second line spinal opioids
    - Hydrophobic
    - Penetrate spine less effectively
    - Rapid redistribution
    - Lower risk of catheter tip granuloma
- Bupivacaine
    - Concentration
        - 0.125% = 1.25mg/ml (pain relief)
        - 0.25% = 2.5mg/ml (pain relief)
        - 0.375% = 3.75mg/ml (sensory/motor block)
        - 0.5% = 5mg/ml (sensory/motor block)
    - Epidural (ED) Bupivacaine 2-6ml/h
    - Intrathecal (IT) Bupivacaine 0.5-2ml/h
    - Side effects: dose-dependent sensory/motor block
    - Sensory/motor block: dose ≥15mg/day
- Clonidine
    - ED Clonidine 150-300mcg/24h
    - IT Clonidine 15-30mcg/24h
    - Side effects: dose-dependent hypotension, bradycardia

Breakthrough pain for spinal analgesia

- Oral or SC Morphine prn
- Oral or SC Ketamine 10-25mg prn

Nerve blocks

- Esophageal visceral pain
  - Interpleural block
- Upper abdominal visceral pain
  - Coeliac plexus block
- Pelvic visceral pain (except ovarian pain)
  - Superior hypogastric block
- Perineal visceral pain
  - Ganglion impar block
- Perineal and perianal pain
  - Saddle block

Peripheral nerve blocks

- Peripheral nerve blocks with proven success rate
  - Gasserian block for trigeminal neuralgia
  - Intercostal block for chest wall or rib metastases
  - Paravertebral block for radicular pain
- Infusion rate
  - Peripheral infusion of lignocaine 1-2% 3-8ml/h
  - Peripheral infusion of bupivacaine 0.125-0.25% 3-8ml/h
  - Peripheral infusion of ropivacaine 0.2-0.3% 3-8ml/h

Breathlessness

Introduction

Breathlessness is a subjective experience of breathing discomfort. It is caused by a mismatch between the need of breathing and the work of breathing.

Sensory information on the need of breathing

- Chemoreceptors
  - Central chemoreceptors
    - Ventrolateral surface of medulla oblongata
      - Detect CSF pH, not plasma pH
        - CO_2 crosses blood-brain barrier
        - Reacts with H_2O
        - Becomes carbonic acid
        - Reduces pH
        - Stimulates central chemoreceptors
      - Cannot detect plasma pH
        - H^+ cannot cross blood-brain barrier
  - Peripheral chemoreceptors
    - Carotid bodies
      - At common carotid arteries
      - Detect blood O2, CO2 and pH
      - By type I glomus cell
      - To carotid sinus nerve
      - To glossopharyngeal nerve
      - To medulla oblongata
    - Aortic bodies
      - At aortic arch
      - Detect blood O2 and CO2

- By type I glomus cell
- To vagus nerve
- To medulla oblongata
- Cold receptors at upper airway
  - Innervated by vagus nerve
  - Detect change in temperature of upper airway
  - Stimulation reduces dyspnoea
- Juxtacapillary receptors (J receptors)
  - Also called pulmonary C-fiber receptors
  - Located within alveolar wall
  - In juxtaposition to pulmonary capillaries of the lung
  - Innervated by vagus nerve
  - Detect increase in pulmonary interstitial volume
    - Due to pulmonary oedema
  - Detect physical engorgement of pulmonary capillaries
    - Due to left heart failure
- Stretch receptors
  - Slowly adapting stretch receptors (SARs)
    - Located at smooth muscle of larger airway
    - Myelinated afferent fibers of vagus
    - Detect increase in airway wall tension
    - Rhythmic discharge during normal breathing
      - Increased discharge during inspiration
      - Reduced discharge during expiration
    - Stimulation of SARs decreases dyspnoea
  - Rapidly adapting stretch receptors (RARs)
    - Located throughout the respiratory tract
    - Thin myelinated afferent fibers of vagus
    - Detect mechanical and chemical irritant stimuli
    - Irregular discharge
    - Stimulations of RARs causes dyspnoea, cough, bronchospasm, secretion

- Chest wall receptors
    - Muscle spindles in chest wall
    - Detect stretch and tension of respiratory muscles

Motor control on the work of breathing

- Medullary respiratory center
    - Primary respiratory control
    - Groups of respiratory neurons
        - Dorsal respiratory group (DRG)
            - Nucleus tractus solitarius (NTS)
            - Inspiratory neurons
                - Activate phrenic nerve neurons
                - Control diaphragm
                - Control inspiration
                - Inhibit expiratory neurons in VRG, PRG
        - Ventral respiratory group (VRG)
            - Nucleus ambiguous (NA)
                - Inspiratory neurons
                    - Supply external intercostal muscles
                    - Supply accessory muscles
            - Nucleus retroambigualis (NRA)
                - Rostral NRA: inspiratory neurons
                - Caudal NRA: expiratory neurons
                    - Supply internal intercostal muscles
                    - Supply abdominal muscles
                    - Control voluntary forced expiration
                    - Inhibit inspiratory neurons
        - Pre-Botzinger complex (pre-BotC)
            - Pacemaker neurons
        - Botzinger complex (BotC)
            - Nucleus retrofacialis (NRF)
                - Expiratory neurons

- Pontine respiratory center
  - Pneumotaxic center
    - Expiratory neurons
      - Medial parabrachial nucleus
    - Inspiratory neurons
      - Lateral parabachial nucleus
      - Kolliker-Fuse nucleus
    - Inhibits DRG
    - Shortens inspiration
    - Causes phase switching
      - More breaths within a given time
      - Increases respiratory rate
  - Apneustic center
    - Believed to stimulate DRG
    - Not found
- Control of breathing
  - Inspiration
    - 1-2s during normal quiet breathing (eupnoea)
    - Inspiratory neurons in DRG and rVRG send signals to diaphragm and external intercostal muscles
    - Diaphragm pulls downward
    - External intercostals pull ribs upward and outward
  - Expiration (passive)
    - 2-3s
    - Expiratory neurons in BotC terminate inspiration by inhibiting inspiratory neurons
    - Inspiratory muscles relax
    - Ribs return to relaxed position due to compliance
    - Expiratory neurons in cNRA are responsible for forced expiration
    - Send signals to internal intercostal muscles and abdominal muscles

Measuring Breathlessness

Introduction

Unidimensional tools are suitable for the rapid assessment of breathlessness and treatment response. Multidimensional tools are best reserved for quality of life assessment.

Definition of dyspnoea

A subjective experience of breathing discomfort that is comprised of qualitatively distinct sensations that vary in intensity. (American Thoracic Society 1999)

Unidimensional tools

- Numerical rating scale (NRS)
  - Scores breathlessness from 0 to 10
  - 0 = breathlessness
  - 10 = worst possible breathlessness
  - Types of NRSs
    - NRS0: breathlessness score right now
    - NRS24 average: average score last 24h
    - NRS24 best: best score last 24h
    - NRS24 worst: worst score last 24h
- Visual analogue scale (VAS)
  - Scores breathlessness from a 10cm line on a ruler
  - 0 = no breathlessness
  - 10 = worst possible breathlessness
  - Ask patient to mark a point that best describes his or her breathlessness
  - VAS24: average score last 24h
  - ESAS: combined VAS and NRS from 0 to 10

- Modified Borg scale
  - Categorical scale with ratio properties
  - Can be used over the phone
  - Nothing at all = 0
  - Very, very slight (just noticeable) = 0.5
  - Very slight = 1
  - Slight = 2
  - Moderate = 3
  - Somewhat severe = 4
  - Severe = 5
  - Very severe = 7
  - Very, very severe (almost maximal) = 9
  - Maximal = 10

Multidimensional tools

- Breathlessness-specific
  - Modified MRC Dyspnoea Scale
  - Baseline/Transition Dyspnoea Index
  - Feinstein's Index of Dyspnoea
- Disease-specific
  - Cancer Dyspnoeic Scale
  - MND Dyspnoeic Rating Scale
  - Clinical COPD Questionnaire

Treating Causes of Breathlessness

Introduction

Disease-directed management can be helpful in the management of breathlessness. Decision making should be based on autonomy, risk-benefit proportionality, performance status, prognosis and quality of life.

Specific treatment of causes of breathlessness

- Upper airway obstruction
    - Steroids
    - Tracheostomy
    - Stenting
    - Radiotherapy
    - Brachytherapy
    - Laser treatment
- Bronchospasm
    - Bronchodilators
    - Steroids
- Pneumonia
    - Antibiotics
    - Steroids if infective exacerbation of COAD
- Heart failure
    - Diuretics
    - Nitrates
    - Digitalis
    - ACE inhibitors
- Lung cancer
    - Radiotherapy
    - Chemotherapy

- Pleural effusion
  - Pleural drainage
  - Pleurodesis
- Lymphangitis carcinomatosis
  - Steroids
  - Bronchodilators
  - Diuretics
- Pulmonary embolism
  - Low molecular weight heparin
- SVCO
  - Steroids
  - Stenting
  - Radiotherapy
  - Chemotherapy
- Anemia
  - Blood transfusion
  - Erythropoietin

Non-pharmacological Management of Breathlessness

Introduction

Focus more on non-drug approach in the early part of illness. Recognize the increasing role of drug approach as disease progresses.

Breathing environment

- Fan
    - To increase airflow
    - Reduces sensation of breathlessness via trigeminal nerve
    - Types
        - Ceiling fan
        - Table fan
        - Stand fan
        - Hand-held fan
    - Tailor distance, airflow direction, speed and duration according to preferences
    - Could be small battery-operated hand-held or clip-on fan from the night market
- Cool temperature
    - Reduces sensation of breathlessness via trigeminal nerves and thoracic nerves
    - Types
        - Air-conditioner
        - Hand-held small portable air-conditioner
        - Cooling mask for eyes
        - Cold cucumber slices for eyes

- Open space
  - Near-window bed
  - Open window if appropriate
  - Draw curtain according to preferences
  - Avoid overcrowding of visitors
- Loose comfortable clothing

Breathing positions

- Ask patients for their most comfortable positions
- Common positions
  - Lying position
    - High lying: lying supine with more pillows
    - High side lying: lying laterally with more pillows
  - Sitting position
    - Upright: sitting upright
    - Leaning forward: arms supported by a cardiac table
    - Leaning backward: back supported by pillows
  - Standing position
    - Leaning forward: arms supported by a ledge
    - Leaning backward: back against the wall

Breathing techniques

- Educate patients about different breathing techniques
- Deep breathing
  - Breathe in as much air as possible slowly
  - Breathe out as much air as possible slowly
- Pursed-lip breathing
  - Breathe in through the nose
  - Breathe out through partially closed lips
- Abdominal breathing
  - Breathe in and feel the rising of abdomen
  - Breathe out and feel the falling of abdomen

Supportive therapy

- Three main components of supportive therapy
    - Open-ended questions
    - Active listening
    - Empathy
- Explore the breathlessness experience
    - Tell me a little about your experience of breathlessness
    - What are the things that make it better?
    - What are the things that make it worse?
    - What are your feelings when you are breathless?
    - What are your thoughts when you are breathless?
    - How is your breathlessness affecting your daily life?
- Common negative emotions
    - Fear
    - Panic attack
    - Anxiety
    - Sadness
- Common negative thoughts
    - I will suffocate to death
    - I will choke to death
    - I am going to die
- Communicate empathy verbally and non-verbally
    - Acknowledge the experience
    - Validate the experience
    - Normalize the experience

Cognitive-behavioural therapy

- Cognitions
    - Address negative automatic thoughts, eg:
        - Filtering: focusing on the negative
        - Magnifying: exaggerating the negative
        - Catastrophizing: overestimating negative outcome

- Cognitive restructuring
  - Filtering: help patient to focus on the positive
  - Magnifying: help patient to see the reality as it is
  - Catastrophizing: help patient to understand that it is very unlikely to suffocate to death
  - Tell patient that fear, anxiety and panic can make the breathlessness worse
- Behaviours
  - Relaxation
    - Teach patient how to relax during breathlessness
      - Mindful breathing
      - Body scan
      - Visualization
      - Progressive muscular relaxation
  - Panic management
    - Give patient a plan of action in advance of the attack
      - Non-pharmacological plan
      - Pharmacological plan
    - Write down the instructions step by step
  - Goal setting
    - Set a realistic goal for the patient
    - Work with the patient to achieve it
    - Indoor activities: talking, eating, drinking, dressing, walking, bathing, toileting
    - Outdoor activities: gardening, strolling, exercising, shopping, travelling
  - Activity pacing
    - Change routine to suit energy level
    - Sit down while dressing, bathing, toileting if possible
    - Reserve energy for important activities
    - Rest more after certain activities

Supporting the family

- Explore understanding of the situation
    - Give proper information about the situation
- Explore thoughts and emotions
    - Empathic communication
    - Address fear and anxiety
    - Address negative thoughts
    - Cognitive restructuring
    - Teach family to relax
    - Teach family to help patient to relax
- Explore coping skills
    - Remind family of self-care
        - Eat
        - Sleep
        - Relax
    - Involve family in:
        - Relaxation
        - Panic management
        - Goal setting
        - Activity pacing

Little teaching from Thich Nhat Hanh

In Vietnam, there are many people, called boat people, who leave the country in small boats. Often the boats are caught in rough seas or storms, the people may panic, and boats may sink. But if even one person aboard can remain calm, lucid, knowing what to do and what not to do, he or she can help the boat survive.

Pharmacological Management of Breathlessness

Introduction

This chapter focuses on the symptomatic management of breathlessness irrespective of the pathology.

Oxygen

- Hypoxic patients are not necessarily breathless
- Breathless patients are not necessarily hypoxic
- Benefits of oxygen therapy
    - Improves resting and exertional hypoxia, hence reducing the need of breathing
    - Produces a facial or nasal cooling effect, hence reducing breathlessness, even in normoxic patient
    - May act as a placebo in reducing breathlessness
- Harms of oxygen therapy
    - Not comfortable for some patients
    - Costly in certain settings
    - Patients may become psychologically dependent
    - Blocks communication
    - Makes eating and drinking difficult
    - Dries the nasal mucosa
    - Causes pressure sores over the face or the ears
- Normoxic patients
    - Breathless: cooling hand-held or electrical fan
    - Still breathless: oxygen nasal prong 2-3L/min for 15min
        - Improvement: continue and reassess after 24h
        - No improvement: stop oxygen

- Hypoxic patients SaO2 <90%
  - Baseline: oxygen nasal prong 2-3L/min for 15min
    - Improvement: continue and reassess after 24h
    - No improvement: stop oxygen
  - Breakthrough: oxygen face mask ± reservoir
    - During acute attack of breathlessness
      - Incident breathlessness
      - Acute pneumonia
      - Acute bronchospasm
      - Acute pulmonary oedema
      - Acute pulmonary embolism
- Dying patients
  - Many dying patients do not need oxygen
  - Many semi-comatose patients do not tolerate oxygen via face mask or even nasal prong
  - Consider a cooling fan before prescribing oxygen
  - Some do not tolerate even a cooling fan
  - Use oxygen only if there is hypoxia and an absolute improvement in comfort after instituting it
  - Use oxygen nasal prong 2-3L/min prn
  - Take off the continuous saturation monitoring
  - Check saturation prn if really necessary
  - Do not restrain patients when they attempt to pull away the delivery device
  - Stop if patients are not tolerating the device
  - Focus on pharmacological management of breathlessness like opioid or benzodiazepines

Opioids in breathlessness

- Use of opioid in cancer and non-cancer breathlessness is supported by systematic review (Jennings 2002)

- Opioid reduces the sensation of breathlessness and associated anxiety
- Breathlessness improves with doses that do not cause clinically significant respiratory depression
    - Bruera 1990, 1993
    - Mazzocato 1999
    - Abernethy 2003
    - Allen 2005
    - Clemens 2008
- Breathlessness in opioid-naïve patients
    - Mild breathlessness NRS 1-3
        - PO Dihydrocodeine 30-60mg tds-qid or
        - Syrup morphine 2.5mg prn/q1h
    - Moderate breathlessness NRS 4-6
        - Syrup morphine 2.5mg q4h and
        - Syrup morphine 2.5mg prn/q1h for breakthrough
    - Severe breathlessness NRS 7-10
        - Syrup morphine 5mg q4h and
        - Syrup morphine 5mg prn/q1h for breakthrough
- Breathlessness in opioid-tolerant patients
    - Mild breathlessness NRS 1-3
        - Give 25% of the q4h analgesic dose
    - Moderate breathlessness NRS 4-6
        - Give 50% of the q4h analgesic dose
    - Severe breathlessness NRS 7-10
        - Give 100% of the q4h analgesic dose
    - Consider increasing baseline opioid dose by 25-50%
- Breathlessness in patients who are too breathless to swallow
    - No renal failure
        - Stat: SC/IV Morphine 2.5mg
        - Infusion: CSCI/CIVI Morphine 0.5mg/h
        - Breakthrough: SC/IV Morphine 2.5mg prn/q1h

- Renal failure
    - Stat: SC/IV Fentanyl 10mcg
    - Infusion: CSCI/CIVI Fentanyl 10mcg/h
    - Breakthrough: SC/IV Fentanyl 10mcg prn/q1h
- Breathlessness crisis
    - When breathlessness is severe (NRS $\geq$7) and patient is acutely distressed, consider rapid parenteral opioid titration, like in pain crisis
- Nebulized opioid
    - Evidence does not support the use of nebulized morphine (Jennings 2002)
    - Nebulized morphine 10-20mg in 5ml normal saline q4h
    - Nebulized fentanyl 25-50mcg in 5ml normal saline q4h

Phenothiazines in breathlessness

- Second line agents
- Use in persistent breathlessness despite opioid titration
- Benefits
    - Reduce breathlessness
    - Reduce anxiety
    - Reduce secretions
    - Reduce nausea
- Dose
    - PO Promethazine 12.5-25mg tds-qid (Viola 2008)
    - PO Chlorpromazine 12.5-25mg tds-qid (McIver 1994)
    - PO Levomepromazine 6-12mg on
    - SC Levomepromazine 6.25-12.5mg on
- Side effects
    - Sedation
    - Hypotension
    - Dysphoria
    - Extrapyramidal side effects

Anxiolytics in breathlessness

- Benzodiazepines
    - No direct anti-breathlessness effect
    - Mechanism of action: bind benzodiazepine receptors between α and γ subunits of GABA-A receptors, enhance GABA effect
    - Benefit: reduce anxiety
    - Indications
        - Short-term relief (2-4 weeks) of severe anxiety
        - Panic attack
    - Consider non-pharmacological approaches first
        - Supportive therapy
        - Cognitive-behavioural therapy
    - Types of benzodiazepines
        - Short acting: half-life <12h
            - PO Midazolam 7.5-15mg prn/tds
            - Buccal Midazolam 2.5-5mg prn/tds
        - Intermediate acting: half-life 12-24h
            - PO/SL Alprazolam 0.25-0.5mg prn/tds
            - PO/SL Lorazepam 0.5-1mg prn/tds
        - Long acting: half-life >24h
            - PO Diazepam 2.5-5mg on
            - PO Clonazepam 0.5-1mg on
    - Selection of benzodiazepines
        - Sustained anxiety: long acting
        - Episodic anxiety: intermediate acting
- Buspirone
    - 5-HT1A receptor partial agonist
    - Reduces anxiety, but not panic attack
    - No sedative or respiratory depressant effect
    - Anxiolytic effect after 2-4 weeks
    - PO Buspirone 5mg tds, up to 10-20mg tds

Steroids in breathlessness

- Indications
    - Multiple lung metastases
    - Upper airway obstruction
    - Lymphangitis carcinomatosis
    - Superior vena cava obstruction
    - Bronchospasm
    - Radiation pneumonitis
- Dose: PO/SC/IV Dexamethasone 8-12mg om for 7 days
- Prescribe dexamethasone as a single daily dose in the morning
- Dexamethasone dose in bd or tds is best avoided in palliative care to prevent insomnia
- Stop dexamethasone abruptly if no improvement in 7 days
- Taper dexamethasone gradually if breathlessness improves

Bronchodilators in breathlessness

- Indication: bronchospasm
- Consider metered-dose inhaler (MDI) with an aerochamber if patient cannot tolerate nebulizer
- Types of bronchodilators and doses
    - Short-acting β_2-agonists (SABA)
        - MDI Salbutamol 100mcg/puff
            - Acute breathlessness: 4-6 puffs prn/q10min
            - Stable breathlessness: 2-4 puffs prn/qid
        - Nebulized Salbutamol
            - Acute breathlessness: 2.5-5mg prn/q30min
            - Stable breathlessness: 2.5-5mg prn/qid
    - Long-acting β_2-agonists (LABA)
        - MDI Salmeterol 1 puff (75mcg) daily
        - DPI Salmeterol 1 puff (50mcg) bd
        - DPI Formoterol 1 puff (12mcg) bd
        - MDI Indacaterol 1 puff (75mcg) daily

- Nebulized Arformoterol 15mcg bd
- Short-acting muscarinic antagonist (SAMA)
    - MDI Ipratropium 20mcg/puff
        - Acute breathlessness: 4-6 puffs prn/q10min
        - Stable breathlessness: 2-4 puffs prn/qid
    - Nebulized Ipratropium
        - Acute breathlessness: 0.25-0.5mg prn/q30min
        - Stable breathlessness: 0.25-0.5mg prn/qid
- Long-acting muscarinic antagonist (LAMA)
    - DPI Tiotropium 1 puff (18mcg) daily
    - Nebulized Tiotropium 0.5mg tds-qid
- Combination agents
    - MDI Combivent (Salbutamol + Ipratropium)
        - Acute breathlessness: 4-6 puffs prn/q10min
        - Stable breathlessness: 2-4 puffs prn/qid
    - Nebulized Combivent
        - Acute breathlessness: 3ml prn/q10min
        - Stable breathlessness: 3ml prn/qid
    - MDI Berodual (Fenoterol + Ipratropium)
        - Acute breathlessness: 4-6 puffs prn/q10min
        - Stable breathlessness: 2-4 puffs prn/qid
    - MDI Stiolto Respimat (Olodaterol + Tiotropium)
        - 2 puffs daily
    - DPI Seretide (Salmeterol + Fluticasone)
        - 1 puff bd
- Methylxanthines
    - PO Theophylline SR 150-300mg bd
    - IV Aminophylline
        - In severe bronchospasm with RR ≥25/min
        - Cannot complete sentence in one breath
        - 250mg in 500ml normal saline over 4h
        - May repeat prn/tds

Diuretics in breathlessness

- Indication: breathlessness due to acute heart failure
- Parenteral loop diuretics are preferred initially because of poor oral absorption from bowel oedema
- Initial doses
  - IV/SC Frusemide 20-80mg om-tds
  - IV/SC Bumetanide 0.5-1mg om-tds
- Continuous infusion in advanced chronic kidney disease
  - CIVI/CSCI Frusemide 5-20mg/h
  - CIVI/CSCI Bumetanide 0.5-2mg/h
- Oral maintenance doses
  - PO Frusemide 20-80mg om
  - PO Bumetanide 0.5-2mg om
- Oral maintenance doses in advanced chronic kidney disease
  - PO Frusemide 80-120mg bd-tds
  - PO Bumetanide 2-5mg bd
- Conversion
  - IV/SC Frusemide = PO Frusemide
  - IV/SC Frusemide 40mg = IV/SC Bumetanide 1mg
- Nebulized Frusemide
  - Reduces breathlessness without causing diuresis
    - Kohara 2003
    - Shimoyama 2002
    - Stone 1994
  - Reduces cough
    - Ventresca 1990
  - Nebulized frusemide 20mg qid

Nitrates in breathlessness

- Indication: breathlessness due to acute heart failure
- Contraindication: hypotension
- Can be combined with diuretic

206

- Sublingual glyceryl trinitrate (GTN)
    - 0.5mg prn/q5min
- Oral nitrates
    - PO Isosorbide dinitrate (Isordil) 10-40mg tds-qid
    - PO Isosorbide mononitrate (Imdur) 30-240mg om
    - PO Isosorbide mononitrate (Elantan Long) 50-100mg om
- Parenteral nitrates
    - IV Nitroglycerin (GTN) 0.5-2mg/h, max 6mg/h
    - IV Isosorbide dinitrate (Isoket) 1-2mg/h, max 10mg/h

Mucolytics in loosening thick respiratory tract secretions

- Indication: thick mucous secretions
- Useful for those who can expectorate
- PO N-Acetylcysteine (NAC) 200mg bd-tds
- PO N-Acetylcysteine (NAC) 600mg bd for COPD patients
- Nebulized acetylcysteine 10% 6-10ml tds-qid
- Nebulized saline 2.5-5ml prn/qid
- Steam inhalation tds

Anticholinegics in reducing respiratory tract secretions

- Indication: respiratory tract secretions
- Useful for those who cannot expectorate
- SC Glycopyrrolate 0.2-0.4mg stat
    - Then CSCI Glycopyrrolate 0.6-1.2mg/24h
- SC Hyoscine hydrobromide 0.4mg stat
    - Then CSCI Hyoscine hydrobromide 1.2-2.4mg/24h
- SC Hyoscine butylbromide 20mg stat,
    - Then CSCI Hyoscine butylbromide 60-120mg/24h

Cannabinoid in breathlessness

- Consider cannabinoid if opioid is contraindicated
- PO Nabilone 0.1-0.2mg bd-qid (Ahmedzai 1997)

Chest wall vibration in breathlessness (Sibuya 1994)

- In-phase chest wall vibration reduces breathlessness
- Out-of-phase chest wall vibration increases breathlessness

Retrosternal block in breathlessness (Barak 2005)

- Lignocaine 1% 35-50ml
- 5cm long needle bent at its middle to create a 60° angle
- Direction in very close relation to the manubrium sterni
- As anterior as possible behind the sternum
- Improves breathlessness within minutes
- Bilateral vocal cord palsies reported when needle position was too posterior behind the sternum

Management of Incident Breathlessness

Introduction

Incident breathlessness is breathlessness which occurs during movement or activity. Most incident breathlessness resolves rapidly with rest.

Indications of treatment

- The movement or activity is prolonged
- The incident breathlessness is distressing or incapacitating

Management of incident breathlessness

- Palliative care referral recommended
- Sublingual use of parenteral formulations
- Maximum sublingual volume = 2ml
- Titrate according to the following steps:

Steps	Fentanyl 50mcg/ml		Alfentanil 0.5mg/ml		Sufentanil 50mcg/ml	
	mcg	ml	mg	ml	mcg	ml
Step 1	25	0.5	0.1	0.2	2.5	Too small
Step 2	50	1	0.2	0.4	5	0.1
Step 3	125	Too big	0.5	1.0	12.5	0.25
Step 4	250	Too big	1.0	2.0	25	0.5
Step 5	500	Too big	2.0	Too big	50	1.0
Step 6	1000	Too big	4.0	Too big	100	2.0

Terminal Breathlessness

Introduction

Terminal breathlessness is breathlessness during the terminal phase.

Diagnosis of terminal breathlessness

- Patient is terminally ill
- Patient is breathless
- Patient has respiratory failure
- Patient is not a candidate for ventilation

Communication

- Drowsiness or coma in dying patients (Morita 1998)
  - 1 week before death: 50%
  - 1 day before death: 70%
  - 6 hours before death: 90%
- Opioids in terminal breathlessness
  - Opioids can increase drowsiness in dying patients
  - Patients may not have enough time to develop tolerance
- Sedatives in terminal breathlessness
  - Sedatives can sedate patients
  - Patients may not be able to communicate with family
- Endpoints of titration of opioid or benzodiazepine
  - Primary: dosage is just enough to relieve breathlessness
  - Secondary: dosage is low enough to maintain a reasonable level of consciousness (may not be achieved in all cases)
- Progression of terminal breathlessness
  - Drowsiness or reduced consciousness may happen even in the absence of opioids or sedatives

Opioids in terminal breathlessness (PCT input)

- Opioid-naïve patients without renal failure
  - Consciousness is important
    - CSCI/CIVI Morphine 0.2mg/h
    - SC/IV Morphine 1mg prn/q1h for breakthrough
  - Consciousness is not an issue
    - SC/IV Morphine 2.5mg stat
    - CSCI/CIVI Morphine 0.5mg/h
    - SC/IV Morphine 2.5mg prn/q1h for breakthrough
- Opioid-naïve patients with renal failure
  - Consciousness is important
    - CSCI/CIVI Fentanyl 5mcg/h
    - SC/IV Fentanyl 10mcg prn/q1h for breakthrough
  - Consciousness is not an issue
    - SC/IV Fentanyl 25mcg stat
    - CSCI/CIVI Fentanyl 10mcg/h
    - SC/IV Fentanyl 25mcg prn/q1h for breakthrough

Sedatives in terminal breathlessness (PCT input)

- Add a sedative if breathlessness persists despite opioid
- Midazolam
  - Consciousness is important
    - CSCI/CIVI Midazolam 0.2-0.5mg/h
    - SC/IV Midazolam 1mg prn/q1h for breakthrough
  - Consciousness is not an issue
    - CSCI/CIVI Midazolam 1mg/h
    - SC Midazolam 2.5mg prn/q1h for breakthrough
    - Avoid IV Midazolam boluses
- Alternative benzodiazepines suitable for home administration
  - Sublingual lorazepam 0.5mg tds and prn/tds or
  - Rectal diazepam 5mg on and prn/tds

- If benzodiazepine fails to calm patient down or fear is present, add SC Levomepromazine 12.5-25mg on and prn/bd
- If levomepromazine is unavailable, give rectal chlorpromazine 25mg tds and prn/tds

Nausea and Vomiting

Introduction

Nausea and vomiting affect 30% of palliative care patients. The number increases to 60% at last weeks of life and 70% at last days.

Definitions

- Nausea is an unpleasant sensation experienced over the pharynx or stomach with an urge to vomit
- Vomiting is the forceful expulsion of gastric or gut contents through the mouth or nasal cavity
- Retching is the attempt to vomit without bringing anything up
- Regurgitation is an effortless expulsion of gastric contents through the mouth or nasal cavity

Causes of nausea and vomiting (N & V)

- Gastrointestinal causes
  - Nausea and vomiting are associated with **FOOD**
    - Oropharyngeal candidiasis
      - Vomiting from pharyngeal irritation
      - With or without odynophagia
      - Contents: phlegm
    - Esophageal obstruction
      - Vomiting immediately after swallowing
      - With or without dysphagia
      - Contents: undigested food
    - Gastric stasis
      - Large volume vomiting
      - Low pressure vomiting

- Infrequent vomiting
- Symptoms relieved by vomiting
- Contents
  - Undigested or partially digested food
  - Gastric juices (yellowish fluid)
- Squashed stomach syndrome
  - Small volume vomiting
  - Low pressure vomiting
  - Symptoms relieved by vomiting
  - Contents
    - Undigested or partially digested food
    - Gastric juices (yellowish fluid)
- Proximal bowel obstruction
  - Large volume vomiting
  - High pressure vomiting
  - Symptoms relieved by vomiting
  - Contents
    - Undigested or partially digested food
    - Gastric juices ± bile (greenish fluid)
- Bowel obstruction
  - Abdominal distension
    - May be absent
      - Proximal obstruction
      - Peritoneal carcinomatosis
  - Abdominal colic
  - Constipation
  - Contents
    - Gastric juices in gastric outlet obstruction
    - Bile in small bowel obstruction
    - Feces in large bowel obstruction

- Constipation
    - Nausea is prominent
    - Vomiting is less prominent
    - Symptoms relieved by defecation
- Intracranial causes
    - Causes: brain tumour, brain or meningeal metastases
    - Early **MORNING** nausea and vomiting
    - Worse with head movement
    - Associated with headache
    - Associated with empty retching and regurgitation
- Vestibular causes
    - Causes: cerebellar metastases, opioid, ENT problems
    - Nausea and vomiting are associated with **MOVEMENT**
    - Positional
    - Associated with vertigo or other ENT symptoms
- Chemical causes
    - Drugs
        - Opioids
        - Chemotherapy
        - Antibiotics
        - SSRIs
    - Toxins
        - Infection
        - Organ failure
    - Electrolyte problems
        - Hypercalcemia
        - Hyponatremia
    - **CONSTANT** nausea
    - Not always relieved by vomiting
    - Variable vomiting
    - Temporal relationship with the chemicals

- Emotional causes
  - **WAVES** of nausea
  - Worse during anxiety or fear
  - Temporal relationship with emotional distress
  - May be triggered by sight, smell or thoughts
  - Relieved by distraction

Mechanisms of nausea and vomiting

- Central pathways
  - Vomiting center
    - Site: medulla oblongata
    - Contents
      - Reticular formation
      - Nucleus of tractus solitarius
    - Input from 4 principal areas
      - Higher centers
        - Cerebral cortex (GABA, 5HT)
        - Thalamus
        - Hypothalamus
        - Higher brainstem
      - Vestibular system
      - Chemoreceptor trigger zone
      - Gastrointestinal tract (5HT3)
        - Vagus nerves
        - Splanchnic nerves
    - Output to 3 principal areas
      - Upper GIT via 5, 7, 9, 10, 12 cranial nerves
      - Lower GIT via 10 and sympathetic nerves
      - Diaphragm and abdominal muscles via spinal nerves
    - Activation produces the vomiting reflex

- Principal receptors
  - Muscarinic cholinergic receptors (M1)
  - Histamine receptors (H1)
- Other receptors
  - Serotonin receptors (5HT3, 5HT2)
  - Neurokinin receptors (NK1)
- Chemoreceptor trigger zone (CTZ)
  - Site: medulla oblongata
  - Specific site: area postrema, floor of fourth ventricle
  - No blood-brain barrier
  - Input
    - Input in bloods
    - Vagus nerve
  - Output
    - Vomiting center
  - Principal receptors
    - Dopamine receptors (D2)
  - Other receptors
    - Muscarinic cholinergic receptors (M1)
    - Histamine receptors (H1)
    - Serotonin receptors (5HT3)
    - Neurokinin receptors (NK1)
    - Opioid receptors
  - Activation stimulates vomiting center
- Afferent pathways
  - Descending fibers from higher centers
  - Vestibular system (H1, M1)
  - Vagus nerves
  - Glossopharyngeal nerves
  - Splanchnic nerves
  - Sympathetic ganglias

The act of vomiting

- Inputs
    - Toxins and drugs activate CTZ (D2, 5HT)
        - CTZ activates vomiting center (H1, M1)
    - Motion sickness activates vestibular nuclei (H1, M1)
        - Vestibular nuclei activate CTZ
        - CTZ activates vomiting center
    - Chemotherapy activates gut (5HT3)
        - Vagal afferents activate vomiting center and CTZ
    - Pain, anxiety, sight and smell activate higher centers
        - Higher centers activate vomiting center
- Parasympathetic output
    - Increases salivation to protect tooth enamel from acid
    - Retroperistalsis pushes contents of small intestines to stomach through relaxed pyloric sphincter
- Motor output
    - Contraction of inspiratory muscles
        - Lowers intrathoracic pressure
        - Deep breathing to prevent aspiration
        - Coordination with abdominal contraction to retch
    - Contraction of abdominal muscles
        - Increases abdominal pressure
        - Expels stomach contents into esophagus and mouth through relaxed esophageal sphincter
- Sympathetic output
    - Sweating
    - Palpitation

Feeling good after vomiting

- Release of abdominal pressure
- Release of endorphins

Non-pharmacological Management of Nausea and Vomiting

Introduction

Non-pharmacological management of nausea and vomiting includes simple measures to modify the sensory inputs and the autonomic and motor outputs of the vomiting center.

Simple measures to modify the sensory inputs

- Sight: keep visual inputs of nausea away from the sight of patient, such as food, vomitus and other repulsive sight
- Hearing: keep auditory inputs of nausea away from the hearing of patient, such as food talk, noise and other repulsive sound
- Smell: keep olfactory inputs of nausea away from the smell of patient, such as food smell, vomitus and other repulsive odour
- Touch: keep tactile triggers of nausea away from the body of patient, such as tight fitting clothing and abdominal pillow
- Feeling: address the fear and anxiety of patient and family, establish a calm environment with fresh air
- Thoughts: address automatic negative thoughts which worsen the symptoms of nausea and vomiting

Dietary modifications

- Follow patient as the lead in eating and drinking
- Patient can eat and drink whatever he or she can tolerate
- Small, frequent meals
- Avoid fatty food
- Avoid overly sweet food
- Avoid favourite food during nausea

- Certain food or drink that can be offered:
    - Bland food at room temperature
    - Salty food
    - Sour food
    - Clear soup
    - Flavoured gelatin
    - Cold, carbonated drink
    - Popsicles and ice cubes
    - Dairy product
    - Sandwiches
    - Fruits
- Separate eating time and drinking time if appropriate
- Eat and drink slowly
- Stop eating and drinking when the feeling of nausea arises
- Sit up for 1-2h after meals if appropriate

Alternatives

- Body scan
- Progressive muscular relaxation
- Guided imagery
- Systematic desensitization
- Hypnosis
- Music
- Acupuncture or acupressure

Simple measures to modify the motor outputs

- Avoid retching
- Hold abdomen while vomiting
- Prepare the 3 essential items for vomiting
    - A vomit container
    - Water for gargling
    - Tissues

Attending to a vomiting episode

- Urgent attention
- Calm presence
- Supply the 3 essential items of vomiting
- Institution of anti-emetics
- Immediate cleaning and changing of stained clothes and bed-sheet

Antiemetics

Introduction

Narrow spectrum antiemetics act on single or limited receptors of vomiting. Broad spectrum antiemetics act on multiple receptors.

Antiemetics and receptor affinities

Drugs	D2	H1	M1	α1	5HT2	5HT3	5HT4
Levomepromazine	-	-	-	-	-		
Olanzapine	-	-	-	-	-	-	
Risperidone	-	-		-	-		
Quetiapine	-	-		-	-	-	
Chlorpromazine	-	-	-	-	-		
Promethazine	-	-	-	-			
Prochlorperazine	-	-		-			
Cyclizine		-	-				
Diphenhydramine		-	-				
Metoclopramide	-					-	+
Domperidone	-						+
Cisapride							+
Haloperidol	-			-			
Hyoscine			-				
Ondansetron						-	
Mirtazapine					-	-	

- Antagonist   + Agonist

Narrow spectrum antiemetics

- Prokinetics
- Haloperidol
- Antihistamines
- 5HT3 antagonists

Broad spectrum antiemetics

- Phenothiazines
- Atypical antipsychotics

Prokinetics

- Metoclopramide
    - Commonly used antiemetic
    - Works on stomach and proximal small bowel
    - Little effect on colonic motility
    - Mechanisms of action
        - 5HT4 agonist at GIT: prokinesis
        - D2 antagonist at GIT
        - D2 antagonist at CTZ
        - 5HT3 at CTZ and GIT at high doses
- Domperidone
    - Does not cross blood-brain barrier
    - Negligible risk of extrapyramidal side effects
    - Antiemetic of choice for Parkinson's disease
    - Mechanisms of action
        - D2 antagonist at GIT
        - D2 antagonist at CTZ
- Cisapride
    - More potent than metoclopramide
    - Increases motility of entire length of GIT
    - Can induce arrhythmia due to class III antiarrhythmic properties
    - Mechanism of action
        - Pure 5HT4 agonist at GIT
- Erythromycin
    - Most potent prokinetic when given intravenously
    - Effective after subtotal gastrectomy
    - Not effective after total gastrectomy

- Not effective for postoperative ileus
- Mechanism of action
  - Motilin receptor agonist at upper GIT
- Levosulpiride
  - Superior to metoclopramide in one RCT (Corli 1995)
  - Effective in 80% of patients
  - Mechanism of action: D2 antagonist

Butyrophenone

- Haloperidol
  - Potent antiemetic
  - Causes less drowsiness compared to chlorpromazine
  - >5mg/day: higher risk of extrapyramidal side effects
  - Mechanism of action: D2 antagonist at CTZ
  - No RCT reported in a Cochrane review (Perkins 2009)

Antihistamines

- Phenothiazines
  - Promethazine
- Piperazines
  - Buclizine
  - Cyclizine
  - Cinnarizine
  - Meclizine
- Monoethanolamines
  - Diphenhydramine
  - Dimenhydrinate
- Mechanisms of action
  - H1 antagonist at vomiting center and vestibular system
  - M1 antagonist at vomiting center and vestibular system
- No RCT reported (Keeley 2008)

Anticholinergics

- Mechanism of action
    - M1 antagonist at vomiting center and GIT
        - Hyoscine hydrobromide
    - M1 antagonist at GIT
        - Hyoscine butylbromide
        - Glycopyrrolate

5HT3 antagonists

- Examples
    - Ondansetron
    - Granisetron
    - Tropisetron
    - Dolasetron
    - Palonosetron
- Mechanism of action
    - 5HT3 antagonist at CTZ, vomiting center and GIT
- Sources of excess 5HT3
    - Enterochromaffin cells after gut mucosa damage
        - Chemotherapy
        - Radiotherapy
        - GI Surgery
    - Enterochromaffin cells because of bowel distension
        - Malignant bowel obstruction
    - Leaky platelets
        - Uremia
    - Raphe nucleus
        - Head injury
        - Brainstem radiotherapy
        - Multiple sclerosis affecting brainstem
- Side effects: headache, giddiness, constipation
- High level of evidence in chemotherapy-induced emesis

Phenothiazines

- Chlorpromazine, prochlorperazine and levomepromazine are broad spectrum antiemetics
- Second or third line antiemetics in palliative care
- Levomepromazine
    - Acts on most receptors involved in vomiting
    - Has analgesic effect
    - Mechanisms of action
        - D2 antagonist at CTZ and GIT
        - H1 antagonist at vomiting center and vestibular sys
        - M1 antagonist at vomiting center and vestibular sys
        - 5HT2 antagonist at vomiting center
        - α1-Adrenergic receptors at CTZ

Atypical antipsychotics

- Olanzapine, risperidone and quetiapine are broad spectrum antiemetics
- Second or third line antiemetics in palliative care
- Olanzapine
    - Mechanisms of action
        - D2 antagonist at CTZ and GIT
        - H1 antagonist at vomiting center and vestibular sys
        - M1 antagonist at vomiting center and vestibular sys
        - 5HT2 antagonist at vomiting center
        - 5HT3 antagonist
        - α1-Adrenergic receptors at CTZ
    - 100% effective in prevention of nausea and vomiting caused by moderate to highly emetogenic chemotherapy when combined with palonosetron and dexamethasone (Navari 2007)

Miscellaneous antiemetics and mechanisms of action

- Dexamethasone
    - Reduces permeability of blood-brain barrier at CTZ
    - Reduces GABA in brainstem
    - Reduces leu-enkephalin release in brainstem
    - Reduces cerebral oedema
    - Reduces tumoral oedema
    - Reduces obstruction at GIT
- Aprepitant (neurokinin 1 receptor antagonist)
    - NK1 antagonist at vomiting center, CTZ, cortex, GIT
- Nabilone (cannabinoids)
    - Cannabinoid receptor agonist (CB1)
- Benzodiazepines
    - $GABA_A$ receptor agonist
- Octreotide
    - Somatostatin receptor agonist
- Propofol
    - $GABA_A$ receptor agonist
        - Inhibits 5HT3 at CTZ

Five Principles of Using Antiemetics

Introduction

The five principles of using antiemetics can serve as an initial guide to manage nausea and vomiting in palliative care.

The five principles

- Prescribe antiemetic regularly for baseline N&V
- Prescribe antiemetic for breakthrough N&V
- Prescribe antiemetic based on the causes of N&V
- Prescribe parenteral antiemetic
- Provide antiemetic education

Baseline N&V

- Prescribe antiemetic regularly, not prn
- Examples
    - SC/IV Metoclopramide 10mg tds
    - SC/IV Haloperidol 1.5mg bd

Breakthrough N&V

- Prescribe antiemetic for breakthrough N&V
- Examples
    - SC/IV Metoclopramide 10mg prn/tds
    - SC/IV Haloperidol 1.5mg/tds

Choice of antiemetics

- Prescribe antiemetic based on the likely causes of N&V
- Step 1: narrow spectrum antiemetic
- Step 2: combination of narrow spectrum antiemetics
- Step 3: broad spectrum antiemetics

- Step 1
  - Narrow spectrum antiemetic ± dexamethasone
    - Gastroparesis: metoclopramide
    - Chemicals: haloperidol
    - Vestibular: antihistamine
    - Chemotherapy: 5HT3 antagonist
  - Increase dose if improvement in 24h
  - Increase step if no improvement in 24h
- Step 2
  - 2 narrow spectrum antiemetics ± dexamethasone
  - Choose combination with additive actions
    - Prokinetic + haloperidol
    - Prokinetic + antihistamine
    - Haloperidol + antihistamine
  - Avoid combination with antagonism
    - Prokinetic + anticholinergic
  - Increase dose if improvement in 24h
  - Increase step if no improvement in 24h
- Step 3
  - Broad spectrum antiemetic ± dexamethasone
    - Phenothiazine: levomepromazine
    - Atypical antipsychotic: olanzapine

Route of antiemetics

- Prescribe parenteral antiemetic
- Oral antiemetic is indicated in:
  - Nausea per se
  - No vomiting
  - No bowel obstruction
  - No swallowing difficulties
- Switching from parenteral to oral antiemetic is recommended only after 72 hours of good control with parenteral antiemetic

Antiemetic education

- Information
    - Causes of N&V
    - Baseline and breakthough N&V
    - Baseline and breakthrough antiemetic prescription
    - Timing of antiemetic with meals
    - Common side effects of prescribed antiemetic
    - Conversion to oral antiemetic after 72h emetic control
    - Aim for complete control of nausea
    - Aim for partial control of vomiting if mechanical causes

Management of Nausea and Vomiting

Introduction

Two different approaches are available in the management of nausea and vomiting: the mechanistic approach (antiemetic selection based on causes of N&V) and the empirical approach (antiemetic selection based on physician preference). Mechanistic approach is practiced in most palliative care settings. However, no study has directly examined the effectiveness of one approach over the other.

Gastrointestinal causes

- Oropharyngeal and esophageal candidiasis
  - Non-pharmacological
    - Mouth care
      - Prevention: drink water immediately after food
      - Treatment: brush teeth and dentures with soft toothbrush and rinse with water
      - Dying patients: swab with gauze dipped in sodium bicarbonate
      - Moisturize mouth regularly with water
      - Consider artificial saliva for dry mouth
  - Pharmacological
    - Antifungals
      - Syrup Nystatin 100,000-500,000 unit qid
      - Treat for 7-14 days
      - Swish and swallow
      - Paint over tongue and mouth if cannot swallow
      - Can make small popsicles with toothpicks to suck on

- Triazole antifungals
  - Indications
    - Resistant infection
    - Esophageal involvement
    - Laryngeal involvement
  - PO Fluconazole 150mg single dose
  - PO Fluconazole 100mg daily
  - PO Itraconazole 100mg bd: with food
  - Syrup Itraconazole 100mg bd: empty stomach
  - Short prognosis: treat with a single dose
  - Longer prognosis: treat for 7-14 days
- Parenteral antifungals for systemic infections
  - IV Fluconazole 100mg daily for 7-14 days
  - IV Itraconazole 100mg bd 7-14 days
- Antiemetics
  - Antihistamines
- Gastric stasis
  - Non-pharmacological
    - Small, frequent meals (4-6x/day)
    - Low fat diet
    - Low fiber diet
    - Liquid diet in severe cases
    - Stop eating once feeling uncomfortable
  - Pharmacological
    - First line prokinetics (30min pre-meals for tds dose)
      - SC/IV/PO Metoclopramide 10-20mg tds
      - CSCI/CIVI Metoclopramide 30-120mg/24h
      - PO Domperidone 10-20mg tds
    - Second line prokinetics
      - IV/PO Erythromycin 250-500mg tds
      - PO Cisapride 10-20mg tds
      - PO Levosulpiride 25mg tds

- Alternative antiemetics to reduce nausea
  - Prochlorperazine
  - Antihistamines
- Antisecretory agents to reduce emetic volume
  - H2 antagonists
  - PPIs
  - SC Octreotide 50-100mcg on
- Anti-foaming agent to reduce bloatedness
  - Syrup Simethicone (Maalox Plus) 10-20ml tds
  - PO Simethicone (Maalox Plus) 2-4 tablets tds
- Antidepressants in refractory cases
  - PO Mirtazapine 15mg on
  - PO Amitriptyline 25-50mg on
  - PO Nortriptyline 25-50mg on
- Interventions for refractory cases
  - Venting nasogastric tube
  - Venting gastrostomy
  - Feeding jejunostomy
  - Botulinum toxin injection into pyloric sphincter
  - Gastric electrical stimulation
- Constipation
  - Refer to chapter of constipation
- Malignant bowel obstruction
  - Refer to chapter of malignant bowel obstruction

Chemical causes

- Opioid-induced nausea and vomiting (OINV)
  - CTZ stimulation
    - Constant nausea during rising opioid level
    - SC/IV/PO Haloperidol 1.5-5mg bd
    - CSCI/CIVI Haloperidol 1.5-20mg/24h

- Gastric stasis
  - Associated with post-prandial stomach fullness >2h
  - SC/IV/PO Metoclopramide 10-20mg tds
  - CSCI/CIVI Metoclopramide 30-120mg/24h
- Increased vestibular sensitivity
  - Associated with vertigo
  - IV/PO Promethazine 25-50mg tds
  - CSCI Promethazine 50-150mg/24h
- Constipation
  - Treat constipation
- Anticipatory nausea and vomiting
  - Associated with sight, smell and thoughts of opioid
  - PO Alprazolam 0.25-0.5mg prn/tds
  - PO Lorazepam 0.5-1mg prn/tds
- Refractory nausea and vomiting
  - IV/SC Dexamethasone 8mg at 8am and 12pm
  - IV/PO Granisetron 1mg bd
  - CSCI Granisetron 1-3mg/24h
  - SC Levomepromazine 6.25-25mg on-bd
  - CSCI Levomepromazine 6.25-50mg/24h
  - PO Levomepromazine 6-25mg on-bd
  - IV/PO Chlorpromazine 25-50mg tds
  - SL Olanzapine 2.5-10mg on
- Chemotherapy-induced nausea and vomiting (CINV)
  - Types of CINV
    - Acute: within first 24h after chemotherapy
      - Serotonin release from enterochromaffin cells
    - Delayed: 1-5 days after chemotherapy
      - Substance P-mediated disruption of blood-brain barrier, GI motility and adrenal hormone
    - Anticipatory: prior to chemotherapy
      - Classical conditioning

- Highly emetogenic chemotherapy HEC (>90%)
    - AC/FAC/FEC combinations for breast cancer
    - Anthracycline + cisplatin combinations
    - Carmustin
    - Cisplatin 5 days regimen
    - Cyclophosphamide >1500mg/m^2
    - Dactinomycin
    - Streptozocin
- Moderately emetogenic chemotherapy MEC (30-90%)
    - CHOP/CHOMP/BEACOPP/ABVD for lymphoma
    - FOLFOX/FOLFIRI/XELOX/XELIRI
    - Carboplatin/oxaliplatin
    - Cyclophosphamide <1500mg/m^2
    - Ifosfamide
    - Oral etoposide/imatinib/temozolomide/vinorelbine
    - Methotrexate
- Low emetogenic chemotherapy LEC (10-30%)
    - Capecitabine
    - Catumaxomab/cetuximab/panitumumab
    - Docetaxel/paclitaxel
    - Fluorouracil
    - Gemcitabine
    - IV Etoposide
    - Pemetrexed
    - Topotecan
- Minimally emetogenic chemotherapy (<10%)
    - Alemtuzumab/bevacizumab/gemtuzumab
    - Erlotinib/gefitinib/sorafenib/sunitinib
    - Hydroxyurea
    - IV Vinorelbine
    - Lenalidomide/thalidomide
    - Vinblastine/vincristine

- Prevention of acute CINV
    - HEC: 5HT3 antagonist + NK1 antagonist + dexa
    - MEC: 5HT3 antagonist + dexa
    - LEC: dexa
    - Minimal: no routine prophylaxis
- Prevention of delayed CINV
    - HEC: NK1 antagonist + dexa
    - MEC: no routine prophylaxis
    - LEC: no routine prophylaxis
    - Minimal: no routine prophylaxis
- Prevention of anticipatory CINV
    - Psychological techniques
    - Low dose benzodiazepine before chemotherapy
- Doses of prophylactic antiemetics
    - 5HT3 antagonists at D1 for HEC and MEC
        - PO Ondansetron 24mg (HEC), 16mg (MEC)
        - IV Ondansetron 8mg
        - PO Granisteron 2mg
        - IV Granisetron 1mg
        - PO/IV Tropisetron 5mg
        - PO/IV Dolasetron 100mg
        - PO Palonosetron 0.5mg
        - IV Palonosetron 0.25mg
    - Dexamethasone
        - PO Dexamethasone 12mg at D1 (HEC, MEC)
        - PO Dexamethasone 8mg at D2-4 (HEC)
        - PO Dexamethasone 8mg at D1 (LEC)
    - NK1 antagonists
        - PO Aprepitant 125mg at D1 (HEC)
        - PO Aprepitant 80mg at D2-3 (HEC)
        - IV Fosaprepitant 150mg at D1 only (HEC)

- Radiotherapy-induced nausea and vomiting (RINV)
  - High risk
    - Total body irradiation
    - 5HT3 antagonist prophylaxis + dexamethasone
  - Moderate risk
    - Upper abdomen
    - 5HT3 antagonist prophylaxis
  - Low risk
    - Brain, head and neck, lower thorax, spine, pelvis
    - 5HT3 antagonist rescue
  - Minimal Risk
    - Breast, extremities
    - D2 antagonist or 5HT3 antagonist rescue
- Toxin-induced nausea and vomiting
  - Causes
    - Drugs: opioids, chemo, antiepileptics, antibiotics
    - Metabolic: hypercalcemia, hyponatremia, uremia
    - Toxin: bacterial toxins, tumour necrosis
  - Antiemetics
    - Block D2 receptors at CTZ
      - SC/IV/PO Metoclopramide 10-20mg tds
      - CSCI/CIVI Metoclopramide 30-120mg/24h
      - SC/IV/PO Haloperidol 1.5-5mg bd
      - CSCI/CIVI Haloperidol 1.5-20mg/24h
    - Block H1, M1 receptors at vomiting center
      - Antihistamines
    - Block multiple receptors
      - SC Levomepromazine 6.25-25mg on-bd
      - CSCI Levomepromazine 6.25-50mg/24h
      - PO Levomepromazine 6-25mg on-bd
      - IV/PO Chlorpromazine 25-50mg tds
      - SL Olanzapine 2.5-10mg on

- Increased intracranial pressure
  - Antiemetics
    - First line: reduce vasogenic cerebral oedema
      - SC/IV/PO Dexamethasone 12mg om 1/52
    - Second line: block H1, M1 at vomiting center
      - IV/PO Cyclizine 50-100mg tds
      - CSCI Cyclizine 150-300mg/24h
      - IV/PO Promethazine 25-50mg tds
      - CSCI Promethazine 50-150mg/24h
    - Third line: block multiple receptors
      - SC Levomepromazine 6.25-25mg on-bd
      - CSCI Levomepromazine 6.25-50mg/24h
      - PO Levomepromazine 6-25mg on-bd
      - SL Olanzapine 2.5-10mg on
- Vestibular causes
  - Antiemetics
    - Antihistamines
      - SC boluses can cause tissue necrosis
      - IV boluses have to be given slowly
      - IV/PO Cyclizine 50-100mg tds
      - CSCI Cyclizine 150-300mg/24h
      - IV/PO Promethazine 25-50mg tds
      - CSCI Promethazine 50-150mg/24h
      - IV/PO Diphenhydramine 25-50mg tds
      - IV/PO Dimenhydrinate 50-100mg tds
    - Anticholinergics
      - SC/SL Hyoscine hydrobromide 0.2-0.4mg tds
      - CSCI Hyoscine hydrobromide 1.2-2.4mg/24h
      - Scopolamine patch 1.5mg q72h to mastoid
    - Phenothiazines
      - IV Prochlorperazine 5-10mg tds slow bolus
      - PO Prochlorperazine 5-10mg tds

- Psychogenic causes
    - First line: non-pharmacological treatment
        - Body scan
        - Progressive muscular relaxation
        - Guided imagery
        - Systemic desensitization
        - Hypnosis
        - Music
    - Second line: benzodiazepines
        - PO/SL Alprazolam 0.25-0.5mg prn/tds
        - PO/SL Lorazepam 0.5-1mg prn/tds
        - PO Diazepam 2.5-5mg on
- Intractable nausea and vomiting
    - Step 1: 2 narrow spectrum antiemetics ± dexamethasone
    - Step 2: 1 broad spectrum antiemetic ± dexamethasone
    - Step 3: intravenous propofol (Lundström 2005)
        - IV Propofol 0.5mg/kg/h
        - Titrate 0.25-0.5mg/kg/h q30-60min till better
        - Optimal dose: 0.5-1.0mg/kg/h for most patients
        - Sedation may happen with doses >1mg/kg/h
        - Monitor sedation and RR at 1, 2, 6, 12h, then bd
        - Stop 2-3min if too drowsy, then restart at lower dose
        - Reduce dose within 24h if patient is better
    - Alternative
        - ABHR suppositories
            - Lorazepam (Ativan) 0.5mg
            - Diphenhydramine (Benadryl) 12.5mg
            - Haloperidol (Haldol) 0.5mg
            - Metoclopramide (Reglan) 10mg

Constipation

Introduction

Constipation is difficulty in passing motion. It is fundamentally defined by the patient.

Characteristics of constipation (≥1 of the following)

- Hard stools
- Infrequent bowel movement
- Difficult bowel movement with excessive straining
- Painful bowel movement
- Absent bowel movement
- A sense of incomplete evacuation

Assessment of constipation (3Ds)

- Diet history
  - Daily dietary history
  - Fibre intake
  - Water intake
  - Coffee, tea and alcohol ingestion
  - Milk products
- Drug history
  - Opioids
  - Laxatives
  - Anticholinergics
  - 5HT3 antagonists
  - Antidepressants
- Defecation history
  - Explore the whole defecation process, from the intention to move bowels till completion and back to activities

- Need of assistance
- Site of defecation
    - Toilet
    - Commode
    - Bedpan
    - Diapers
- Process of defecation
    - Effort in defecation
    - Manoeuvres in facilitating defecation
    - Excessive straining
    - Pain during or after defecation
    - Incomplete evacuation
    - Duration of defecation
    - Frequency of defecation
- Stool characteristics
    - Consistencies
    - Volume
    - Shape
    - Colour
    - Odour
- Patient's expectation of bowel movement

Examination of constipation

- Hydration status
- Abdominal examination
    - Signs of bowel obstruction
    - Signs of constipation: left-sided indentable fecal masses
    - Bowel sounds
- Rectal examination
    - Perianal excoriation
    - Haemorrhoids or fissures
    - Anal tone

- Stool consistencies
- Stool colour
- Ballooned rectum: suggesting higher impaction
- Steps in performing a rectal examination for constipation
  - Step 1: preparation of gloves and lubricant
  - Step 2: positioning of patient
  - Step 3: inspection of perianal area
  - Step 4: touch the anus with lubricated gloved finger
  - Step 5: wait for the anus to relax
  - Step 6: advance the finger slowly following the curve
  - Step 7: circumferential palpation of rectal vault
  - Step 8: remove the finger and inspect stools
- Avoid rectal examination
  - Refusal
  - Neutropenic sepsis
  - Abdominoperineal resection

Bristol stool chart

- Type 1: separate hard lumps – constipation
- Type 2: sausaged-shaped, lumpy – constipation
- Type 3: sausaged-shaped, cracked surface – normal
- Type 4: sausaged-shaped, smooth surface – normal
- Type 5: soft blobs – diarrhoea
- Type 6: mushy – diarrhoea
- Type 7: watery – diarrhoea

Investigations

- Abdominal x-ray in suspected malignant bowel obstruction

Mechanisms of Constipation

Introduction

Normal intenstinal function depends on the control of intestinal motility and fluid handling by neural, endocrine and paracrine factors.

Neural control of intestinal activity

- Enteric nervous system (ENS): the second brain
  - 100 million neurons
  - Embedded in GI lining from esophagus to anus
  - Comprises 2 interconnected networks
    - Myenteric ganglia (Auerbach's plexus)
      - Within muscular layer
      - Parasympathetic and sympathetic input
      - Innervate muscular layer: inner and outer
      - Regulate GI motility
      - 30% sensory neurons (myenteric IPANs)
        - IPAN = intrinsic primary afferent neurons
        - Detect intraluminal chemistry
        - Mediate GI reflexes
    - Submucosal ganglia (Meissner's plexus)
      - Within submucosal layer
      - Parasympathetic input only
      - Derived from Auerbach's plexus
      - Regulate fluid and electrolyte transport
      - 14% sensory neurons (submucosal IPANs)
        - Detect intraluminal chemistry
        - Mediate mucosally driven peristaltic and secretory reflexes

- Autonomic nervous system (ANS)
  - Parasympathetic nervous system
    - Vagus: innervates ENS
      - Foregut: celiac plexus
      - Midgut: superior mesenteric plexus
    - Pelvic splanchnic nerves: innervate ENS
      - Hindgut: inferior mesenteric plexus
    - Stimulates GI motility and secretion
  - Sympathetic nervous system
    - Inhibits GI motility and secretion

Neurotransmitters

- Excitatory neurotransmitters
  - Acetylcholine (primary)
    - Binds muscarinic receptors (GPCR)
    - Increases cytosolic Ca^{2+}
    - Causes secretion and smooth muscle contraction
  - Substance P
    - Binds neurokinin 1 receptors (NK1)
    - Causes secretion of saliva and pancreatic enzymes
    - Causes smooth muscle contraction
    - Promotes inflammation and tissue repair
  - Serotonin
    - 95% of body's serotonin is found in the gut
    - Source: enterochromaffin cells
    - 5HT1P
      - Stimulates submucosal IPANs
      - ↑ peristalsis and secretion
      - Agonist: causes diarrhoea
      - Antagonist: causes ileus
      - Not the best target for treatment of GI motility compared to 5HT4

- 5HT3
    - Stimulates extrinsic sensory nerves and sends sensory signals like N&V to CNS
    - Stimulates myenteric IPANs
    - ↑ reflexes such as giant migratory contractions, but not peristaltic and secretory reflexes
    - 5HT3 antagonists
        - Reduce CINV
        - Reduce visceral hypersensitivity of IBS, particularly bloating sensation
        - Cause constipation
        - Do not paralyze bowels
- 5HT4
    - Stimulates submucosal IPANs presynaptically
    - Enhances release of acetylcholine and CGRP
    - Promotes transmission in prokinetic pathways
    - Depends on natural stimuli to evoke peristaltic and secretory reflexes
    - Will not induce overwhelming motility
    - But not effective if damaged enteric nerves
    - 5HT4 agonists: safe compared to 5HT1P
- Inhibitory neurotransmitters
    - Nitric oxide
        - Binds NO receptors
        - Increases cGMP
        - Causes smooth muscle relaxation
    - ATP
        - Causes smooth muscle relaxation
    - Vasoactive intestinal peptide (VIP)
        - Binds VIP receptors (GPCR)
        - Increases cytosolic Ca^{2+}
        - Causes secretion and smooth muscle relaxation

Endocrine control of intestinal activity

- Gastrin
    - Source: G cells of stomach
    - Receptors: CCK-B receptors
    - Function: ↑ acid secretion from parietal cells
- Cholecystokinin (CCK)
    - Source: I cells of duodenum and jejunum
    - Receptors: CCK-A receptors
    - Function: ↑ pancreatic enzyme secretion
- Secretin
    - Source: S cells of duodenum
    - Receptors: secretin receptors
    - Function: ↑ pancreatic and biliary HCO_3^- secretion
- Glucose dependent insulinotropic peptide (GIP)
    - Source: K cells of duodenum and jejunum
    - Receptors: GIP receptors
    - Function: ↑ insulin secretion from pancreatic β cells

Paracrine factors

- Histamine
    - Source: enterochromaffin cells of stomach
    - Receptors: H2 receptors
    - Function: ↑ acid secretion from parietal cells
- Somatostatin
    - Source: D cells of stomach
    - Receptors: somatostatin receptors
    - Function: inhibits gastrin secretion from G cells

Intestinal motility

- Small intestine motility
    - Peristalsis
        - Pattern of intestinal motility after meals

- Forward movement of small intestine contents
- Orad smooth muscle contraction via acetylcholine
- Caudad smooth muscle relaxation via NO, ATP, VIP
  - Segmentation
    - Pattern of intestinal motility after meals
    - Mixing of small intestine contents
  - Migrating motor complexes
    - Pattern of intestinal motility in between meals
    - A wave of peristalsis from stomach to ileum
    - Initiated by motilin from duodenum
    - Occur every 1.5-2 hours
    - Clear stomach and small intestines of residue
    - Reduce bacterial growth
    - Responsible for rumbling when hungry
- Large intestine motility
  - Segmentation and haustral migration
    - Mixing of large intestine contents
    - Facilitate water absorption
    - Move feces gradually to rectum
  - Mass movement
    - 1-3/day
    - High-amplitude propagated contractions
    - Stimulated by gastrocolic and duodenocolic reflexes after food
    - Pushes feces into rectum

Intestinal fluid handling

- Dynamic state of secretion and absorption
  - Secretion
    - Secreted intestinal fluid: 7L/day
      - Saliva: 1.5L/day
      - Gastric secretions: 2L/day

- Pancreatic juices: 1.5L/day
- Bile: 0.5L/day
- Small intestine secretions: 1.5L/day
- Dietary fluid: 2L/day (8 x 8 ounces glasses)
- Absorption
  - Small bowel transit: 2-4 hours
  - Large bowel transit: 1-2 days
  - Small bowel absorption 8.5L/day
  - Large bowel absorption 0.4L/day
  - Fecal excretion 0.1L/day
- Gut fluid balance
  - In: 9L/day
  - Out: 9L/day
  - Normal stool: 75% water (100ml)
  - Diarrhoea: >85% water
  - Constipation: <65% water

Defecation

- Feces stored in rectal ampulla
- Distension of rectum
- Stimulation of stretch receptors
- Reflex contraction of rectum
- Relaxation of internal anal sphincter
- Urge to defecate
- Relaxation of external anal sphincter
- Defecate

Common causes of constipation in cancer patients

- Chemotherapy (neurotoxicity)
  - Platinum compounds
  - Vinca alkaloids
  - Taxanes

- Thalidomide/lenalidomide
- Bortezomib
- 5HT3 antagonists
- Opioids
  - Motility: prevent integration needed for propulsive contractions by inhibiting enteric interneurons
  - Fluid handling: increase water absorption by slowing of passage of luminal contents, reduce secretion by inhibiting secretomotor neurons
  - Defecation: precipitate fecal impaction by reducing sensations of rectal distention
  - Opioids that are less constipative
    - Fentanyl
    - Alfentanil
    - Buprenorphine
    - Methadone
    - Tramadol
- Drugs with anticholinergic effects
  - Anticholinergics
  - Antihistamines
  - Tricyclics
  - Neuroleptics
- Direct tumour effect
  - Invasion of gut wall
  - Infiltration of enteric nerves
  - Compression of extrinsic nerves
  - Spinal cord compression
- Paraneoplastic constipation
  - Small cell lung cancer
  - Carcinoid tumour
- Hypercalcemia of malignancy
- Age-related loss of enteric neurons (>65 years old)

- Agre-related reduction in rectal sensitivity
- Reduced mobility
- Reduced dietary fluid intake

Five Principles of Using Laxatives

Introduction

There is no one single correct way in using laxatives in palliative care.

5 principles

- Rule out bowel obstruction
- Regular oral laxatives based on mechanisms
- PRN Rectal laxatives for fecal impaction
- PAMORA for unsuccessful laxation in OIC
- Laxatives and lifestyle education

Rule out bowel obstruction

- Most laxatives are not suitable in bowel obstruction
- Risk of worsening obstruction with bulk-forming laxatives
- Risk of worsening colic with stimulant laxatives
- Risk of perforation with stimulant laxatives
- Use softening laxatives if in doubt

Regular oral laxatives based on mechanisms

- Prescribe softening laxatives for hard stools
- Prescribe stimulating laxatives for no bowel movement
- Often a combination of both is necessary

PRN Rectal laxatives for fecal impaction

- Prescribe rectal softeners for hard impaction
- Prescribe rectal pushers for soft impaction
- Prescribe high enema for high impaction
- Consider manual evacuation for unsuccessful disimpaction

PAMORA for unsuccessful laxation in OIC

- Prescribe peripherally acting μ-opioid receptor antagonists for unsuccessful laxation in OIC
- Use PAMORA to clear accumulation of stool
- Then restart conventional laxatives and establish new regime

Laxatives and lifestyle education

- Laxatives education
  - Types
  - Actions
    - Softening laxatives: soften stools
    - Stimulating laxatives: move stools
  - Titration
  - Rectal measures
- Lifestyle education
  - Target cortex
    - Ensure time, privacy and favourable environment
  - Target intestinal fluid handling
    - Encourage adequate fluid intake as preferred
    - Encourage dietary fiber if appropriate
    - Drink barley – fiber
  - Target gut motility
    - Encourage regular toilet habits
      - Recognize urge of defecation
      - Do not ignore the urge
      - Make use of gastrocolic reflex
        - Toilet sitting after meals
    - Encourage exercise and mobility as preferred
    - Encourage gentle abdominal massage
    - Drink prune juice – mild stimulant laxative

Laxatives

Introduction

Laxatives can be divided into predominantly softening laxatives and predominantly stimulating laxatives.

Classification

- Stool lubricants   Predominantly softening
- Bulk-forming agents
- Macrogols
- Stool surfactants
- Osmotic agents
- Saline laxatives
- Anthranoids
- Phenolics   Predominantly stimulating

Stool lubricants

- Seldom used in palliative care
- Types
  - Mineral oil
  - Liquid paraffin
  - Liquid paraffin + magnesium hydroxide (Milpar)
- Doses
  - Mineral oil 10-20ml pre-breakfast and pre-bed
  - Liquid paraffin 10-20ml pre-breakfast and pre-bed
  - Milpar 10-20ml pre-breakfast and pre-bed
- Mechanisms
  - Lubricate stool surface
  - Soften stool

- Onset of action: 1-3 days
- Side effects
    - Leakage of oily fecal material
    - Perianal irritation
    - Lipoid pneumonia – not with Milpar

Bulk-forming agents

- Not suitable for most palliative care patients
    - Need to drink 200-300ml of water each time
    - Unpalatable
- Types
    - Wheat bran
    - Psyllium or Ispaghula (Fybogel)
    - Methylcellulose (Celevac)
    - Sterculia (Normacol)
    - Malt soup extract (Maltsupex)
- Doses
    - Wheat bran 10g bd with 250ml water after meals
    - Fybogel 1 sachet bd with 150ml water after meals
    - Celevac 3-6 tablets bd with 250ml water after meals
    - Normacol 1-2 sachets bd with 250ml water after meals
    - Maltsupex 15ml bd with 250ml water after meals
- Mechanisms
    - Normalizers: soften hard stool, make loose stool firmer
    - Increase stool bulk: shorten transit
    - Fermentation: shorten transit
- Onset of action: 2-4 days
- Side effects
    - Inadequate water intake
        - Form viscous mass
        - Obstruct bowels

Macrogols

- Polyethylene glycol
- Short term use in palliative care to flush bowels
- Brand names
  - Forlax
  - Movicol
  - Fortrans
  - Others: MiraLAX, SoftLAX, ClearLAX, GoLYTELY etc
- Doses in constipation
  - Forlax 2 sachets dly-bd in 250ml water
  - Movicol 2 sachets dly-bd in 250ml water
- Doses in fecal impaction
  - Forlax 8 sachets dly in 1L water
  - Movicol 8 sachets dly in 1L water
  - Fortrans 1 sachet dly in 1L water
- Mechanisms
  - Osmotic laxative
  - Non-absorbable polymer solution
  - Soften stool
  - Accelerate transit
- Onset of action: 1-3 days
- Side effects
  - Abdominal distension
  - Abdominal pain
  - Diarrhoea

Stool surfactants (emollients)

- Useful stool softeners in partial bowel obstruction
- Combinations: laxatives of choice in many palliative centers
- Types
  - Docusate sodium (Coloxyl tablets)
  - Poloxamer (Coloxyl drops)

- Doses
    - Docusate sodium 100-200mg bd
    - Coloxyl drops: for infants
- Mechanisms
    - Reduce surface tension of stool
    - Increase water penetration of stool
    - Soften stool
    - Stimulate secretion
    - Stimulate peristalsis at higher doses
- Onset of action
    - Coloxyl tablets: 12-72h
    - Coloxyl drops: 12-24h
- Side effects
    - Abdominal cramps
    - Diarrhoea
    - Nausea

Osmotic agents

- Lactulose is a common osmotic agent used in palliative care
- Useful for those who can drink ≥ 2L of water per day
- With less water, it ferments and causes bloating and colic
- Types
    - Lactulose
    - Sorbitol
    - Mannitol
- Doses
    - Syrup lactulose 10-30ml bd, max 30ml qid
    - Syrup sorbitol 10-30ml bd
    - Syrup mannitol 10-30ml bd
- Mechanisms
    - Osmotic laxatives: small bowel flushers
    - Non-absorbable sugars

- Increase water in intestinal lumen
- Soften stool
- Fermentation produces acetic, formic, lactic acids that stimulate peristalsis
- These acids are absorbed so the osmotic effect does not extend throughout the colon
- Onset of action: 1-2 days
- Side effects
  - Sweet taste (does not affect diabetic control)
  - Flatulence
  - Colic
- Contraindication
  - Anuria (risk of fluid overload)

Saline laxatives

- Last option in palliative care because of strong purgative action
- Types
  - Magnesium hydroxide (Milk of Magnesia)
  - Magnesium sulphate (Epsom salt)
  - Magnesium citrate (Citroma)
  - Sodium phosphate (Fleet Phospho-Soda solution)
- Doses
  - Milk of Magnesia 15-30ml bd
  - Epsom salt 2-4 teaspoons in 8oz water bd
  - Citroma 150-300ml single dose with 8oz water
  - Fleet solution 45ml stat, then 45ml 6h later
- Mechanisms
  - Osmotic laxatives: small and large bowels
  - Osmotic influence throughout the gut
  - Soften stool
  - Increase secretion
  - Stimulate peristalsis

- Onset of action: 1-6h
- Side effects
    - Sudden passage of offensive liquid feces
- Contraindications
    - Chronic kidney disease
    - Heart failure (sodium phosphate)

Anthranoids

- Senna is a common anthranoid used in palliative care
- Types
    - Dantron – small and large bowel pusher
    - Senna – large bowel pusher
    - Cascara sagrada – large bowel pusher
    - Casanthranol – large bowel pusher
- Doses
    - Dantron 50-150mg bd
    - Senna 15-30mg bd, max 30mg qid
    - Cascara sagrada 300mg dly ($\geq$ 1/52: hepatotoxicity risk)
    - Casanthranol: available in combination with docusate
- Senna
    - Derived from plants
    - Inactive glycosides
    - Hydrolyzed by bacterial glycosidases in large bowel to active aglycone compound
    - Effect on large bowel but no effect on small bowel
- Dantron
    - Synthetic anthranoid
    - Direct action on small and large bowel
- Mechanisms
    - Stimulant laxatives: stool pushers
    - Stimulate Meissner's plexus: ↑ secretion
    - Stimulate Auerbach's plexus: ↑ motility

- Onset of action: 6-12h
- Side effects
  - Abdominal cramp
  - Diarrhoea
  - Red urine (Dantron)
  - Perianal excoriation (Dantron)
  - Pseudomelanosis coli with chronic use
    - Reversible in 12 months after stopping laxative
    - Association with colon cancer not established

Phenolics

- Bisacodyl is a common phenolic used in palliative care
- Types
  - Bisacodyl – small and large bowel pusher
  - Sodium picosulphate – large bowel pusher
  - Phenolphthalein – withdrawn from market
- Doses
  - Bisacodyl 10-20mg on-bd, max 20mg qid
  - Sodium picosulphate 5-10mg on, max 15mg bd
- Bisacodyl
  - Hydrolyzed to active metabolites by intestinal esterases
  - Acts on small and large bowels
- Sodium picosulphate
  - Hydrolyzed to active metabolites by colonic bacteria
  - Acts on large bowel
- Mechanisms
  - Similar laxative effect to anthranoids
  - Stimulant laxatives: stool pushers
- Onset of action: 6-12h
- Side effects
  - Abdominal cramp
  - Diarrhoea

Miscellaneous oral and parenteral laxatives

Ricinoleic

- Vegetable oil obtained from seeds of Ricinus communis
- Type: Castor oil – small bowel pusher
- Dose: Castor oil 15-30ml daily
- Mechanisms
    - Hydrolysed by lipase in small bowel to ricinoleic acid
    - Release of neurotransmitters from enterochromaffin cells
    - Inhibits water absorption
    - Increases mucosal permeability
    - Stimulates motility
- Onset of action: 2-6h
- Side effects
    - Cramp
    - Severe diarrhoea

Chloride channel activator

- Bicyclic fatty acid derived from PGE1
- Type: Lubiprostone (Amitiza)
- Dose: Lubiprostone 24mcg bd
- Mechanisms
    - Acts on type 2 chloride channels on apical surface of luminal epithelium
    - Increases secretion without affecting serum Na^{2+} and K^+
    - Accelerates small and large bowel transits
- Onset of action: within 24h
- Side effects
    - Nausea
    - Diarrhoea
    - Headache
    - Flatulence

Prokinetics

- Use: constipation with intestinal hypomotility or gastroparesis
- Types
    - Metoclopramide
    - Domperidone
    - Cisapride
    - Tegaserod
    - Neostigmine
- Doses
    - Metoclopramide 10-20mg tds before meals
    - Domperidone 10-20mg tds before meals
    - Cisapride 10-20mg tds before meals
    - Tegaserod 6mg bd before meals
    - SC Neostigmine 0.5mg prn/tds
- Mechanisms
    - 5HT4 agonists
        - Metoclopramide
        - Domperidone
        - Cisapride
        - Tegaserod
    - Acetylcholinesterase inhibitor
        - Neostigmine
- Onset of action
    - Metoclopramide: 15-60min
    - Domperidone: 30min
    - Cisapride: 30-60min
    - Tegaserod: within 4 weeks
    - Neostigmine: minutes to 10h
- Side effects
    - Extrapyramidal effects (Metoclopramide, domperidone)
    - Cardiac arrhythmias (Cisapride)
    - Heart attack or stroke (Tegaserod)

Peripherally acting μ-opioid receptor antagonists (PAMORA)

- Use: opioid-induced constipation (OIC)
- Types
    - Oral naloxone
    - Methylnaltrexone
    - Alvimopan
    - Naloxegol
- Doses
    - PO Naloxone 0.8mg bd
        - Double the dose q2-3 day
        - Till bowel movement or adverse effect
    - SC Methylnaltrexone 8mg EOD if 40-60kg
    - SC Methylnaltrexone 12mg EOD if 60-120kg
    - PO Alvimopan 0.5-1.5mg dly, max 12mg bd
    - PO Naloxegol 25mg om
- Onset of action
    - Methylnatrexone: 30-60min
    - Alvimopan: 4-7h
    - Naloxegol: 1-3h
- Side effects
    - Diarrhoea
    - Cramp
    - Nausea and vomiting
    - Opioid withdrawal symptoms

Combination laxatives

- Benefits: dual mechanisms, compliance
- Types
    - Liquid paraffin and magnesium hydroxide (Milpar)
    - Docusate sodium and casanthranol (Peri-Colace)
    - Docusate sodium and senna (Senna-Plus)
    - Dantron and docusate (Co-Danthrusate)

- Dantron and poloxamer (Co-Danthramer)
- Doses
  - Milpar 10-20ml bd
  - Peri-Colace 2-4 cap on-bd
  - Senna-Plus 2-4 tab on-bd
  - Co-Danthrusate 2-4 cap on-bd
  - Co-Danthramer 2-4 cap on-bd

Rectal laxatives

- Indications
  - Unsuccessful oral laxatives
  - Cannot swallow oral laxatives
  - Cannot tolerate oral laxatives
  - Fecal impaction
  - Neurogenic bowel
- Stool lubricants
  - Arachis oil enema (peanut oil) 130ml prn
  - Olive oil enema 250ml prn
  - Mineral oil enema 100ml prn
  - Give overnight for hard stools
  - Then give stool flusher enema next day
  - Can give as high enema for ballooned rectum
- Stool softener
  - Docusate sodium (Norgalax micro-enema) 1 tube prn
  - Onset: 15-30min
- Stool flushers
  - Glycerin enema (Ravin enema) 2 tubes prn
  - Sodium citrate enema 2 tubes prn
  - Sodium phosphate enema (Fleet enema) 133ml prn
  - Tap water enema 500ml prn: risk of fluid overload
  - Onset: 15-30min (glycerin), 5-15min (sodium citrate), 2-5min (sodium phosphate)

- Fleet enema: can give as high enema for ballooned rectum
- Stool pusher
  - Bisacodyl suppository 10-20mg prn
  - Onset: 20-60min
  - Contact: rectal mucosa
  - Converted by colonic flora to desacetyl form
  - Stimulates colonic peristalsis

Malignant Bowel Obstruction

Introduction

In the past, surgery was the treatment of choice for malignant bowel obstruction. In 1985, Baines and colleagues reported in Lancet the first successful medical management of 38 patients with malignant bowel obstruction without surgery or NG tube. Since then, medical palliation of symptoms of malignant bowel obstruction was increasingly reported in the literature.

Survival of patients with malignant bowel obstruction (MBO)

- Median survival
    - 1 month (Woolfson 1997)
    - 2 months (Chan 1992)
    - 3 months (Jong 1995)
    - 6 months (Lau 1993)
- Median survival according to ECOG (Wright 2010)
    - ECOG 0-1: 7 months
    - ECOG 2: 2 months
    - ECOG3-4: 1 month
- Surgical vs medical Rx: no survival difference (Woolfson 1997)

Good surgical candidates

- Good performance status
- Good nutritional status
- Ascites <3L
- Unifocal obstruction
- Absence of palpable abdominal or pelvic masses
- Options of future disease-modifying treatments
- Life expectancy > 2months

Absolute contraindications to surgery (EAPC 2001)

- Recent laparotomy demonstrated inoperability
- Previous abdominal surgery showed diffuse metastatic cancer
- Involvement of proximal stomach
- Intraabdominal carcinomatosis demonstrated radiologically
- Diffuse palpable intra-abdominal masses
- Massive ascites which rapidly recurred after drainage

Relative contraindications to surgery (EAPC 2001)

- Advanced age with cachexia
- Poor performance status
- Poor nutritional status
- Previous abdominal or pelvic radiotherapy
- Symptomatic extra-abdominal metastases
- Asymptomatic extensive extra-abdominal metastases

Candidates for stenting

- Unifocal obstruction
- Advanced metastatic disease
- Poor surgical candidate
- Patients for surgery once medically optimized

Traditional conservative management

- Drip and Suck Therapy
    - Not suitable in the palliative care setting
    - Vigorous hydration
        - ↑ bowel secretions
        - ↑ bowel oedema
        - ↑ peripheral oedema
        - Best replaced with judicious hydration PRN
        - Hydration for comfort and preference
        - Example: SC hydration 5-10ml/h, max 20ml/h

- Nasogastric (NG) tube insertion (Pictus 1988)
    - Nasopharyngeal irritation
    - Nasal cartilage erosion
    - Occlusion necessitating flushing or replacement
    - Spontaneous expulsion
    - Best replaced with temporary PRN NG for symptoms
    - Temporary NG insertion for large volume vomiting
    - Aim to remove NG as soon as possible

Palliative management

- Medical resolution
    - Spontaneous resolution occurs in 1/3 within 48h
    - Medical resolution if no spontaneous resolution in 5 days
    - Steroids
        - Shrink bowel oedema
        - SC Dexamethasone 8-16mg om for 1/52 or
        - CSCI Dexamethasone 8-16mg/24h for 1/52
        - NNT = 6 (Cochrane Review 2000)
        - Statistically non-significant trend in resolution
    - Metoclopramide
        - Pushes bowel contents
        - SC Metoclopramide 10-20mg tds
        - CSCI Metoclopramide 30-120mg/24h
        - Can worsen colic
        - Combined with opioid to control colic
        - Contraindicated in complete bowel obstruction
        - Risk of perforation with complete obstruction
- Symptomatic management
    - Pain
    - Nausea and vomiting
    - Constipation
    - Abdominal distension

Pain management

- Treat abdominal pain according to WHO ladder
- Prescribe parenteral opioid during initial titration
- Opioid-naïve patients
  - CSCI/CIVI Morphine 0.5mg/24h
  - SC/IV Morphine 2.5mg prn/q1h for breakthrough pain
- Opioid-naïve patients with renal failure CC<30ml/min
  - CSCI/CIVI Fentanyl 10mcg/h
  - SC/IV Fentanyl 20mcg prn/q1h for breakthrough pain
- Switch to fentanyl patch once pain is stable for 2-3 days
- Stop opioid infusion 8h after application of fentanyl patch
- Fentanyl and methadone may have less constipating effects in comparison with morphine
- Non-opioids for additional analgesia
  - IV Paracetamol 1g over 15min q6h
  - CSCI Dclofenac 75-150mg/24h
  - CSCI Ketorolac 60-90mg/24h
- Anticholinergics for colic
  - Use breakthrough opioid as first line analgesia for colic
  - Use anticholinergic as second line
  - SC/IV Hyoscine butylbromide 20mg prn/q1h for colic
  - CSCI/CIVI Hyoscine butylbromide 60-120mg/24h if ≥3 doses/day + irreversible bowel obstruction

Management of nausea and vomiting

- Targets
  - Complete relief of nausea
  - Partial relief of vomiting (1-2 vomit/day)
- Steps
  - Step 1: haloperidol or metoclopramide
  - Step 2: step 1 + antihistamine
  - Step 3: broad spectrum antemetic

- Haloperidol
  - Antiemetic of choice in complete bowel obstruction
  - SC/IV Haloperidol 1.5-5mg bd or
  - CSCI/CIVI Haloperidol 1.5-10mg/24h
  - Partial response to 10mg/24h : titrate to max 20mg/24h
  - No response to 10mg/24h: add antihistamine
- Metoclopramide
  - Antiemetic of choice in functional or partial obstruction
  - Avoid in the presence of colic
  - Avoid combining with hyoscine butylbromide because they antagonize each other
  - SC/IV Metoclopramide 10-20mg tds
  - CSCI/CIVI Metoclopramide 30-120mg/24h
  - Stop if patient develops colic
- Antihistamines
  - SC boluses can cause tissue necrosis
  - IV boluses have to be given slowly
  - CSCI is the preferred route of administration
  - Dilute with water for injection (WFI), not saline
  - Stop if patient complains of burning
  - SC Cyclizine 50-100mg tds
  - CSCI Cyclizine 150-300mg/24h
  - SC Promethazine 25-50mg tds
  - CSCI Promethazine 50-150mg/24h
  - SC Diphenhydramine 25-50mg tds
  - SC Dimenhydrinate 50-100mg tds
- Broad spectrum antiemetics
  - SL Olanzapine 2.5-10mg on
  - SC Levomepromazine 6.25-25mg on-bd
  - SC Levomepromazine 6.25-50mg/24h
- 5HT3 antagonists
  - Consider adding a 5HT3 antagonist after step 3

- SC/IV Granisetron 1mg dly-bd
- SC/IV Ondansetron 8mg dly-tds
- CSCI/CIVI Ondansetron 8-24mg/24h
- Neostigmine
  - Functional obstruction despite metoclopramide
  - SC Neostigmine 1-2.5mg test dose
  - Then CSCI Neostigmine 5-20mg/24h if tolerated
- Rectal antiemetics
  - No access to parenteral medications
  - ABHR suppositories tds
    - Lorazepam (Ativan) 0.5mg
    - Diphenhydramine (Benadryl) 12.5mg
    - Haloperidol (Haldol) 0.5mg
    - Metoclopramide (Reglan) 10mg
  - Gralla suppositories tds
    - Diphenhydramine 25mg
    - Dexamethasone 5mg
    - Metoclopramide 20mg
  - PR Prochlorperazine 25mg tds
  - PR Chlorpromazine 50-100mg tds
- Venting nasogastric tube
  - Use: large volume vomiting or proximal obstruction
  - Remove NG when vomitus <100ml/day
  - Use antisecretory agents to expedite removal
- Venting gastrostomy
  - Use: long term decompression
  - 84% had symptom resolution and return of ability to consume liquids or soft food for a median of 74 days (Campagnutta 1996)
  - Contraindications
    - Significant ascites
    - Tumour infiltration of stomach

Management of constipation

- Rectal measures
  - Options
    - Glycerin enema 2 tubes prn
    - Fleet enema 133ml prn
    - Olive oil enema 250ml prn
  - High fleet enema may be tried with special care with the gentle insertion of urinary catheter and instillation of fleet enema with or without olive oil
  - Enema may be given through stoma with care
- Oral laxatives
  - Complete bowel obstruction
    - Little role
    - Can worsen the situation
  - Partial bowel obstruction
    - Liquid paraffin or sodium docusate may be used
    - Osmotic and stimulant laxatives
      - Used with extreme care if no colic
      - Osmotic: lactulose
      - Stimulant: senna
      - Stop if colic or no response

Management of abdominal distension

- Food
  - Fasting is usually unnecessary
  - Patients will stop eating if they are very uncomfortable
  - Allow orally as tolerated
  - Inform patients that vomiting may occur
  - Liquid-based low fiber diet is preferred
  - Juices are preferred for vegetables and fruits
  - Balance between QOL and symptom control as decided by patients

- Temporary venting NG tube for large volume vomitus
- Parenteral nutrition may be useful for selected MBO patients with good performance status ECOG1-2 who are unable to take oral or enteral nutrition adequately
- Fluid
  - Oral fluid few ml prn/q1-2h as tolerated
  - Small ice cube if cold fluid is preferred
  - IV/SC fluid 250-1000ml/day prn
  - Regular review for peripheral oedema
  - Anticholinergics for high volume vomitus
    - CSCI Hyoscine butylbromide 60-120mg/24h
    - CSCI Hyoscine hydrobromide 1.2-2.4mg/24h
  - Octreotide for high volume vomitus
    - Very expensive
    - Onset of action: 24-48h
    - Use: failed maximal dose of anticholinergics
    - Starting dose: CSCI Octreotide 100-300mcg/24h
    - Usual dose: CSCI Octerotide 300-600mcg/24h
    - Maximal dose: CSCI Octreotide 900mcg/24h
    - Diluent: normal saline
  - Depot injection
    - Use: favourable response to octreotide
    - Octreotide (Sandostatin LAR)
      - Deep IM 10-30mg monthly
    - Lanreotide (Somatuline LA)
      - IM 30mg every 2 weeks
    - Lanreotide (Somatuline Autogel)
      - Deep SC 60-120mg every 28 days
  - PPI and H2 antagonists for gastric secretions
- Air
  - Simethicone: coalesces air bubbles
    - Syrup Maalox Plus 10-20ml tds

- PO Maalox Plus 2-4 tablets tds
- Carbonated drinks: induce burping
  - Coke or 100 Plus
  - May increase air inside bowels

3-step protocol for inoperable MBO (Laval 2006)

- Step 1: symptomatic management for 5 days
  - Corticosteroids
  - Antiemetics
  - Anticholinergics
  - Analgesics
  - IV fluids
  - ± NG tube
- Step 2: somatostatin analogue for 3 days if vomiting persists
  - Stop corticosteroids
  - Start octreotide for 3 days
  - Response: find lowest effective dose of octreotide
- Step 3: definitive procedure if vomiting persists
  - Venting gastrostomy or stenting
- Symptom control
  - Step 1: 62%
  - Step 1 + 2: 76%
  - Step 1 +2 + 3: 90%

Sleep

Introduction

Sleep is a naturally recurring state with reduced consciousness and diminished sensory and muscular activities.

Two-process model of sleep regulation

- Two main processes involved in sleep regulation
- Process C (Circadian rhythm)
    - Function: regulates alertness level by circadian clock
    - Site: suprachiasmatic nucleus (SCN) in hypothalamus
    - Reset: using Zietgebers (environmental cues)
    - Most important Zietgeber: daylight
    - Coordinated with day-night cycle
    - Hormone: melatonin from pineal gland
    - Control of timing of sleep
    - Independent of amount of preceding sleep or wakefulness
    - Peripheral clock: heart, lung, liver, kidneys, intestines etc
- Process S (Sleep homeostasis)
    - Function: regulates sleepiness level by homeostatic sleep drive due to accumulation of hypnogenic substances
    - Best known hypnogenic substance: adenosine
    - Adenosine: byproduct of using energy ATP
    - Control of sleep duration and intensity
    - Correlate of sleep intensity: slow-wave sleep
    - Dependent on amount of preceding sleep or wakefulness: sleep debt
    - Adenosine antagonists
        - Caffeine in tea, coke, coffee
        - Theophylline in tea, chocolate

Neurological mechanisms of sleep

- Sleep center
    - Site: anterior hypothalamus (VLPO)
    - VLPO
        - Ventrolateral preoptic nucleus
        - Sleep switch
        - Neurotransmitters: GABA and galanin
        - Function: inhibits arousal systems
- Arousal systems (wakefulness center)
    - Site: brainstem, hypothalamus, basal forebrain
    - Reticular activating system (RAS) of brainstem
        - Cholinergic system
            - Pedunculopontine nucleus (PPT)
            - Laterodorsal tegmental nuclei (LDT)
        - Serotonergic system
            - Dorsal raphe nuclei (DR)
            - Median raphe nuclei (MR)
        - Noradrenergic system
            - Locus coeruleus (LC)
        - Dopaminergic system
            - Ventral periaqueductal gray matter (vPAG)
    - Orexinergic system of lateral hypothalamus
        - Perifornical region
    - Histaminergic system of posterior hypothalamus
        - Tuberomammillary nucleus (TMN)
    - Cholinergic system of basal forebrain
        - Magnocellular nuclei (basal nuclei of Meynert)
- Flip-flop switch model of sleep
    - Mutual inhibition between VLPO and arousal systems
    - Either sleep neurons or arousal neurons are active
    - No intermediate state
    - Similar to the electrical flip-flop circuit

- Wakefulness
  - Monoaminegic systems inhibit VLPO
    - TMN inhibits VLPO
    - LC inhibits VLPO
    - DR inhibits VLPO
  - Orexinergic system reinforces monoaminergic tone
    - Stabilizes the switch
    - No direct inhibition of VLPO
- Sleep
  - VLPO inhibits monoaminergic systems
  - VLPO inhibits orexinergic system
- Reciprocal interaction model of NREM-REM cycle
  - Interaction between REM-ON and REM-OFF neurons
  - Anticholinergic mechanisms: REM-OFF
  - Cholinergic mechanisms: REM-ON
  - REM-OFF: LC/DR inhibits PPT/LDT
  - REM-ON: PPT/LDT inhibits LC/DR

Types of sleep

- Non-rapid eye movement sleep (NREM)
  - Synchronized sleep
  - R&K scoring (Rechtschaffen and Kales 1968)
    - Stage 1: light sleep
    - Stage 2: medium sleep
    - Stage 3: deep sleep
    - Stage 4: deep sleep
  - AASM stages (American Academy of Sleep Medicine 2004)
    - N1: stage 1
    - N2: stage 2
    - N3: stage 3 and 4
- Rapid eye movement sleep (REM)
  - Unsynchronized sleep

Stages of sleep (R&K scoring)

- Alert awake state
  - Gamma waves: 30-40Hz
    - Fastest brainwaves
    - Smallest amplitude
    - Occurrence
      - Extreme focus
      - Ecstasy
      - Compassion meditation
  - Beta waves: 12-30Hz
    - Dominate normal waking state
    - Called awake waves
    - Fast and small
    - Occurrence
      - Focused mental activity
      - Problem solving
      - Decision making
      - Judgment
    - Types
      - High beta waves: 20-30Hz
      - Beta waves: 16-20Hz
      - Low beta waves: 12-16Hz
- Relaxed state with eyes closed
  - Alpha waves: 8-12Hz
    - Predominantly from occipital area
    - Called drowsy waves
    - Occurrence
      - Drowsiness
      - Daydreaming
      - Mindfulness meditation
  - Hypnagogic hallucination and myoclonic jerk may occur

- Stage 1 sleep
  - Light sleep
  - Theta waves: 4-8Hz
  - Called light sleeping waves
  - Slower frequency, greater amplitude
  - 5-10min
  - Conscious awareness of external environment reduces
- Stage 2 sleep
  - Medium sleep
  - Sleep spindles
    - Sigma waves
    - Short burst of 12-14Hz brain activity
    - Lasting 0.5s
    - Produced by thalamic reticular nucleus (TRN)
      - Phenomena: oscillation
      - Spontaneous burst-firing of TRN neurons
      - Surround inhibition of thalamocortical neurons
  - K-complexes
    - Short negative high-voltage peak
    - Followed by a slower positive complex
    - Then a final negative peak
    - Lasting 1-2min
    - Often followed by bursts of sleep spindles
  - Sleep spindles and K complexes
    - Protect sleep
    - Suppress cortical arousal in response to stimuli
  - 20min
  - Conscious awareness of external environment disappears
- Stage 3 sleep
  - Deep sleep or slow-wave sleep (SWS)
  - Delta waves: 0.5-4Hz
  - Called deep sleeping waves

- Slowest frequency, greatest amplitude
- Initiated in the preoptic area
- 20-50% delta waves
- Most restful form of sleep
- Important in declarative memory (conscious memory)
- Stage 4 sleep
  - Deep sleep or slow-wave sleep (SWS)
  - >50% delta waves
  - 30min
  - Combined with stage 3 in AASM stages
  - Parasomnias: night terror, sleep walking, sleep talking and bed wetting occur during the end of this period
- REM sleep
  - Dreaming sleep, active sleep or paradoxical sleep
  - Very similar to awake brain with beta waves
  - Fast, small, random with sawtooth waves
  - Body is paralyzed with atonia
  - Most dreams occur during this stage
  - Important in procedural memory (unconscious memory)

Sleep cycles

- Frequency: 4-5 sleep cycles per night
- Duration for first cycle: 90min
- Duration for subsequent cycles: 100-120min
- 1-2-3-4-3-2-REM-2-3-4-3-2-REM-2-3-4-3-2-REM-2-3-2-REM
- Best illustrated by hypnogram (not shown)
- Characteristics:
  - Light to deep sleep, then deep to light sleep, then REM
  - Stage 1: only in the beginning
  - Duration of deep sleep reduces with each cycle
  - Duration of REM sleep increases with each cycle

Sleep Terms

Introduction

Sleep disorders can be primary or secondary.

Primary sleep disorders

- Dyssomnias
    - Insomnia is difficulty in initiating or maintaining sleep
        - Early insomnia (sleep-onset insomnia)
            - Also called initial insomnia
            - Difficulty in falling asleep
            - Increase in sleep latency
            - Association: anxiety
        - Middle insomnia (sleep-maintenance insomnia)
            - Difficulty in maintaining sleep
            - Decrease in sleep efficiency
            - Fragmented unrestful sleep
            - Frequent awakening during sleep
            - Association: medical illness, pain, depression
        - Late insomnia (end-of-sleep insomnia)
            - Also called terminal insomnia
            - Early morning awakening
            - Inability to return to sleep
            - Association: major depression
    - Hypersomnia is excessive daytime sleepiness
- Parasomnias
    - Sleep disorders that occur during sleep or arousal
        - Sleep transition disorders
            - Hypnic jerks (at sleep onset)
            - Sleep talking (during sleep)

- Nocturnal leg cramps (during sleep)
  - Arousal disorders
    - Sleep walking (during deep sleep)
    - Sleep terrors (sudden arousal from deep sleep)
    - Confusional arousal (arousal from deep sleep)
- REM parasomnias
  - Nightmares
  - Sleep paralysis

Secondary sleep disorders

- Associated with psychological disorders
- Associated with neurological disorders
- Associated with other medical disorders

Sleep terminology

- Sleep onset: the transition from awake to sleep
- Sleep latency: the duration of time from bedtime to sleep onset
- Sleep fragmentation: repetitive interruptions of sleep by arousals or awakenings
- Sleep efficiency: the ratio of total sleep time to time in bed
- Early morning awakening: early termination of sleep, accompanied by an inability to return to sleep
- Arousal: an abrupt change from a deeper stage of NREM sleep to a lighter stage, or from REM to wakefulness, with the possibility of awakening as the final outcome
- Awakening: the return to the awake state
- Sleep inertia: feeling groggy after abrupt awakening
- Sleep hygiene: the conditions and practices that promote continuous and effective sleep
- Zeitgeber: an environmental cue, such as sunlight, noise, social interaction, that usually helps an individual entrain to the 24-hour day

Sleep Assessment

Introduction

A comprehensive sleep assessment is necessary before managing sleep disorders.

Determining the type of sleep disorders

- Early insomnia: difficulty falling asleep
- Middle insomnia: difficulty staying asleep
- Late insomnia: early morning awakening
- Non-restorative sleep: sleep with poor quality
- Parasomnia: abnormal behaviour during sleep

Determining the risk factor of sleep disorders

- Predisposing factors
  - Young cancer patients
  - Female
  - History or family history of insomnia
  - History of anxiety or depressive disorders
  - Medical comorbidities
- Precipitating factors
  - Physical symptoms
    - Pain
    - Breathlessness
    - Cough
    - Nausea and vomiting
    - Diarrhoea
    - Urinary frequency
    - Fever
    - Delirium

- Psychological reactions to bad news
  - Anxiety
  - Depression
  - Fear
  - Anger
  - Automatic negative thoughts
- Cancer treatment
  - Surgery
  - Radiotherapy
  - Chemotherapy
  - Hormonal therapy
- Diet
  - Caffeine
  - Nicotine
  - Alcohol
- Drugs
  - Steroids
  - Bronchodilators
  - Psychostimulants
  - Antihypertensives
    - Methyldopa
    - Propranolol
  - Antidepressants
    - Fluoxetine
    - MAOIs
    - Protriptyline
    - Bupropion
- Hospitalization
  - Unfamiliar environment
  - Change of pre-sleep routine
  - Lighting at night
  - Noise from other patients

- Noise from healthcare staff
- Noise from beeping machines
- Night time vital signs checking
- Night time medication dispensing
- Perpetuating factors
  - Cognitive distortions about sleep
  - Maladaptive sleep behaviours
    - Poor sleep hygiene
      - Irregular sleeping time
      - Lying on bed during the day
      - Frequent nap during the day
      - Spending time on bed other than sleeping

Taking a sleep history

- Daytime activities
- Afternoon nap
- Sleep hygiene
- Pre-sleep routine and changes
- Pre-sleep emotions and thoughts
- Sleep environment
- Sleep partner
- Sleep time
- Sleep latency
- Sleep duration
- Sleep efficiency
- Nocturnal awakening
- Reasons of difficulty falling asleep
- Reasons of nocturnal awakening
- Aggravating and relieving factors
- Dreams
- Freshness after waking up
- Impact of sleep disorder on patient or caregivers

Sleep Architecture

Introduction

Various factors influencing sleep architecture are mentioned here.

Age

- Sleep latency: ↑
- Light sleep: ↑
- Deep sleep: ↓
- REM sleep: ↓
- Nocturnal awakening: ↑
- Circadian rhythm: phase advance (sleep and wake up earlier)

Pain

- Light sleep: ↑
- Deep sleep: ↓
- REM sleep: ↓
- Nocturnal awakening: ↑
- Alpha waves intrusion into SWS: fibromyalgia

Depression

- Deep sleep: ↓
- REM latency: ↓ (biological marker of depression)
- REM sleep: ↑ in early night
- Nocturnal awakening: ↑

Anxiety

- Sleep latency: ↑
- Light sleep: ↑
- Deep sleep: ↓

- Nocturnal awakening: ↑
- REM parasomnia: nightmares

Delirium

- Circadian rhythm: reversed

Opioids (Studies based on healthy subjects not in pain)

- Sleep latency: ↓ (chronic use)
- Deep sleep: ↓
- REM sleep: ↓ (initial use)
- Nocturnal awakening: ↑

Benzodiazepines

- Sleep latency: ↓
- Light sleep: ↑
- Deep sleep: ↓ (especially long-acting benzodiazepines)
- REM latency: ↑
- REM sleep: ↓ (especially long-acting benzodiazepines)
- Nocturnal awakening: ↓
- Benzodiazepine-induced sleep is not as restful as natural sleep
    - Reduction of slow-wave sleep
    - Reduction in REM sleep
        - Reduced daytime performance
            - REM sleep: learning and memory
        - Reduced sleep quality
            - REM sleep: resting of all muscles except eyes
- Hangover effect: sleepiness and reduced cognitive performance during the next day

Non-benzodiazepines

- Longer SWS compared to benzodiazepines
- Less hangover effect compared to benzodiazepines

Non-pharmacological Management of Sleep Disorders

Introduction

Cognitive-behavioural therapy (CBT) is the mainstay of non-pharmacological intervention for sleep disorders.

CBT components

- Cognitive therapy
    - Address dysfunctional thoughts
        - My sleep problem will get worse and worse
        - If I cannot sleep, my cancer will progress faster
        - I am going to die with a lot of suffering
    - Cognitive restructuring
        - My sleep problem will improve if I worry less
        - I know poor sleepers who are in remission
        - My suffering can be relieved
- Sleep hygiene education (American Sleep Association 2007)
    - Maintain a regular sleep routine
    - Avoid naps if possible
    - Do not stay in bed awake for more than 5-10minutes
    - Do not drink caffeine inappropriately
    - Do not watch TV or read in bed
    - Avoid substances that interfere with sleep
    - Exercise regularly
    - Have a quiet, comfortable bedroom
    - If you are a "clock-watcher" at night, hide the clock
    - Have a comfortable pre-bedtime routine

- Stimulus control therapy
  - Behavioural therapy to reassociate stimulus and sleep
  - Goal: establish regular circadian sleep-wake rhythm
  - Stimulus: bed
  - Use bed for sleep only
  - No reading, eating, watching TV, listening to radio on bed
  - Go to bed only when sleepy
  - Get out of bed if cannot sleep within 15-20min
  - Return to bed only when sleepy
  - Avoid napping during the day
- Sleep restriction therapy
  - Behavioural therapy to curtail the time in bed to the actual sleep time
  - Goal: create mild sleep debt
  - Restrict total time spent in bed to actual amount of time asleep based on completed sleep diaries
  - Avoid fixing sleep window <5 hours
  - Adjust bedtime weekly according to sleep efficiency
    - Sleep efficiency >85%: sleep 30min earlier
    - Sleep efficiency 80-85%: keep similar bedtime
    - Sleep efficiency <80%: sleep 30min later
- Relaxation therapy
  - Progressive muscular relaxation
  - Guided imagery
  - Hypnosis
  - Body scan
  - Meditation

Pharmacological Management of Sleep Disorders

Introduction

Benzodiazepine and nonbenzodiazepine hypnotics are standard medications of choice for insomnia.

Benzodiazepine hypnotics

- Mechanism of action: bind benzodiazepine receptors between α1 and γ2 subunits of GABA-A receptors, increase Cl⁻ influx, hyperpolarize neurons, enhance GABA effect

Drugs	Onset	Half-life
Short acting		
PO Triazolam	Intermediate	1-5h
PO Midazolam	Fast	2-5h
Intermedate acting		
PO Oxazepam	Slow	5-15h
PO Alprazolam	Intermediate	6-20h
PO Bromazepam	Fast	10-20h
PO Temazepam	Fast	10-20h
PO Lorazepam	Intermediate	10-20h
Long acting		
PO Nitrazepam	Fast	24h
PO Clonazepam	Intermediate	20-40h
PO Clobazam	Fast	36-42h
PO Quazepam	Fast	29-73h
PO Chlordiazepoxide	Intermediate	3-100h
PO Flurazepam	Fast	47-100h
PO Diazepam	Fast	24-120h

- Onset of action of benzodiazepines
  - Fast onset = <15min
  - Intermediate onset = 15-30min
  - Slow onset = 30-60min
- Duration of action of benzodiazepines
  - Short acting: half-life <12h
  - Intermediate acting: half-life 12-24h
  - Long acting: half-life >24h
- Doses of short acting benzodiazepines
  - PO Triazolam 0.25-0.5mg on
  - PO Midazolam 7.5-15mg on
- Doses of intermediate acting benzodiazepines
  - PO Oxazepam 15-30mg on
  - PO Alprazolam 0.25-0.5mg on
  - PO Bromazepam 1.5-12mg on
  - PO Lorazepam 0.5-2mg on
  - PO Temazepam 7.5-30mg on
- Doses of long acting benzodiazepines
  - PO Nitrazepam 5-10mg on
  - PO Clonazepam 0.5-2mg on
  - PO Clobazam 20-30mg on
  - PO Quazepam 7.5-15mg on
  - PO Chlordiazepoxide 5-10mg on
  - PO Flurazepam 15-30mg on
  - PO Diazepam 5-10mg on
- Short acting benzodiazepines
  - Best used for sleep-onset insomnia
  - Least hangover effect
  - Suitable for active person and elderly
  - Highest risk for rebound insomnia
  - Highest risk for tolerance and dependence
  - For short term use: < 1 week

- Intermediate acting benzodiazepines
  - Best used for sleep-maintenance insomnia
  - More hangover effect
  - Less rebound insomnia
  - Less tolerance and dependence
  - For short term use: < 1 month
- Long acting benzodiazepines
  - Best used for insomnia with concomitant daytime anxiety
  - May be effective for 2 nights or more
  - Accumulation of active metabolites is most problematic in elderly and in those with impaired liver function
  - Most hangover effect
  - Least rebound insomnia
  - Least tolerance and dependence
- Using benzodiazepines in insomnia
  - Fast onset is preferred
  - Intermediate acting is preferred
  - First line: bromazepam, temazepam, lorazepam
  - Second line: nitrazepam, flurazepam, diazepam
  - Half the recommended doses in elderly
  - Sublingual administration can be used in palliative setting
- Stopping benzodiazepine
  - Reduce dose gradually within several weeks or months, or eliminate doses at certain nights, such as Friday and Saturday night
- Switching benzodiazepine to nonbenzodiazepine
  - Overlap with administration of non-benzodiazepine
  - Reduce benzodiazepine dose gradually within 10 days

Nonbenzodiazepine hypnotics

- Mechanism of action: benzodiazepine receptor agonists with selectivity for $\alpha 1$ subunit of GABA-A benzodiazepine-1 receptor

- Promote physiological sleep
- Sleep latency: ↓
- Deep sleep: ↑
- Nocturnal awakening: ↓ except zaleplone (no change)
- Total sleep time: ↑ except zaleplone (no change)
- Little hangover effect
- Little rebound insomnia except eszopiclone
- Less tolerance and dependence
- For short term use: < 1 month except eszopiclone
- Action can be reversed by flumazenil
- Zolpidem (Stilnox)
    - Class: imidazopyridine
    - Onset: <30min
    - Half-life: 2-3h
    - Use: sleep-onset insomnia
    - Dose: 10mg on, 5mg on (elderly)
    - For short term use: < 1 month
- Zaleplone (Sonata)
    - Class: pyrazolopyrimidine
    - Onset: <30min (faster than zolpidem)
    - Half-life: 1h
    - Use: sleep-onset insomnia, breakthrough awakening
    - Dose: 10-20mg on, 5mg on (elderly)
- Zopiclone (Imovane)
    - Class: cyclopyrrolone
    - Onset: <30min
    - Half-life: 3-5h
    - Use: sleep-onset and sleep-maintenance insomnia
    - Dose: 7.5-15mg on, 3.75mg on (elderly)
- Eszopiclone (Lunesta)
    - S-enantiomer of zopiclone
    - Class: cyclopyrrolone

- Onset: <30min
- Half-life: 6h
- Use: sleep-onset and sleep-maintenance insomnia
- Dose: 1-3mg on
- Potential hangover effect with 2-3mg
- Potential rebound insomnia
- For use up to 6 months

Melatonin receptor agonist

- Ramelteon
  - Mechanism: binds MT1 and MT2 receptors in SCN
  - Sleep latency: ↓
  - Total sleep time: ↑
  - Onset: 30min
  - Half-life: 1-2h
  - Use: sleep-onset insomnia, delayed sleep phase syndrome
  - Dose: 8mg on
  - No hangover effect
  - No rebound insomnia
  - No tolerance and dependence
  - Approved for long term use

Clomethiazole

- Also called chlormethiazole
- Positive allosteric modulator at barbiturate/picrotoxin site of GABA-A receptor, and glycine receptor
- Enhances both GABA effect and glycinergic effect
- Onset: rapid
- Half-life: 3-5h
- Best used for insomnia in elderly
- Dose: 192-384mg on
- Little hangover effect

- Rebound insomnia
- Tolerance and dependence
- Limit use to <9 days to avoid dependence

Chloral hydrate

- Enhances GABA effect
- Modest short term efficacy
- Onset: 20-60min
- Half-life: 8-12h (metabolites)
- Dose for adult: 0.5-1g on
- Dose for children: 25-50mg/kg on
- More toxic than benzodiazepines
- Hangover effect
- Tolerance and dependence

Antidepressants with sedative effects

- Trazodone 25-100mg on
    - Sedating heterocyclic antidepressant
    - Serotonin antagonist and reuptake inhibitor (SARI)
    - Milder anticholinergic side effects than TCA
    - Onset: 30-60min for insomnia
    - Half-life: 7h, shorter than most TCA
    - Best used for insomnia with depression
    - Can be administered over a longer period for insomnia
- Amitriptyline 25-100mg on
    - Sedating tricyclic antidepressant (TCA)
    - Serotonin and noradrenaline reuptake inhibitor (SNRI)
    - Onset: 20-45min for insomnia
    - Half-life: 9-25h (metabolite nortriptyline 15-39h)
    - Best used for insomnia with pain or depression
    - Dose for insomnia per se: 10-50mg on
    - Side effects: anticholinergic effects, daytime sedation

- Mirtazapine 15-30mg on
  - Sedating tetracyclic antidepressant
  - Noradrenergic and specific serotonergic antidepressant
  - NaSSA
  - Sleep latency: ↓
  - SWS: ↑ (5HT2A/C antagonism)
  - REM sleep: unchanged
  - Total sleep time: ↑
  - Onset: 2 weeks
  - Half-life: 20-40h
  - Best used for insomnia with depression
  - Hangover effect in 10% with rapid tolerance

Antipsychotics with sedative effects

- Best used for insomnia with delirium
- Haloperidol 1.5-5mg on (useful for unpleasant dreams)
- Olanzapine 2.5-10mg on
- Risperidone 0.5-2mg on
- Quetiapine 25-100mg on

Antihistamines with sedative effects

- Best used for insomnia with pruritus or cough
- Chlorpheniramine (Piriton) 4-8mg on
- Hydroxyzine (Atarax) 25-50mg on
- Diphenhydramine (Benadryl) 25-50mg on
- Promethazine (Phenergan) 25-50mg on

Barbiturates

- Bind GABA-A receptors
- Enhance GABA effect
- Effective hypnotics
- Onset: 20-60min for phenobarbital

- Half-life: 2-6 days for phenobarbital
- Dose: PO Phenobarbital 100-200mg on
- Hangover effect
- Rapid development of tolerance after about 2 weeks
- Risk of dependence
- Serious or fatal consequences with overdose, esp with alcohol
- Gradual withdrawal recommended

Medication adjustment to avoid insomnia

- Give steroid as a single morning dose
- Give diuretic as a single morning dose
- Give fluoxetine as a single morning dose
- Give sertraline as a single morning dose
- Give methylphenidate at 8am and 12pm

Delirium

Introduction

Delirium is a syndrome of acute brain failure characterized by disturbances in consciousness. The disturbances can be a change in the content of consciousness (attention), a change in the level of consciousness (arousal), or both.

Types of delirium

- Hyperactive delirium (agitated delirium): patient is agitated, restless and confused
- Hypoactive delirium (lethargic delirium): patient is lethargic, withdrawn and confused
- Mixed delirium: patient has a mixture of hyperactive and hypoactive delirium

Causes of delirium

- Check for simple reversible causes of delirium before thinking about the complicated ones
- Symptom distress: pain, breathlessness, nausea and vomiting, acute urinary retention, fecal impaction, insomnia, fatigue
- Psychosocial distress: fear of pain, fear of dying, fear of being alone, witnessing death of another patient
- Hospital causes: blood-taking, nasogastric tube insertion, urinary catheter insertion, continuous vital sign monitoring, physical restraint, change of bed, soiled bed sheets, folded bed sheets, uncomfortable bed
- Organ failure causes: respiratory failure, cardiac failure, liver failure, renal failure, brain failure (brain metastases, stroke, encephalopathy)

- Metabolic and toxin causes: hypoglycaemia, hyponatremia, hypercalcemia, septic encephalopathy
- Drug causes: opioid, steroid, benzodiazepine, anticholinergic, antihistamine, antidepressant, antipsychotic, anticonvulsant
- Antibiotic causes: penicillin, cephalosporin, fluoroquinolone, sulfonamide, metronidazole
- Chemotherapy causes: asparaginase, bleomycin, carmustin, cisplatin, cytarabine, 5-fluorouracil, gemcitabine, ifosfamide, methotrexate, procarbazine, vincristine, vinblastine

Delirium assessment

- Confusion Assessment Method (CAM)
    - Acute onset and fluctuating course
    - Inattention
    - Disorganized thinking
    - Altered level of conscious
- Memorial Delirium Assessment Scale (MDAS)
    - Reduced level of consciousness
    - Disorientation
    - Short-term memory impairment
    - Impaired digit span
    - Reduced ability to maintain and shift attention
    - Disorganized thinking
    - Perceptual disturbance
    - Delusions
    - Decreased or increased psychomotor activity
    - Sleep-wake cycle disturbance

Pathophysiology of delirium

- Multifactorial
- Not fully understood
- Decreased cerebral oxidative metabolism

- Neuroanatomical structures
    - Level of consciousness (Arousal)
        - Ascending reticular activating system (ARAS)
            - Dorsal mesencephalic reticular formation
            - Mesencephalic nucleus
            - Locus ceruleus and raphe nuclei
            - Thalamic intralaminar nucleus
            - Dorsal hypothalamus
            - Tegmentum
            - Basal forebrain
    - Content of consciousness (Attention)
        - Alerting network: maintaining alertness
            - Same areas for arousal: ARAS
            - Main neurotransmitter: noradrenergic system of locus ceruleus
        - Orienting network: orienting to sensory information
            - Pulvinar
            - Superior colliculus
            - Superior parietal lobe
            - Temporoparietal junction
            - Frontal eye field
            - Main neurotransmitter: cholinergic system of basal forebrain
        - Executive network: resolving conflicts between multiple competing attention cues
            - Anterior cingulate gyrus
            - Dorsolateral prefrontal cortex (DLPRC)
            - Main neurotransmitter: dopamine system of mesocortex
- Neurotransmitters
    - Acetylcholine-dopamine hypothesis
        - Acetylcholine insufficiency

- Dopamine excess
  - Other neurotransmitters
    - Serotonin, noradrenaline, histamine, hypocretin, glutamate, endorphins, GABA
- Cytokines: IL-1, IL-6, IL-8, IFN, TNF
- Chronic hypercortisolism

Non-pharmacological management of delirium

- Environmental interventions
  - Avoid over and understimulation
  - Visual interventions
    - Adequate lighting during daytime
    - Minimal lighting during night-time
    - Huge calender and clock
    - Make the environment familiar
      - Photographs
      - Personal objects
  - Auditory interventions
    - Keeping a quiet environment
    - Silent monitoring
    - Slow music if appropriate
    - Slow electronic chanting if appropriate
  - Physical interventions
    - Familiar objects
    - Home pillows and blankets
    - Bed sheet rearrangement
    - Avoid restraints
    - Avoid continuous vital signs monitoring
    - Minimize tubes and lines
  - Social interventions
    - Family staying in
    - Familiar staff if possible

- Sleep interventions
    - Facilitate normal sleep
    - Exposure to sunlight during daytime
    - Encourage activities during daytime
    - Keep room dark during night-time
    - Minimize interruption during night-time
    - Avoid vital signs checking at night if appropriate
- Patient support
    - Maintain communication
    - Active listening
    - Explore patient's ideas, concerns and expectations
    - Explore patient's emotions
    - Explore reasons behind hallucination or delusion
    - Explore reasons behind patient's behaviour
    - Explain to patient about each procedure and intervention
- Family support
    - Taking care of a delirious patient is stressful
    - Do not forget to support the family member
    - Give simple explanation of the nature of delirium
    - Explore family's ideas, concerns and expectations
    - Acknowledge family distress
    - Educate family in consoling patient
    - Educate family in re-orientating patient
    - Facilitate the linking of the content of hallucination and delusion with past experiences
    - Provide respite care if needed

Pharmacological management of delirium (PCT input)

- Review of meditations
    - Stop deliriogenic drugs if appropriate
    - Consider opioid rotation for opioid neurotoxicity
    - Consider steroids for brain metastases

- Typical antipsychotics
  - Haloperidol
    - Gold standard treatment for delirium
    - Onset: 1h (PO), 10-15min (SC)
    - Half-life: 0.5-1.5 days
    - Duration: 24h
    - Less sedating compared to chlorpromazine
    - Less anticholinergic effect
    - Extrapyramidal effect more likely when ≥ 7.5mg/day
    - Mild delirium (10 < MDAS score ≤ 15)
      - PO Haloperidol 0.75-1.5mg bd
      - SC Haloperidol 0.5-1.5mg bd
    - Moderate delirium (15 < MDAS score ≤ 22)
      - PO Haloperidol 2.5-5mg bd
      - SC Haloperidol 2.5-5mg bd
    - Severe delirium (MDAS score > 22)
      - PO Haloperidol 5-10mg bd
      - SC Haloperidol 5-10mg bd
    - Rapid titration of haloperidol for severe agitation
      - PO/SL/SC Haloperidol 0.5-2.5mg prn/q1h
      - Administer until delirium is controlled in 24h
    - 30-minute haloperidol titration schedule
      - 0.5, 0.5, 0.5, 1, 1, 1, 2, 2, 2, 5, 5, 5mg prn
      - Administer q30min
    - Maximum reported dose 50mg/day
  - Chlorpromazine
    - Onset: 30-60min (PO), 15-30min (SC)
    - Half-life: 1.25 days
    - Duration: 4-6h
    - PO/SC/PR Chlorpromazine 12.5-50mg q4-6h
    - Risk of skin irritation with SC
    - Preferred in agitated delirium (sedation)

- Levomepromazine
  - Onset: 30min
  - Half-life: 0.5-1.25 days
  - Duration: 12-24h
  - PO Levomepromazine 5-25mg bd
  - SC Levomepromazine 6.25-25mg bd
  - Preferred in agitated delirium (sedation)
- Atypical antipsychotics
  - Less extrapyramidal side effects
  - PO Olanzapine 2.5-10mg on, max 20mg bd (agitation)
  - PO Quetiapine 12.5-100mg bd, max 200mg bd (agitation)
  - PO Risperidone 0.25-1mg bd, max 3mg bd
  - PO Ziprasidone 10-40mg bd, max 80mg bd
  - PO Aripiprazole 5-30mg dly, max 30mg dly
- Benzodiazepines
  - Second line treatment of agitated delirium
  - Usually added if haloperidol dose has reached 20mg/day
  - SC Midazolam 2.5mg prn/q1h
  - CSCI Midazolam 0.5-1mg/h
  - SL Lorazepam 1-2mg prn/q1h
  - SC Lorazepam 0.5-2mg prn/q4h
  - CSCI Lorazepam: risk of precipitation
  - CIVI Lorazepam 4mg/24h
  - Risk of paradoxical reactions: < 1% (Mancuso 2004)
- Miscellaneous agents
  - Trazodone
    - Sedating heterocyclic antidepressant
    - Serotonin antagonist and reuptake inhibitor (SARI)
    - Less anticholinergic effects than TCA
    - PO Trazodone 25-50mg tds or 25-100mg on
    - Maximum dose: 300mg/day
    - Maximum use: 7 days

- Mianserin
  - Tetracyclic antidepressant
  - Noradrenergic and specific serotonergic antidepressant (NaSSA)
  - Use: delirium in elderly
  - Dose: PO Mianserin 10-30mg on
  - Effects
    - Controls behavioural symptoms
    - Improves sleep
    - Reduces hallucinations
    - No change in cognition
- Clomethiazole (Chlormethiazole)
  - GABA-A and glycine agonist
  - Use: restlessness in elderly
  - Dose: PO Clomethiazole 192mg tds or 192-384mg on
  - Maximum use: 7 days
- Psychostimulants
  - PO Methylphenidate 5-10mg at 8am and 12pm
  - PO Modafinil 100-200mg om
  - Use: hypoactive delirium
  - Evidence: case reports
- Cholinesterase inhibitors
  - PO Donepezil 5-10mg on
  - PO Rivastigmine 1.5-6mg bd
  - Rivastigmine patch 4.6, 9.5, 13.3mg q24h
  - Evidence: no evidence from RCT

Terminal Delirium

Introduction

Terminal delirium is delirium that occurs in some patients during their last few days of life.

Communication with patients and family members

- Involve palliative care specialists
- Initiate discussion with family members and patient (if patient has lucid moments)
- Discuss goals of care
- Discuss palliative sedation
    - Level of sedation
        - Conscious sedation: partially responsive
        - Deep sedation: unresponsive
    - Temporal
        - PRN sedation
        - Night sedation
        - Respite sedation
        - Continuous sedation
    - Goals of sedation
        - Palliate symptoms
        - Not hastening of death
- Elicit wishes and concerns
    - Wish to maintain consciousness
    - Wish to reverse sedation
    - Address concern about reversibility of sedation
    - Address concern about hastening of death
- Shared decision making
- Respect dignity and values of patient and family

Management of terminal delirium in palliative care

- Wait-and-see approach
    - Hypoactive or lethargic delirium
    - Pleasant confusion
    - Pleasant hallucinations or delusions
    - Natural part of the dying process
    - Anticipatory prescription for agitation
        - SC Haloperidol 1-2mg prn/q1h
        - SC Midazolam 2.5-5mg prn/q1h
- Pharmacological interventions
    - Hyperactive or agitated delirium
    - Synonyms
        - Terminal restlessness
        - Terminal agitation
        - Terminal anguish
        - Pre-death restlessness
    - Clinical features
        - Restlessness
        - Fidgeting
        - Purposeless movements
            - Pulling tubes and lines
            - Snatching the air
            - Plucking bedsheets
            - Taking off clothes
            - Getting out of the bed
            - Pacing to and fro
            - Going to toilet repetitively
    - First line treatment for terminal restlessness
        - Benzodiazepines
        - Goal: sedation just enough to palliate restlessness
        - Also useful for delirium with seizures
        - Risk of paradoxical agitation, esp elderly

- Midazolam
  - SC Midazolam 2.5-5mg stat, then 1-2.5mg/h
    - Titrate up to 5mg/h if necessary
  - SC Midazolam 2.5-5mg stat, then 30-60mg/24h
    - Titrate up to 120mg/24h if necessary
  - Maximum reported midazolam dose: 50mg/h
- Alternative benzodiazepines
  - SL Lorazepam 1-2mg q4-6h
  - SC Lorazepam 1-2mg q4-6h
  - CSCI Lorazepam: risk of precipitation
  - CIVI Lorazepam 4-20mg/24h
  - SL Clonazepam 1-4mg q12h
  - CSCI Clonazepam 2-8mg/24h
  - PR Diazepam 10-20mg q6-8h
  - IV Diazepam 5-10mg q6-8h
- Rapid titration
  - IV Midazolam 0.5mg q5min till settled
  - SC Midazolam 1mg q15min till settled
  - SL Lorazepam 1-2mg q1h till settled
    - Usual dose: 2-10mg/day
    - Up to 20-50mg/day for extreme agitation
- Second line treatment for terminal restlessness
  - Neuroleptics
  - Add haloperidol if CSCI Midazolam 1.5mg/h fails or
  - Add haloperidol if paradoxical agitation with benzo
  - SC Haloperidol 2.5-5mg stat, then 10-30mg/24h
  - Alternative neuroleptics
    - PR Chlorpromazine 25-50mg q4-6h
      - Max dose 200mg q4h
    - SC Levomepromazine 12.5-25mg stat
      - Then 50-75mg/24h
      - Max dose 300mg/24h

- Rapid titration
  - IV Haloperidol 0.5-2mg q10min till settled
  - SC Haloperidol 0.5-2mg q30min till settled
  - PR Haloperidol 0.5-2mg q60min till settled
    - Then give total dose at night or
    - Divide total dose by 4 for q6h dosing
  - IV/SC Chlorpromazine 12.5-25mg q30min
  - PO/PR Chlorpromazine 12.5-25mg q60min
    - Then give total dose at night or
    - Divide total dose by 4 for q6h dosing
- Third line treatment for terminal restlessness
  - Failed CSCI Midazolam 60-120mg/24h +
    - Failed CSCI Haloperidol 30mg/24h or
    - Failed CSCI Levomepromazine 200mg/24h
  - Phenobarbital (single agent)
    - Onset: 5min (IV)
    - Half-life: 2-6 days
    - Duration: 4 hours to 2 days
    - Concentration: 200mg/ml
    - Do not mix with another drug
    - Local necrosis: SC bolus or IV extravasation
    - IM Phenobarbital 100-200mg undiluted stat or
    - IV Phenobarbital 100-200mg with 10ml WFI in rate of 50mg/min
    - Then CSCI Phenobarbital 600-1600mg/24h
    - Max 2400mg/24h
    - Dilute 1ml phenobarbital with 10ml WFI
      - Phenobarbital 600mg with 30ml WFI
      - Phenobarbital 800mg with 40ml WFI
      - Phenobarbital 1200mg with 60ml WFI
      - Phenobarbital 1600mg with 80ml WFI
      - Phenobarbital 2400mg with 120ml WFI

- Propofol (single agent)
  - Onset: 0.5min
  - Half-life: 3-12h
  - Duration: 3-10min
  - Concentration: 10mg/ml (1%), 20mg/ml (2%)
  - Aim: conscious sedation (open eyes to call)
  - IV Propofol 1mg/kg/h via forearm vein
  - Increase 0.5mg/kg/h q5-10min till sedation
  - Usual dose 1-2mg/kg/h
  - Max dose 4mg/kg/h
  - Bolus: 1mg/kg/min for 2-5min
  - RR and sedation assessment q1h for 24h
  - Then q12h review
  - No response to call or RR<8/min: stop 2-3min, restart at lower dose
  - Replenish infusion immediately once empty
  - No response to 4mg/kg/h: add CSCI Midazolam
  - No analgesic property: continue analgesia
- Dexmedetomidine (Precedex)
  - α2 agonist with analgesic properties
  - Onset: <5min
  - Half-life: 2h
  - Duration: 4h
  - Dilute 400mcg in 100ml normal saline
  - IV Dexmedetomidine 0.2mcg/kg/h
  - Increase 0.1mcg/kg/h q30min till sedation
  - Usual dose 0.2-0.7mcg/kg/h
  - Max dose 1.5mcg/kg/h
  - RR and sedation assessment q1h for first 24h
  - Then q12h review
  - Side effects: hypotension, bradycardia
  - Reduce opioid dose gradually during titration

Prognostication

Introduction

Prognostication is the act of predicting how much time is left for a patient to live.

Benefits of prognostication

- Clinical decision making
- Advance care planning
- Prioritization in life
- Preparation for dying

Components of prognostication (Lamont, Christakis 1999)

- Foreseeing: formulating a prognosis
- Foretelling: communicating prognosis

The optimism of physicians

- Physicians tend to overestimate life expectancy by a factor of 5 on average (Christakis 1996)

Little thoughts

First sign of dying: when we were born

Second sign of dying: when we are told of having a life-limiting illness

Third sign of dying: when we see the palliative care team

Fourth sign of dying: when we see distant relatives coming back to see us

Fifth sign of dying: when we hear people saying prayers around our bed

---

Clinical Prediction of Survival (CPS)

- Overly optimistic: 3-5x actual survival
- Actual survival: 30% shorter than CPS
- Horizon effect: more accurate for shortest survival
- Most effective when added to other prognostic tools

Foreseeing prognosis of months

- GSF Prognostic Indicator Guidance 2011
- Step 1: surprise question
    - Ask ourself the one year surprise question
    - Would you be surprised if patient dies within one year?
    - Not surprised: prognosis < 1 year
    - Sensitivity 69%, specificity 84% (Moroni 2014)
- Step 2: general indicators of poor prognosis
    - Functional decline
    - Comorbidities
    - Increasing symptom burden
    - Decreasing response to treatment
    - Repeated crisis admissions
- Step 3: specific indicators of poor prognosis
    - Cancer
        - Metastatic cancer
        - ECOG 3-4
    - Heart failure
        - NYHA Class III/IV
        - Difficult symptoms despite optimal therapy
        - Multiple admissions for heart failure
    - Chronic obstructive pulmonary disease
        - FEV1 <30%
        - Breathless after 100m or house-bound
        - On LTOT
        - Multiple admission for COPD exacerbation

- Renal failure
  - Stage 4/5 CKD
  - Symptomatic renal failure
  - Difficult symptoms despite optimal therapy
  - Withholding or withdrawal of dialysis
- Neurological diseases
  - Progressive functional and cognitive decline
  - Difficult symptoms despite optimal therapy
  - Speech and swallowing problems
- Geriatric diseases
  - Poor functional and cognitive status
  - Multiple comorbidities
  - Multiple symptoms
  - Recurrent infections
- HIV disease (not in GSF)
  - Age > 65
  - ADL dependent
  - Poor performance status
  - HAART withdrawal

Foreseeing prognosis of weeks to short months

- Eastern Cooperative Oncology Group (ECOG)
  - ECOG 3 (>50% bed-ridden): prognosis < 3 months
  - ECOG 4 (total bed-ridden): prognosis < 1 month
- Karnofsky Performance Scale (KPS)
  - KPS 30-40 (total dependence): prognosis < 2 months
  - KPS 10-20 (very sick): prognosis < 2 weeks
- Palliative Performance Scale (PPS)
  - PPS 50 (total dependence): prognosis < 2 months
  - PPS 30-40 (reduced oral intake): prognosis < 1 month
  - PPS 10-20 (sips or no oral intake): prognosis < 2 weeks

- Palliative Prognostic Score (PaP) (Pirovano 1999)
    - Prognosis < 1 month
    - Score 0-17.5
    - Higher score = higher likelihood for prognosis < 1 month
        - CPS < 1 year
        - KPS 10-20
        - Dyspnoea
        - Anorexia
        - Leucocytosis
        - Lymphocytopenia
- Palliative Prognostic Index (PPI) (Morita 1999)
    - Prognosis < 3-6 weeks
    - Score 0-15
    - PPI >4 = prognosis < 6 weeks
    - PPI ≥6 = prognosis < 3 weeks

Palliative Prognostic Index	
Prognostic factors	Score
Performance status	
■ PPS 10-20	4
■ PPS 30-50	2.5
■ PPS > 50	0
Oral intake	
■ Mouthfuls or less	2.5
■ Moderately reduced	1
■ Normal	0
Edema	1
Dyspnoea at rest	3.5
Delirium	4

- 3-Variable Model for Advanced Cancer (Chow 2002)
    - 1 risk factor = prognosis < 14 months
    - 2 risk factors = prognosis < 5 months
    - 3 risk factors = prognosis < 3 months

- Risk factors
  - Non-breast cancer
  - Non-bone metastases
  - KPS ≤ 60

Foreseeing prognosis of days

10 Clinical signs of impending death within 7 days (Hui 2014)	Prognosis (days)	Frequency* (%)
Liquid dysphagia	7	90
Reduced consciousness	7	90
PPS ≤ 20	4	93
Peripheral cyanosis	3	59
Cheyne-Stokes breathing	2	41
Urine output<100ml in 12h	1.5	72
Apnoea periods	1.5	46
Respiration with mandibular movement	1.5	56
Death rattle	1.5	66
Pulselessness of radial artery	1	38

7 Clinical signs of impending death within 3 days (Hui 2015)	Prognosis (days)	Frequency* (%)
Decreased response to visual stimuli	3	70
Hyperextension of neck	2.5	46
Drooping of nasolabial fold	2.5	78
Non-reactive pupil	2	38
Decreased response to verbal stimuli	2	69
Grunting of vocal cords	1.5	54
Inability to close eye lids	1.5	57

*Frequency of sign in last 3 days of life

Foretelling prognosis

- Please refer to the chapter of communicating prognosis

Dying trajectories

Introduction

While prognostication deals with the "when" of dying, dying trajectory deals with the "how" of dying.

Dying trajectories (Lynn 2003)

Sudden death trajectory

Function

- Little or no time to help the patient
- Intense bereavement support for the family

Cancer trajectory

Function

- Rapid functional decline during last few months of life
- Anticipatory grief support for the patient and family

Organ failure trajectory

Function

Time

- Sine-waving
- Not sure which dip is final
- Advance care planning

Frailty trajectory

Function

Time

- Lingering death
- Advance care planning while patient is compos mentis
- Caregiver support – prolonged caregiving

Symptom Management in the Last Days of Life

Introduction

The most important step in the management of patients in their last days of life is to recognize dying. If dying is unrecognized, patients will continue to receive useless treatment.

Diagnosing dying

- The process of dying can be seen as a process of deterioration of the different organ systems of a person   •
- The sequence of deterioration depends on the dynamic process of ongoing multiple organ failure
- Pre-active phase of dying (days to short weeks before death)
  - Musculoskelatal system
    - Rapidly increasing weakness and fatigue
    - Difficulty getting out of bed or sitting up
    - Bed-ridden
    - Total dependent in activities of daily living
  - Gastroiñtenstinal system
    - Rapid decline in oral intake
    - Reduced or absence of hunger or thirst
    - Fecal incontinence
  - Cardiovascular system
    - Tachycardia
    - Low blood pressure
  - Renal system
    - Peripheral oedema
    - Urinary incontinence

- Neurological system
  - Limited attention span
  - Delirium
  - Restlessness
  - Sleepy most of the time
  - Loss of interest in surroundings
- Respiratory system
  - Reduced communication
  - Grunting or moaning
- Active phase of dying (hours to short days before death)
  - Gastrointenstinal system
    - Inability to swallow tablets
    - Inability to swallow fluid
  - Cardiovascular system
    - Peripheral mottling or cyanosis
    - Pulselessness of radial artery
    - Cold extremities
  - Renal system
    - Reduced urine output
    - Anuria with urine output <100ml in 12h
  - Neurological system
    - Reduced consciousness
    - Reduced or absent response to call
    - Inability to close eyelids
    - Reduced or no blinking
  - Respiratory system
    - Inability to speak
    - Death rattle
    - Abnormal respiratory patterns
      - Cheyne-Stokes breathing
      - Apnoea periods
      - Respiration with mandibular movement

Communicating the diagnosis of dying

- Assess patient's ability to communicate
- Assess insight into situation
- Involve family members
- Provide relevant information sensitively
- Explain the significance of signs and symptoms of dying
- Allow time for digestion of the information
- Provide support for emotional and cognitive reactions
- Respect all psychological reactions, including non-acceptance
- Explore what is important to patient and family at this time
- Discuss goals of care
- Discuss management plan
- Explore preference of place of dying if appropriate
- Allow time and space for patient and family to grieve
- Encourage family and friends to talk to patient
- Tell them patient may still be hearing even though unconscious
- Encourage expressions of intimacy
- Tell them patient may still be feeling
- Encourage family to stay with patient if possible
- Discuss the process of dying if appropriate
- Discuss what to do after death if appropriate
- Address spiritual needs

Little story

I was stopped by my boss as I attempted to rush through a crowd of family members to see a dying patient. My boss asked me to wait. After a while the family moved aside spontaneously. It was a beautiful experience. Remember. The most important person at the deathbed is the patient, not us. Second is the family.

Stopping unnecessary investigations and treatments

- Do no harm
- Stop monitoring of vital signs
- Stop all unnecessary blood-taking
- Stop all unnecessary investigations
- Stop all unnecessary medications
- Stop all unnecessary medical and nursing interventions
- Review the need of artificial hydration and nutrition
- Deactivate implantable cardiac defibrillator if present
- Document Do Not Resuscitate (DNR) order

Symptom management of a dying patient

- Continue essential symptom medications
    - Analgesics
    - Antiemetics
    - Anxiolytics
- Continue some symptom medications as PRN if appropriate
    - Anticonvulsants
    - Antibiotics
    - Insulin
- Convert to an appropriate route
    - Subcutaneous
    - Intravenous
    - Sublingual
    - Suppository

Anticipatory prescriptions for symptoms

- SC Morphine 2.5mg prn/q1h for pain or breathlessness
- SC Hyoscine butylbromide 20mg prn/q1h for secretions
- SC Haloperidol 1.5mg prn/q1h for nausea and vomiting
- SC Midazolam 2.5mg prn/q1h for sleeplessness or agitation

Pain and breathlessness

- Misconception: pain will increase at the end of life
- Reality: pain may increase, stabilize or decrease (Sykes 2003)
- Conscious patient: assess symptoms by asking patient
- Unconscious patient: assess pain by using FLACC scale

<u>FLACC scale</u>

Criteria	0	1	2
Face	Normal	Grimace	Clenched jaw
Legs	Normal	Restless	Kicking
Activity	Normal	Squirming	Arched
Cry	Normal	Moaning	Screaming
Consolability	Normal	Reassurable	Nonreassurable

- Unconscious patient: assess breathlessness by looking for signs of respiratory distress, such as RR ≥ 25 breaths/min, laboured breathing
- Pain or breathlessness in opioid-naïve patient
    - CSCI Morphine 0.5mg/h
    - SC Morphine 2.5mg prn/q1h for breakthrough symptoms
- Pain or breathlessness in opioid-naïve renal failure patient
    - CSCI Fentanyl 10mcg/h
    - SC Fentanyl 25mcg prn/q1h for breakthrough symptoms
- Pain or breathlessness in opioid-tolerant patient
    - Consult palliative care team for opioid conversion
- Alternative drugs
    - SL Morphine: moribund patients at home
    - SL Buprenorphine: moribund patients at home
    - SL Methadone: moribund patients at home
    - SL Dextromoramide 5-20mg prn/q3h: procedural pain
    - Fentanyl patch: stable pain
    - Buprenorphine patch: stable pain

Respiratory tract secretions

- Death rattle: gurgling noise from secretions during last days
- Median prognosis: 1.5 days
- Patients are usually unconscious
- Type I death rattle (true death rattle)
    - Secretions from salivary glands
    - Failure of swallowing reflex
    - During final hours
    - Responsive to anticholinergics
- Type II death rattle (pseudo death rattle)
    - Secretions from bronchial glands
    - Failure of cough reflex
    - Less responsive to anticholinergics
- Victoria Respiratory Congestion Scale (VRCS)
    - 0 = inaudible
    - 1 = audible only very close to patient
    - 2 = clearly audible from end of bed in quiet room
    - 3 = audible at 9.5m or at door of room
- VRCS 0-1: reassurance
- VRCS 2-3: positioning + antisecretory agents
- Antisecretory agents
    - SC Glycopyrrolate 0.2-0.4mg q4h or
        - CSCI Glycopyrrolate 0.6-1.2mg/24h
    - SC Hyoscine hydrobromide 0.4-0.6mg q4h or
        - CSCI Hyoscine hydrobromide 1.2-2.4mg/24h
    - SC Hyoscine butylbromide 20mg q4h or
        - CSCI Hyoscine butylbromide 60-120mg/24h
- Alternative drugs
    - SL Atropine eyedrops 1% 3-4 drops tds-qid
    - Scopolamine patch 1.5-4.5mg q72h to mastoid
        - Onset: 8h after application
        - Effect: continues 12h after removal

Nausea and vomiting (N&V)

- Determining the precise cause of N&V can be difficult
- Treat N&V empirically
- Antiemetics
    - SC Haloperidol 1.5-5mg bd or
        - CSCI Haloperidol 1.5-20mg/24h
    - SC Metoclopramide 10-20mg tds or
        - CSCI Metoclopramide 30-120mg/24h
    - IV Promethazine 25-50mg tds or
        - CSCI Promethazine 50-150mg/24h
    - SC Levomepromazine 6.25-25mg on-bd or
        - CSCI Levomepromazine 6.25-50mg/24h
- Do not combine metoclopramide and antisecretory agents
- Alternative drugs
    - SL Olanzapine 2.5-10mg on
    - PR Chlorpromazine 50-100mg tds
    - ABHR suppositories tds
        - Lorazepam (Ativan) 0.5mg
        - Diphenhydramine (Benadryl) 12.5mg
        - Haloperidol (Haldol) 0.5mg
        - Metoclopramide (Reglan) 10mg

Sleeplessness

- Most patients will sleep more during their final days
- Some may experience reversal of sleep pattern
- Treatment of insomnia in last days of life
    - SC Midazolam 2.5-5mg on or
        - CSCI Midazolam 1-2.5mg/h during nighttime
- Alternative drugs
    - SL Lorazepam 1-2mg on
    - PR Diazepam 10-20mg on

Agitation or restlessness

- Common
- Sometimes can be reversed by simple measures
  - Breakthrough medications for symptoms
  - Re-positioning for positional discomfort
  - Urinary catheter insertion for retention of urine
  - Fecal disimpaction for retention of feces
- Treatment of agitation or restlessness
  - CSCI Midazolam 1-2.5mg/h
    - SC Midazolam 2.5mg prn/q1h for agitation
  - CSCI Haloperidol 10-30mg/24h
    - SC Haloperidol 2.5-5mg prn/q1h for agitation
  - CSCI Levomepromazine 50-75mg/24h
    - SC Levomepromazine 12.5-25mg prn/tds
- Alternative drugs
  - SL Lorazepam 1-2mg tds
  - PR Diazepam 10-20mg tds
  - PR Chlorpromazine 50-100mg tds

Nursing care for a dying patient

- Oral care
  - Keep the mouth moist
    - Frequent sips of water, ice chips, pineapple chunks
    - Artificial saliva
    - Moisturizing gel with aloe vera
    - Cooking oil for lips
  - Keep the mouth clean
    - Soft toothbrush and bland toothpaste if able to rinse
    - Soft-cotton or sponge-tipped swabs moistened with a solution of water and baking powder
    - Gentle swabbing q30-60min prn for comfort
  - Encourage family participation in oral care

- Skin care
  - Ripple mattress
  - Gentle turning with a draw sheet
  - Reduce turning to bd-tds
  - Incident pain: SC Morphine 30min before turning
  - Re-position prn for comfort
  - Smoothen bed surface and draw sheet
  - Moisturize the skin
- Eye care
  - Artificial tears for dry eyes
  - Gentle swabbing with moistened cotton
- Feeding
  - Explain reduced to no eating and drinking at final days
  - Explain reduced to no sensation of hunger and thirst
  - Discuss natural dehydration in the dying process
  - Benefit of endorphin release in natural dehydration
  - Discuss futility of artificial hydration and nutrition
  - Risks of secretions, ascites and oedema
  - Respect individual and sociocultural beliefs
  - Allow orally as tolerated
  - Consider sips or droplets of oral feeding prn
- Bladder and bowel care
  - Urinary catheter if appropriate
  - Incontinence pad if appropriate
  - Change pad immediately after soiling
  - Switch oral laxatives to glycerin enema prn

Psychosocial and spiritual care

- Ensure supportive physical environment
- Ensure well-being of family or caregiver
- Address psychosocial and spiritual needs of patient and family
- Regular review irrespective of patient's situation

Care after death in the hospital

- Confirm death
- Notify family member gently
- Allow time for family to come to see patient
- Allow time for family to grieve
- Respect spiritual or religious rites and rituals
- Perform last office according to policy when family is ready
- Explain to family what to do next
- Notify primary team or community hospice if appropriate

Hydration and Nutrition at the End-of-life

Introduction

One of the most difficult issues to deal with at the end of life is hydration and nutrition. Patients will consume less and less up to a stage when they consume near-nothing or nothing. Witnessing this diminishing of oral intake can be a hard time for the family.

Goals of hydration and nutrition

- Sustain life by provision of calories, nutrients and water
- Sustain function
- Alleviate suffering by reducing thirst and hunger
- Enhance pleasures in life
- Enhance social activities: nurturing and being nurtured

Types of feeding

- Natural feeding (basic care)
  - Unassisted
  - Assisted
    - Spoon-feeding
    - Syringe-feeding
- Artificial feeding (medical treatment)
  - Artificial hydration
    - Subcutaneous hydration
    - Intravenous hydration
  - Artificial nutrition
    - Tube feeding
    - Parenteral nutrition

Tube feeding

- Prevention of aspiration pneumonia
    - Benefit
        - Non-bedridden stroke
    - No benefit
        - Bedridden stroke
        - Other neurological disorders
        - Advanced dementia
        - Aspiration risk demonstrated with videofluoroscopy
        - Cancer
- Prevention of pressure sores
    - No benefit
        - Advanced dementia
        - Nursing home residents
- Prolongation of life
    - Benefit
        - Non-bedridden head & neck cancer with dysphagia
        - Non-bedridden malignant proximal GI obstruction
        - Proximal GI cancer receiving chemo or radiotherapy
        - Reversible illness in catabolic state: eg acute sepsis
        - Motor neuron disease
        - Nursing home residents < 40 years
        - AIDS with wasting syndrome
    - No benefit
        - Advanced cancer except above conditions
        - Advanced dementia
- Quality of life
    - Benefit
        - True hunger and thirst: eg proximal GI cancer
    - No benefit
        - Active dying
        - Dry mouth

Hunger in terminal illnesses (McCann 1994)

- 64% did not experience hunger
- 34% experienced hunger only initially
- 3% experienced hunger throughout their stay
- When hunger was reported, it was ameliorated by providing small amounts of food

Tube feeding and harm

- Denied pleasure of eating if kept nil by mouth (NBM)
- Distress of NG tube insertion
- Nasopharyngeal discomfort
- Nausea and vomiting
- Delirium
- Restraint
- Aspiration
- Complications of PEG/PEJ

Weissman's triad of a dying patient in the hospital

- Triad: feeding tube, restraints and pulse oximetry
- Death spiral
    - Hospital admission
    - Poor oral intake
    - Swallowing evaluation
    - Feeding tube placement
    - Increased agitation
    - Self-removal of feeding tube
    - Restraint
    - Re-insertion of feeding tube
    - Aspiration pneumonia
    - Intravenous antibiotics and pulse oximetry
    - Few cycles of release-remove-restraint-reinsert
    - Death

Recognition of dying

- Poor or no oral intake in the setting of a chronic life-limiting illness and declining function: marker of the dying process

Golden rule of eating at the end of life

- Let the patient be the lead
    - When to eat
    - What to eat
    - What amount to eat

Artificial hydration

- Benefit
    - Delirium
    - Opioid toxicity, esp in renal failure
- No benefit
    - Thirst
- Harm
    - ↑ respiratory tract secretions
    - ↑ ascites
    - ↑ oedema
    - Inhibits mobility further
    - Impedes family involvement
    - Medicalization of death

Treatment of thirst or dry mouth at the end of life

- Regular mouth care
- Small amounts of fluids
- Ice chips
- Small pineapple chunks
- Artificial saliva
- Moisturizing mouth gel

Natural dehydration

- Benefit
    - ↓ cerebral oedema: more lucid
    - ↓ respiratory secretions: less cough, choking, rattles
    - ↓ GI secretions: less vomiting
    - ↓ peritumoural oedema: less pain
    - ↑ endorphins: less pain

Summary of hydration and nutrition at the end of life

- Conventional nutritional care
    - Earlier stages of illness
    - Allows patient to cope with illness and treatment
- Palliative nutritional care
    - Later stages of illness
    - Focuses on symptom control and quality of life
    - Supplementation as appropriate
    - Relaxes dietary restriction
    - Emotional support
    - Family support

Communication

- Family: He is not eating. He is getting weaker.
- Staff: You are right. It is common for patients to eat less and less as the disease progresses. Someday they eat a little; someday they eat a bit more. But overall their interest in food will gradually decline. They may even reach a stage of eating nothing. It can be difficult for family to see them eating so little.
- Family: He is going to starve to death.
- Staff: We need to continue offering him small amounts of food as he wishes. Most of the time the sensation of hunger will gradually disappear when the disease progresses.

- Family: What can we do to help him?
- Staff: At this stage, it is common for family to encourage them to eat more. Some even force them to eat, resulting in a so-called "food battle". Patient may then suffer more or vomit. The best thing you can do for him is to let him be the lead. Let him choose when to eat, what to eat and what amount to eat. You can offer him his favourite food but do not pressurize him too much.

Withholding and Withdrawal of Life-Sustaining Treatment

Introduction

Withholding and withdrawal of life-sustaining treatment are medical procedures. All healthcare staff should be equipped with the knowledge and skills in the practice of withholding and withdrawal of medical treatment.

Clinical situations (mostly in ICUs)

- Refusal of treatment
  - Patient has a right to refuse treatment provided:
    - Patient has intact decision-making capacity
    - Patient is fully informed of the risks and benefits of the treatment, and the consequences of refusing it
- Medical futility
  - Medical futility refers to medical treatment which is extremely unlikely to benefit patients
    - Quantitative futility: the likelihood of a medical treatment to benefit patient is extremely unlikely
    - Qualitative futility: the quality of the benefit produced by a medical treatment is extremely poor

Decisional capacity assessment (Appelbaum & Grisso 1988)

- The ability to EXPRESS a choice
- The ability to UNDERSTAND the relevant information
- The ability to APPRECIATE a situation and its consequences
- The ability to REASON rationally

Diagnosing medical futility

- Quantitative definition
  - Physicians conclude that in the last 100 cases a medical treatment has been useless (Schneiderman 1990, 1996)
    - Through personal experiences
    - Through experiences shared with colleagues
    - Through consideration of reported empirical data
  - Objective outcome predictions in ICU
    - Multiple Organ Dysfunction Score
    - MOD >20 = 100% mortality
      - PaO2/FiO2 ratio
        - <300 (1 point)
        - <225 (2 points)
        - <150 (3 points)
        - <75 (4 points)
      - Platelet count
        - <120 (1 point)
        - <80 (2 points)
        - <50 (3 points)
        - <20 (4 points)
      - Serum bilirubin
        - >20 (1 point)
        - >60 (2 points)
        - >120 (3 points)
        - >240 (4 points)
      - Pressure adjusted heart rate (HR x CVP/MAP)
        - >10 (1 point)
        - >15 (2 points)
        - >20 (3 points)
        - >30 (4 points)

- Glasgow Coma Scale
    - <15 (1 point)
    - <13 (2 points)
    - <10 (3 points)
    - <7 (4 points)
- Serum creatinine
    - >100 (1 point)
    - >200 (2 points)
    - >350 (3 points)
    - >500 (4 points)
- Qualitative definition (Schneiderman 2011)
    - The unacceptable likelihood of achieving an effect that the patient has the capacity to appreciate as a benefit
    - None of the effects is a benefit unless the patient has at the very least the capacity to appreciate it, a circumstance that is impossible if the patient is permanently unconscious

Principles of withholding and withdrawal of treatment

- The intention is to remove useless treatment
- The intention is not to hasten death
- Even though hastening of death can be foreseen
- The intention to hasten death is ethically impermissible
- The intention to hasten death is legally impermissible
- Withholding and withdrawal of treatment are ethically similar
- If withholding of treatment is justified, withdrawal is justified
- Withdrawal of treatment is a medical procedure
- Any medical treatment can be withdrawn
- Basic care cannot be withdrawn

The decision-making hierarchy

- Fully informed patient with intact decisional capacity
- Legally appointed surrogate decision maker
- Advance decision to refuse treatment (ADRT)
- Substituted judgment from close family members
    - Patient's previous statement of wishes and preferences
    - Patient's possible wishes and preferences based on values and beliefs if patient is presumed to understand current condition and prognosis
- Best interest of patient
    - Represented by close family members with careful weighing of the risk-benefit explained by the physician
    - Represented by physician if family is unable to represent patient's best interest

The decision-making process

- The first step is to arrive at the decision. If no clear consensus within the health care team, time should be taken to resolve disagreement. Ethical principles and outcome data should be applied rather than personal values and biases.
- If the decision has been made to withdraw treatment by the patient or the senior clinician responsible for the care of the patient, doctors or nurses who have a conscientious objection to the decision may withdraw from the care of patient, with the arrangement of a replacement to take over his or her role.
- Informed consent is needed before withdrawal of treatment. Physician is not obliged to provide futile intervention requested by family but effort should be made to reach an agreement.
- Useful ways include open and sensitive communication, exploration and sensitive handling of misunderstanding, and responding to emotions.

- If family insists on intervention after open communication, then the primary physician should make a decision whether to withdraw treatment, withhold further treatment or to allow a time-limited trial.

Communication with colleagues

- Before discussing with the patient or family, it is crucial for different teams to meet and discuss about patient's prognosis and plan. If there is any difference in opinion, a general consensus needs to be achieved.
- Sometimes it is not uncommon for a clinician to remain hopeful even in the most drastic situation. Giving time for the clinician to accept the situation may be the best solution if condition allows.
- On the other hand, clinician may give up hope early even though there may be a reasonable chance of recovery. Then we should communicate our opinion in a non-confrontational manner.

Communication with patient

- Most patients for withdrawal of treatment are semi-comatose or comatose. If patient is mentally sound, every effort needs to be made to discuss the situation with the patient. Sometimes this will require a long time, especially if the patient has difficulty in communication.

Communication with family members

- Find out the decision maker in the family. If decision making is shared within the family, then try to involve those who can represent the patient.

- Discussion of withdrawal of treatment needs a gentle explanation of patient's condition and prognosis. Discuss prognosis in a way that is meaningful to the family.
- Then, ask the family to focus on what the patient would want, not what the family wants.
- Explain the reasons of withdrawal of treatment. The treatment cannot reverse the disease process. Stopping it allows the disease to take it natural course. Comfort care and nursing care will be continued.
- Respond to family's emotion and thoughts. If family is in denial, allow time for them to sink in if possible.
- If family is ready, explain the steps of withdrawal and what will likely happen after the withdrawal. Explain agonal breathing and respiratory tract secretions and steps in palliation.
- Stress to family that withdrawal of treatment is a medical decision, not a family decision. This is to reduce any feeling of guilt for making this difficult decision.
- Mention organ donation if appropriate.

Little information

Although hastening of death can be foreseen in withdrawal of life-sustaining treatment. The intention to hasten death is wrong. Caution needs to be taken to avoid misunderstanding.

- Allow time for reaching a consensus
- Allow time-limited trial for the lack of consensus
- Consider compassionate continuation of futile treatment for family's non-acceptance if appropriate
- Administer drugs just enough to make patient comfortable
- Continue palliative care if patient survives the withdrawal

Checklist for ventilation withdrawal

- The multidisciplinary team has agreed to withdraw ventilation, and one or more of the following may apply
  - Continuing ventilation has a very small chance of benefiting patient
    - Patient is dying
    - Patient has progressive irreversible multi-organ failure despite intensive treatment
    - Patient is diagnosed to have brainstem death or impending brainstem death
  - Continuing ventilation produces an exceedingly poor quality of benefit
    - Patient is in a coma, persistent vegetative state or minimally conscious state
    - Patient has advanced metastatic cancer with poor prognosis
  - Advance decision of refusal of ventilation or presumed refusal of ventilation
    - Patient has legal document in ADRT
    - Patient has appointed a legal surrogate decision maker for refusal of consent
    - Presumed refusal of ventilation based on substituted judgment from the family, complemented by adequate value history of patient
- Consensus on withdrawal of ventilation has been achieved from ALL of the following
  - The multidisciplinary team
  - Patient (if intact decisional capacity)
  - Family members

- Information on ventilation withdrawal has been communicated
  - Family is aware that decision of ventilation withdrawal is a medical decision
  - Family is aware that ventilation cannot reverse the underlying disease process
  - Family is aware that ventilation withdrawal allows the natural course of the disease to take place
  - Family is aware that ventilation withdrawal is not euthanasia, but the removal of useless treatment
  - Family is aware that palliative care will be continued to ensure patient's comfort
  - Family is aware of the procedures after death
- Discussion of organ or body donation if appropriate
- Family preferences have been elicited in terms of the following
  - Family presence during ventilation withdrawal
  - Time of ventilation withdrawal
  - Place of ventilation withdrawal: hospital or home
  - Religious practices and rituals before, during and after
- Documentation of decision making process and communication has been done
  - Indication of ventilation withdrawal
  - Consensus on ventilation withdrawal
  - Communication on ventilation withdrawal
  - Family preferences
  - Do not resuscitate (DNR) order
- Facilitation of practices that support family grief
  - Ensure privacy if possible
  - Liberalize visitation
  - Ensure access to patient by lowering the side rails
  - Allow family to perform last rites or rituals
  - Allow family to grief
  - Encourage family to speak to patient

- Procedures of ventilation withdrawal
  - Discontinue unnecessary monitoring and treatment, such as cardiac monitoring, inotropes, feeding tubes
  - Initiate or maintain opioid and sedative infusion
    - Ensure patency of intravenous line by flushing
    - Initiate opioid infusion: IV Morphine 2.5-5mg/h
    - Initiate sedative infusion: IV Midazolam 2.5-5mg/h
  - Ensure adequate analgesia and sedation
    - Assess pain with FLACC scale
    - Aim pain score 0 with IV Morphine 2.5-5mg prn
    - Assess sedation with Riker Sedation-Agitation Scale
    - Aim sedation scale 1 with IV Midazolam 2.5-5mg prn
      - Riker Sedation-Agitation Scale
        - 7 = dangerous agitation
        - 6 = very agitated
        - 5 = agitated
        - 4 = calm and cooperative
        - 3 = sedated
        - 2 = very sedated
        - 1 = unarousable
    - Ensure adequate time for patient to has sufficient motor activity for pain and sedation assessment after stopping any paralytic drug
  - Sequential reduction of ventilation settings
    - Titrate FiO2 down to 21% and PEEP to 0 in 5min
    - Titrate PS down to 5 in 5-10min
    - Titrate IMV rate down to 5 in 5-10min
    - Give IV Morphine 5mg and IV Midazolam 5mg for any slightest sign of distress
    - Explain to family about potential secretions sounds
    - Extubate patient
    - Give IV Morphine 5mg and IV Midazolam 5mg prn

- Care after withdrawal of ventilation
    - IV Morphine 5mg prn/q15min for distress
    - IV Midazolam 5mg prn/q15min for distress
    - Reassure family if patient is comfortable
    - Allow family to stay with patient
- Document the steps of withdrawal in the medical notes

Do Not Resuscitate (DNR)

Introduction

Cardiopulmonary resuscitation (CPR) is a life-saving technique useful in many emergencies. But when death is inevitable, CPR negates the possibility of a peaceful death.

Do not resuscitate (DNR)

- Also called "no code"
- A legal order written either in the hospital or on a legal form to respect the wishes of a patient not to undergo CPR or ACLS if their heart were to stop or they were to stop breathing

History of CPR and DNR

- 1960: first introduction of CPR (Kouwenhoven 1960)
- 1970s: implementation of DNR policies in US (Fosbinder 1980)
- 1993: proposal of formal DNR guidelines (Doyal 1993)
- 1989: introduction of DNAR (Hadorn 1989)
- 2005: introduction of AND (Knox 2005)

Differences between DNR, DNAR and AND

- DNR
    - Do not resuscitate
    - Gives misimpression that the attempt is likely to succeed
    - Patients think they are deciding whether to live or die, even though they are in an end-of-life situation
- DNAR
    - Do not attempt resuscitation
    - Indicates a resuscitation attempt
    - Does not indicate that it is likely to succeed

- AND
  - Allow natural death
  - Affirms that patients want nature to take its course
  - Without CPR or ACLS

Variety of terms

- Do not attempt CPR (DNACPR): specific
- Do not intubate (DNI): specific
- Not for active resuscitation (NAR): non-specific
- Best supportive care (BSC): non-specific
- Maximal medical management (MMM): non-specific

CPR statistics

- Outcomes
  - Reversal of spontaneous circulation (ROSC)
  - Survival to discharge: more meaningful
- CPR success rate on television (Diem 1996)
  - Chicago Hope: 36% survival to discharge
  - ER: not applicable (events in emergency room only)
  - Rescue 911: 100% survival to discharge
  - CPR success rate on TV shows was over-optimistic
- National Registry of CPR (Peberdy 2003)
  - 14, 720 resuscitation attempts from 2000-2002
  - ROSC: 44%
  - Survival to discharge: 17%
- Meta-analysis of CPR outcomes (Ebell 1998)
  - 49 publications
  - 9,838 patients
  - ROSC: 41-44%
  - Survival to discharge: 13-15%

- CPR success rate in cancer patients (Reisfield 2006)
    - Meta-analysis of 42 studies
    - Localized cancer: 9.1% survival to discharge
    - Metastatic cancer: 7.8% survival to discharge
- CPR success rate in dialysis patients (Hijazi 2003)
    - 14% survival to discharge
    - 3% survival to 6 months
- CPR success rate in elderly (Kim 2000)
    - < 80 years: 19% survival to discharge
    - 81-90 years: 9% survival to discharge
    - > 90 years: 4% survival to discharge
- In-hospital CPR success rate of different countries
    - UK: 17% survival to discharge
    - Canada: 16% survival to discharge
    - US: 15% survival to discharge
    - Other European countries: 14% survival to discharge
    - Iran: 12%
    - Malaysia: 10% survival to discharge
- Factors which predict a failure to survive to discharge
    - Sepsis the day prior to the CPR event
    - Serum creatinine >130μmol/l
    - Metastatic cancer
    - Dementia
    - Dependent status
- CPR success rate with 0% success rate (O'Keefe 1991)
    - Metastatic cancer ECOG3-4
    - Pneumonia
    - Creatinine >150μmol/l
    - Shock
    - PaO2 <6kPa

DNR facts

- DNR = withholding CPR (+ ACLS + intubation)
- DNR ≠ withholding treatment of reversible causes
- DNR ≠ withholding of artificial hydration and nutrition
- DNR preferences ≠ other end-of-life preferences
- DNR ≠ agreeing to giving up hope
- DNR ≠ agreeing to abandonment
- DNR ≠ agreeing to termination of life

The problems in DNR discussion

- Too little and too late
  - 76% occurred when incapacitated (Bedell 1986)
  - 2-3 days before death (Baker 2003)
- Lack of information for informed consent (Tulsky 1995)
  - 4% residents discussed survival rate
  - Discussion length: 10min
  - Doctors: 8min talking
  - Patients: 2min talking
- Incorrect knowledge (Adams 2006)
  - Assumption of CPR survival rate >50% in 80%
- Depersonalized discussion (Deep 2008)
  - Should we try to restart your heart?
  - Should we shock you, press on your chest?
  - Should we not do anything?
  - Did not discuss values and goals
- Extrapolation of DNR to limit other treatments
  - Withholding blood products in 43%
  - Withholding antibiotics in 32%
  - Withholding diagnostic tests
  - Withholding other life-sustaining treatments

The reasons for the problems in DNR discussion (Yuen 2011)

- Technological-driven medical culture
- Inadequate hospital DNR policies
- Insufficient communication skills training
- Profit-driven

CPR Preferences (Murphy 1994)

- >60 years old and healthy
    - Before learning success rate: 41% wanted CPR
    - After learning success rate: 22% wanted CPR
- >60 years old with chronic illness with life expectancy < 1 year
    - Before learning success rate: 11% wanted CPR
    - After learning success rate: 5% wanted CPR

Decision-making

- Futile CPR
    - Doctors are not obliged to offer futile treatment
    - Sensitive communication is needed
- Not futile
    - Intact decisional capacity: patient can refuse
    - Impaired decisional capacity
        - Legally appointed surrogate decision maker
        - Advance decision to refuse treatment (ADRT)
        - Substituted judgment from the family
        - Best interest

DNR discussion

- DNR discussion is not necessary if
    - CPR is futile
    - Patient does not want to discuss
    - Patient may be excessively distressed by the discussion
    - Patient lacks capacity

- How to discuss DNR
  - Explore insight into illness and prognosis
  - Discuss values
    - Tell me a little about what is important to you now
    - What is your current view about your quality of life?
  - Discuss goals of care
    - What are your preferences in terms of treatment?
    - Explore priority
      - Survival
      - Function
      - Comfort
  - Discuss DNR
    - Futile CPR
      - Discuss end-of-life preferences sensitively
      - Explain futility of CPR if appropriate
      - Respond to emotions
    - Not futile
      - Discuss advance care planning
      - Explore CPR preferences if appropriate
      - Discuss CPR success rate
        - In-hospital: 15% (1 in 6)
        - Out-of-hospital: 5% (1 in 20)
        - Terminal illness: 0%

Palliative Sedation

Introduction

Palliative sedation is a final resort in the relief of refractory suffering. It is an important and necessary medical intervention in selected terminally ill patients with refractory suffering.

Definitions of palliative sedation

- Intentional administration of sedative drugs in dosages and combinations required to reduce the consciousness of a terminal patient as much as necessary to adequately relieve one or more refractory symptoms. (Broeckaert 2002)
- The use of sedative medications to relieve intolerable and refractory distress by the reduction in patient consciousness. (Morita 2002)
- The monitored use of medications intended to induce varying degree of unconsciousness, but not death, for relief of refractory and unendurable symptoms in imminently dying patients. (Hospice and Palliative Nurses Association 2003)
- The use of sedating medications to decrease a patient's level of consciousness to mitigate the experience of suffering, but not to hasten the end of life. (The American Academy of Hospice and Palliative Medicine 2003)
- The primary intention of deliberately inducing a temporary or permanent light-to-deep sleep, but not deliberately causing death, in patients with terminal illness and specific refractory symptoms. (Paul Rousseau 2004)
- The use of specific sedative medications to relieve intolerable suffering from refractory symptoms by a reduction in patient consciousness, using appropriate drugs carefully titrated to the cessation of symptoms. (De Graeff 2007)

- The monitored use of medications intended to induce a state of decreased or absent awareness (unconsciousness) in order to relieve the burden of otherwise intractable suffering in a manner that is ethically acceptable to the patient, family and health-care providers. (European Association of Palliative Care 2009)

Important points from the definitions

- Patient is imminently dying
- Patient has refractory symptoms or suffering not relieved by standard palliative care treatment
- The use of sedative medications is monitored
- The intention is to relieve refractory suffering by reducing consciousness, but not to cause death
- The level of sedation varies from light to deep
- The duration of sedation can be temporary or permanent
- The intervention should be done in an ethically acceptable manner, to patient, family and healthcare providers

Determining intractable or refractory suffering

- All possible treatments have failed, or it has been determined by team consensus, based on repeated and careful assessment by skilled experts, that there is no method for alleviation within the time frame and risk-benefit ratio that the patient can tolerate. (Cherny 1994, Morita 2002, Levy 2005)
- To determine the refractoriness of physical suffering, palliative care consultation is strongly recommended
- To determine the refractoriness of psychoexistential suffering, palliative care consultation is a MUST
- Determined on basis of patient evaluation if possible
- Determined by proxy judgments in collaboration with families and staff if patient evaluation is impossible

Adverse effects of palliative sedation

- Patients
    - Impairment or loss of ability to interact
    - Paradoxical agitation
    - Small risk of hastening of death
        - Respiratory depression
        - Aspiration
        - Hemodynamic compromise
    - Although there are data indicating that palliative sedation does not hasten the death of patients overall, a small risk of hastened death for individual patient exists
    - Prognosis hours to days
        - The risk may be judged to be trivial relative to the goal of relieving otherwise intolerable suffering
    - Longer prognosis
        - The risk of hastened death may have significant, or even catastrophic, consequences
        - Risk-reducing precautions may be indicated
            - Vital sign monitoring and antidotes availability
- Distress among family members or healthcare staff
    - Inability to interact with patient
    - Disagreement regarding the indication for sedation
    - Perception that decision to sedate is precipitous
    - Perception that decision to sedate is delayed
    - Perception that sedation hastens death

Problems of palliative sedation (EAPC 2009)

- Abuse of palliative sedation (illegal practices)
    - The deliberate use of deep sedation in patients without refractory symptoms
    - The deliberate use of high doses of sedation that far exceeds that which is necessary to provide comfort

- Injudicious use of palliative sedation
  - Reversible causes of distress are not being addressed
  - Palliative care experts are not being engaged
  - Decision of sedation affected by frustration in caring of a complex symptomatic patient
  - Sedation is requested by the family, not the patient
- Injudicious withholding of palliative sedation
  - To avoid difficult end-of-life discussion
  - Exaggerated concern of hastening death
- Substandard clinical practice of palliative sedation
  - Inadequate consultation with the patient, family members or staff to ensure understanding of the indication for the intervention, the goals of care, the anticipated outcomes and potential risks
  - Inadequate assessment of psychosocial-spiritual factors
  - Inadequate monitoring of symptom distress and relief
  - Inadequate monitoring of adverse effects
  - Inappropriately rapid dose escalation
  - Inadequate support to family and distressed staff

EAPC framework for palliative sedation 2009

- Pre-emptive discussion of the role of sedation in EOL care
  - Discuss goals of care
  - Discuss end-of-life care preferences
  - Discuss the use of sedation if clinically appropriate
    - In refractory symptoms
    - In catastrophic events: eg terminal bleeding
  - Document outcome of discussion
- Describe the indications of palliative sedation
  - Refractory physical symptoms
    - Agitated delirium
    - Breathlessness

- Pain
- Seizures
- Refractory psychoexistential suffering in rare cases
- Continuous deep sedation only if prognosis hours to days
- Transient or respite sedation may be indicated earlier
- Describe the necessary evaluation and consultation procedures
  - Multi-professional palliative care input
  - Medical evaluation for reversible causes of deterioration
  - Psychosocial-spiritual evaluation
  - Prognostic evaluation
  - Decisional capacity evaluation
  - Document the following:
    - Indication of sedation
    - Decision-making process
    - Aim of sedation
    - Planned depth and duration of sedation
- Specific consent requirement
  - Discuss condition and prognosis
  - Discuss rationale for sedation
  - Discuss aim of sedation
  - Discuss method of sedation
    - Sedative
    - Depth or planned sedation
    - Duration of planned sedation
  - Discuss anticipated outcomes
    - Reduced consciousness
    - Communication impairment
    - Effects on oral intake
  - Discuss potential uncommon risks
    - Paradoxical agitation
    - Delayed or inadequate relief
    - Small risk of hastening of death

- Discuss continuation of palliative and nursing care
- Discuss expected outcome without sedation
- Discuss commitment to the patient's well-being and provision of best possible care irrespective of patient treatment choices
- Involve family members in the discussion if possible
- Documentation of the discussion
- In the care of the terminally ill patients who have no advanced directive and no healthcare proxy and who are in severe distress whilst actively dying, provision of comfort measures (including, if necessary, the use of sedation) is the 'standard of care' and should be the default strategy for clinician treatment decisions
- Indicate the need to discuss the decision-making with family
  - Explain patient's condition and suffering
  - Explain the rationale and aim of sedation
  - Address differences in opinion
  - Support families to relieve them of factors that contribute to conflicts, such as grief and guilt
- Selection of sedation method
  - The level of sedation should be the lowest necessary to provide adequate relief of suffering
  - Mild intermittent sedation should be attempted first unless in emergency situations
  - Down-titration to re-establish lucidity after an agreed interval should be considered and discussed to re-evaluate patient's preferences regarding sedation and for pre-planned famly interactions, with the understanding of the possibility of failure to restore lucidity or the re-appearance of refractory symptoms before death
  - Deep sedation should be adopted when mild sedation is ineffective

- Deep continuous sedation should be selected first if
    - The suffering is intense
    - The suffering is definitely refractory
    - Death is anticipated within hours or a few days
    - The patient's wish is explicit
    - Terminal catastrophic events
        - Massive bleeding
        - Asphyxia
- Present direction for dose titration, monitoring and care
    - Q20min review till adequate sedation
    - Then TDS review
    - Monitor severity of suffering
    - Monitor level of sedation
    - Monitor adverse effects of sedation
        - Paradoxical agitation
        - Aspiration
    - Consider vital signs monitoring for longer prognosis
    - Continue nursing care
- Decision regarding hydration and nutrition and medications
    - The decision about artificial hydration and nutrition is independent of the decision about sedation
    - Comprehensive evaluation of of the patient's wishes and the estimated benefits-harms in palliation of suffering
    - Medications for palliation should be continued
- Care and information needs of family
- Care for healthcare professionals

Level of sedation (Claessens 2011)

- Mild intermittent sedation
    - Intermittent
    - Mild reduction in consciousness
    - Still reacts to stimuli

- Mild continuous sedation
  - Continuous
  - Mild reduction in consciousness
  - Still reacts to stimuli
- Deep intermittent sedation
  - Intermittent sedation to unconsciousness
    - Acute: to treat an acute refractory symptom
    - Non-acute: to treat a non-acute refractory symptom
- Deep continuous sedation
  - Continuous sedation to unconsciousness
    - Acute: to treat an acute refractory symptom
    - Non-acute: to treat a non-acute refractory symptom

Monitoring the severity of suffering

FLACC scale

Criteria	0	1	2
Face	Normal	Grimace	Clenched jaw
Legs	Normal	Restless	Kicking
Activity	Normal	Squirming	Arched
Cry	Normal	Moaning	Screaming
Consolability	Normal	Reassurable	Nonreassurable

Monitoring the level of sedation

- Riker Sedation-Agitation Scale
  - 7 = dangerous agitation
  - 6 = very agitated
  - 5 = agitated
  - 4 = calm and cooperative (easily arousable)
  - 3 = sedated (arousable with verbal stimuli)
  - 2 = very sedated (arousable with physical stimuli)
  - 1 = unarousable

Drugs used for palliative sedation

- Midazolam (IV/SC)
    - Starting dose: 0.5-1mg/h
    - Usual effective dose: 1-20mg/h
    - Boluses: 1-5mg prn/q1h
- Lorazepam (IV)
    - Starting dose: 4mg/h
    - Usual effective dose: 4-20mg/24h
    - Boluses: 0.5-2mg prn/q2h
- Flunitrazepam (IV/SC)
    - Starting dose: 0.2-0.5mg/h
    - Boluses: 1-2mg prn
- Levomepromazine (IV/SC)
    - Starting dose: 50-75mg/24h
    - Maximum dose: 300mg/24h
    - Boluses: 12.5-25mg prn/q1h
- Chlorpromazine (IV/IM/PR)
    - Starting dose
        - 12.5mg q4-12h (IV/IM)
        - 3-5mg/h (IV)
        - 25-100mg q4-12h (PR)
    - Usual effective dose
        - 12.5-50mg q8h (IV/IM)
        - 25-100mg q8h (PR)
- Phenobarbital (IV/IM/SC)
    - Starting dose: 600mg/24h (SC)
    - Usual effective dose: 600-1600mg/24h (SC)
    - Maximum dose: 2400mg/24h (SC)
    - Dilute 1ml phenobarbital with 10ml WFI
        - Phenobarbital 600mg with 30ml WFI
        - Phenobarbital 800mg with 40ml WFI
        - Phenobarbital 1200mg with 60ml WFI

- Phenobarbital 1600mg with 80ml WFI
- Phenobarbital 2400mg with 120ml WFI
  - Boluses
    - IM Phenobarbital 100-200mg undiluted prn/q4-8h
    - IV Phenobarbital 100-200mg with 10ml WFI in rate of 50mg/min prn/q4-8h
- Propofol (IV)
  - Starting dose: 0.5mg/kg/h via forearm vein
  - Increase 0.5mg/kg/h q5-10min till sedation
  - Usual dose 1-2mg/kg/h
  - Max dose 4mg/kg/h
  - Bolus: 1mg/kg/min for 2-5min prn

Palliative sedation for refractory psychoexistential suffering

- Problems
  - Difficult to establish true refractoriness
  - Severity of suffering may be dynamic and idiosyncratic
  - Standard approaches have low intrinsic morbidity
  - Presence of symptoms does not necessarily indicate a far advanced state of physiological deterioration
- Special guidelines
  - Reserved for patients with advanced terminal illness
  - Diagnosis of refractory symptoms
    - By clinicians skilled in psychological care who have established relationship with patient and family
    - Following a period of repeated assessment
    - Trials of routine approaches for anxiety, depression and existential distress
  - Multidisciplinary case conferences, including psychiatry, chaplaincy, ethics, nurses, family members
  - Initiated on a respite basis for 6-24h, then down-titration
  - Continuous sedation after repeated respite sedation trials

Physician-Assisted Suicide and Euthanasia

Introduction

Physician-assisted suicide and euthanasia are illegal practices in Malaysia. However, it is important to understand these practices to avoid confusion with withdrawal of life-sustaining treatment and palliative sedation.

Physician-assisted suicide (PAS)

- Physician-assisted suicide occurs when a physician provides the means, usually a prescription for a large dose of oral barbiturates, by which a patient can ingest by him or herself to end his or her life.
- The practice of PAS is legal in the following country:
  - Colombia
  - Luxembourg
  - Netherlands
  - Switzerland
  - United States (California, Oregon, Vermont, Washington)

Voluntary active euthanasia (VAE)

- Voluntary active euthanasia occurs when a physician administers lethal injections at a patient's request.
- The physician injects a combination of drugs, eg
  - Sodium thiopental to induce coma
  - Pancuronium to paralyze respiratory muscles
  - Potassium chloride to stop the heart
- The practice of VAE is legal in the following country:
  - Belgium
  - Colombia

- Luxembourg
- Netherlands

Intentionality

- In PAS and VAE, the intention of the physician is to relieve suffering by killing or hastening of death.
- In withdrawal of life-sustaining treatment, the intention of the physician is to remove futile treatment to allow natural death. Hastening of death can be foreseen, but not intended. In the unusual event where patient continues to survive, continued support is necessary.
- In palliative sedation, the intention of the physician is to relieve refractory suffering, but not hastening of death. Sedative is titrated to a level just enough to relieve suffering, but no further once suffering is relieved.

Ethics in Palliative Care

Introduction

In the palliative care setting, it is not uncommon for one to face ethical dilemma in decision-making. Therefore, it can be useful for us to know some of the major ethical theories which we can use to analyse a situation and to help us in the decision-making.

Deontological ethics (duty ethics)

- The morality of an action is judged based on the duties of the healthcare professionals
- Deon = duty in Greek
- The term deontology was coined by Charlie Dunbar Broad
- Deontology formulated by Immanuel Kant
- Immanuel Kant described:

Nothing in the world – indeed nothing beyond the world – can possibly be conceived which could be called good without qualification except a good will.

- Duties as identified by William David Ross
  - Duty of beneficence
  - Duty of non-maleficence
  - Duty of justice
  - Duty of self-improvement
  - Duty of reparation
  - Duty of gratitude
  - Duty of promise keeping
- Principlism is the main deontological approach
  - Four basic principles from Beauchamp and Childress
  - Foundation of current medical decision-making

The four principles or duties of biomedical ethics

Autonomy = respect patient autonomy

- Latin: *Voluntas aegroti suprema lex*
- Meaning: free will of the patient is the supreme law
- Secondary principles
    - Shared decision making
    - Informed consent
        - Information
        - Comprehension
        - Voluntariness
    - Informed refusal
    - Advance decision to refuse treatment (ADRT)
    - Truth-telling
    - Confidentiality

Non-maleficence = do no harm

- Latin: *Primum non nocere*
- Meaning: first, do no harm
- Secondary principles
    - Do not kill
    - Do not cause needless pain
    - Do not incapacitate others
- Negligence
    - The professional must have a duty to the patient
    - The professional must breach the duty
    - The patient must experience a harm
    - The harm must be caused by the breach of duty

Beneficence = do good

- Latin: *Salus aegroti suprema lex*
- Meaning: well-being of the patient is the supreme law

- Secondary principles
    - Do no harm
    - Prevent harm
    - Remove harm
    - Do good

Social justice = do justice

- Distributive justice
- Meaning: fair distribution of limited medical resources
- Secondary principles
    - Use medical factors to determine fair distribution
        - Likely benefit to the patient
            - Cure
            - Prolongation of survival
            - Improvement in quality of life
            - Improvement in function
        - Urgency of need
        - Duration of benefit
    - Do not use non-medical factors
        - Age
        - Gender
        - Race
        - Lifestyle
        - Social status or social worth
        - Contribution to society
        - First come first served basis
        - Random pick
- Caveats of deontology
    - Emphasis on rules and duties: inflexibility in applying the rules may do harm
    - Duties ≠ intention: one may not intend to do good, but may act merely out of the duty of doing good

Consequentialism

- The morality of an action is judged based on the consequences
- The term consequentialism was coined by Elizabeth Anscombe
- Utilitarianism is the main consequentialism approach
    - Founder: Jeremy Bentham
    - Expanded by John Stuart Mill
    - Utility = happiness, pleasure, satisfaction
    - Utilitarian calculus (felicific or hedonic calculus)
      = greatest happiness for the greatest number
    - The morality of an action is judged based on its usefulness
      in maximizing utility or minimizing negative utility among
      everyone
- The judged consequences
    - The positive and negative consequences of an action
    - The positive and negative consequences of other options
    - The consequences of such decision on patients, families,
      friends, healthcare professionals, health care institution
      and society
- Caveats of consequentialism
    - Emphasis on consequences and outcome
        - Character of the person can be bad
        - Intention of the person can be bad

Virtue ethics

- The morality of an action is judged based on the characters of
  healthcare professionals
- Emphasizes the character of the person performing the action
- Influence: Plato and Aristotle
- Eudaimonism is the main virtue ethics approach
    - Eudaimonia = happiness, well-being, human flourishing
    - Happiness is achieved through virtue
    - In order to act rightly, one should be a virtuous person

- Caveats of virtue ethics
  - Emphasis on the character of the moral agent
    - A kind person may still do harm to patients

Casuistry

- Casuistry = case-based reasoning
- Casus = case in Latin
- Relies on analysis of individual cases versus paradigm cases
- Useful especially when conflicting rules occur
- Caveats of casuistry
  - Emphasis on individual cases
  - Needs a paradigm case to compare

Doctrine of double effect (DDE)

- Origin: Summa Theologiae written 1265-1274
- Author: Thomas Aquinas
- To judge an action which is intended to achieve a good effect but with the potential of giving rise to an unintended bad effect
- The action must satisfy 4 conditions to be morally permissible
  - The nature-of-the-act condition: the action must be either morally good or indifferent
  - The means-end condition: the bad effect must not be the means by which one achieves the good effect
  - The right-intention condition: the intention must be the achieving of only the good effect, with the bad effect being only an unintended side effect
  - The proportionality condition: the bad effect must not be disproportionate to the good effect
- DDE in pain management of terminally ill patients
  - Irrelevant in most cases
  - Appropriate use of opioids does not hasten death in terminally ill patients (Fohr 1998)

- Use of high dose opioids in terminally ill patients does not hasten death (Morita 2001)
- Deaths during opioid titration are related to disease progression in most patients, not to the use of opioids (Manfredi 1998)
- DDE is not needed to justify the use of high dose opioids in pain management of terminally ill patients
- DDE in sedation of terminally ill patients
    - Irrelevant in most cases
    - Appropriate use of sedatives does not hasten death in terminally ill patients (Morita 2001)
    - Palliative sedation used to relieve refractory symptoms does not hasten death (Maltoni 2009)
    - DDE is not needed to justify the use of sedation in the palliative care setting
- DDE in special cases
    - In rare circumstances when very high doses of opioids or sedatives are needed in a rapidly escalating manner to relieve suffering in terminally ill patients, with the risk of hastening death foreseen but unintended, DDE may be invoked to justify its use

Psychosocial Care

Introduction

The relief of suffering in palliative care patients needs a combination of good symptom control and psychosocial care.

Definition of psychosocial care

- Care concerned with the psychological and emotional well-being of the patient and their family/carers, including issues of self-esteem, insight into and adaptation to the illness and its consequences, communication, social functioning and relationships. (The National Council for Hospice and Specialist Palliative Care Services 1997)

The 5 components of psychosocial care (Tan 2015)

Presence

- Definitions
    - A mode of being available or open in a situation with the wholeness of one's unique being, a gift of self which can only be given freely, invoked or evoked (Paterson 1976)
    - A mode of being available in a situation with the wholeness of one's unique individual being; a process resulting in exchange of authentic meaningful awareness, essence linking, and thus more being (Hines 1991)
    - The physical "being there" and the psychological "being with" a patient with the purpose of meeting the patient's healthcare needs (Gardner 1985)
    - The state achieved when one moves within oneself to an inner reference of stability of being in the moment (Dossey 1995)

- The first and foremost requisite for a therapeutic relationship
- Types of presence (Stiles 1997)
    - Physical presence
        - Being there
        - Body to body contact
        - Skills: seeing, examining, touching, hugging
        - Requisite: recognizing patient as a person, empathy
        - Barrier: rushing, excessively task-orientated
    - Psychological presence
        - Being with
        - Mind to mind contact
        - Skills: listening, communicating, caring, connecting
        - Requisite: attention, empathy
        - Barrier: lack of concern
    - Spiritual presence
        - Therapeutic presence, transcendent presence
        - Spirit to spirit contact
        - Whole being to whole being
        - Skills: meditating, at-one-ment, openness, loving,
        - Requisite: inner quietude, mindfulness
        - Barrier: cognitive and emotional reactivity

Listening

- A crucial component of communication skills
- Goal: to understand the thoughts and feelings of a person
- Active listening
    - Originated from person-centered therapy of Carl Rogers
    - 3 core concepts of person-centered therapy
        - Congruence
            - Relating to another genuinely
            - Not hiding behind a professional façade

- Unconditional positive regard
  - Accepting another as who he or she is
  - Listening without judgment
- Empathy
  - Communicating the desire to understand and appreciate another's perspective and feelings
- Techniques of active listening
  - Encourage expression of thoughts and feelings
    - Use open-ended questions
    - Use silence
    - Use facilitations such as nodding and fillers
    - Pay attention to speech and body language
  - Check for understanding
    - Clarifying
    - Repeating
    - Paraphrasing
    - Summarizing
    - Reflecting
  - Avoid reacting
    - Avoid interrupting
    - Avoid judging
    - Avoid explaining reactively
    - Avoid advising prematurely
    - Avoid blocking of expression

Empathy

- Etymology
  - Empatheia: in passion (Greek)
  - Einfühlung: into feelings (German) by Lipps in 1903
  - Empathy: coined by Edward B. Titchener in 1909 as a "translation" from Einfühlung

- Definitions
    - Empathy means entering the private perceptual world of the other and becoming thoroughly at home in it. It involves being sensitive, moment to moment, to the changing felt meanings which flow in this other person, to the fear or rage or tenderness or confusion or whatever, that he or she is experiencing. It means temporarily living in his or her life, moving about in it delicately without making judgment, sensing meanings of which he or she is scarcely aware... It includes communicating your sensing of his or her world as you look with fresh and unfrightened eyes at elements of which the individual is fearful. It means frequently checking with him or her as to the accuracy of your sensing, and being guided by the responses you receive... to be with another in this way means that for the time being you lay aside the views and values you hold for yourself in order to enter another world without prejudice. (Carl Rogers 1975)
    - The capacity to think and feel oneself into the inner life of another person (Kohut 1984)
    - The ability to understand another's situation, perspective and feelings (Coulehan 2000)
- Types of empathy
    - Emotional empathy: the capacity to respond with an appropriate emotion to another's mental states
    - Cognitive empathy: the capacity to understand another's perspective or mental state
- Stages of empathy
    - Empathic understanding
        - Perceptions
        - Emotions
        - Cognition: beliefs, concerns, hope and meaning

- Communicated empathy
  - Acknowledgment
  - Validation
  - Normalization
- Perception of empathy from patients and families
- Exquisite empathy
  - A highly present, intimate, and heartfelt interpersonal connection in the therapeutic relationship with clients, without fusing or losing sight of the clinician's own perspective (Harrison 2009)
- Sympathy, pity and emotional contagion
  - Pity and sympathy: feeling sorry
  - Emotional contagion: the tendency to automatically mimic and synchronize expressions, vocalizations, postures, and movements with those of another person's and, consequently, to converge emotionally

Compassion

- Definitions
  - The sincere wish to alleviate the suffering of another. The desire to alleviate another's pain includes not only their present experience of discomfort but also the cause of their suffering, the underlying reasons they are not well. (Nyima 2006)
  - The feeling that arises when witnessing another's suffering and that motivates a subsequent desire to help (Goetz 2010)
- Types of compassion (Nyima 2006)
  - Conceptual compassion
    - Arises from concepts
    - Deliberate
    - Requires conscious effort

371

- Unstable
- Selective
- Situational
- Goal-orientated
- Fatigable
- Non-conceptual compassion
  - Arises from a concept-free state of mind
  - Natural
  - Effortless
  - Stable
  - Non-selective: embraces everyone without prejudice
  - Non-situational
  - Process-orientated
  - Non-fatigable
- Developing a compassionate attitude (Nyima 2006)
  - On waking up, make the first thought a noble one – a very sincere and strong thought of doing good
  - Remind ourselves of that noble thought every so often throughout the day
  - Before falling asleep, make the final thought a noble one
- Steps to becoming more compassionate (Nyima 2006)
  - Reduce negative habits: judgment of others
  - Increase positive habits: being kind and helpful to others
  - Free oneself from clinging to concepts

Boundary awareness

- The mutually understood, unspoken, physical, and emotional limits of the relationship between the trusting patient and the caring physician or provider (Farber 1997)
- Examples of potential boundary issues
  - Receiving gifts from patients
  - Giving out phone number to patients

- Socializing with patients outside of the clinical setting
- Revealing excessive personal information to patients
- Examples of definite boundary issues
  - Accepting money from a patient or family member
  - Attending to patient to fulfil a personal need
  - Attempting a deathbed conversion
  - Giving in to request for futile treatment
  - Giving in to request for hastening of death
- Although sometimes crossing boundaries can enhance patient care, boundary awareness is essential to avoid boundary issues that are harmful to the therapeutic relationship and boundary violation

Communication

Introduction

Communication is an indispensable component of psychosocial care. To communicate effectively, first, make a connection.

Making a connection (Dalai Lama & Howard Cutler 2009)

- Contemplating our basic human nature
    - Recognize that every person is basically a social person
    - Cultivate a deep appreciation of this basic human nature, which is to connect with each other and to cooperate together in improving the situations
- Contemplating our interconnectedness
    - Reflect on how human beings depend on each other for survival in the society
    - Reflect on how our welfare is closely connected to the welfare of others
- Contemplating our common humanity
    - Reflect on the fact that human beings share the same basic wish to be happy and free from suffering
    - Cultivate an empathic attitude towards others
    - Connect with others on a human-to-human level, based on our common humanity, our basic wish
- Connecting with others
    - Interact exactly the same with every person
    - Exhibit the same level of interest and warmth
    - Give every person the same level of full attention
    - Speak with every person as if they are the most important person in the world at that moment, as if they are the only person

The three crucial components of communication

- Non-verbal communication
    - Body language (kinesics)
        - Microkinesics
            - Oculesics: study of eye behaviour
            - Facial kinesics: study of facial expressions
        - Macrokinesics
            - Appearance
            - Artifacts
            - Postures
            - Gestures
            - Body movement
    - Paralanguage: study of non-lexical component of speech
    - Haptics: study of touch
    - Proxemics: study of space and distance
    - Chronemics: study of time
- Listening
    - Language
    - Paralanguage
- Empathy
    - Diagnostic empathy
    - Therapeutic empathy

Comparison of verbal and non-verbal communication

Verbal communication	Non-verbal communication
- $\approx 35\%$	- $\approx 65\%$
- By words	- By cues
- Conveys information	- Conveys feeling
- Intermittent	- Continuous
- Unichanneled	- Multichanneled
- May not be reliable	- More reliable

Non-verbal communication

Emotional recognition from oculesics (Straker 2008)

- Anger: eyes wide open and staring
- Disgust: eyes turned away rapidly
- Fear: eyes wide or looking downward, or closed
- Anxiety: eyes wet, blinking more
- Sadness: eyes looking downward, possibly wet with tears
- Happiness: eyes sparkling

Signs of crying

First sign: a sudden pause in communication
Second sign: eyes shiny
Third sign: tears lining lower eyelids (silver line sign)
Fourth sign: tears filling medial canthus
Fifth sign: tears falling

Emotional recognition from facial expressions (Paul Ekman 2003)

- Anger
  - Lowered and drawn-together brows
  - Raised upper eyelids: the glare
  - Tightened upper and lower eyelids
  - Pressed lips or open in square or rectangular shape
  - Red margin of lips becomes narrower
  - Lips become thinner
  - Clenched jaw
  - Jaw thrust forward
  - Exposed teeth

- Disgust and contempt
  - Lowered brows
  - Pushed up lower eyelids
  - Crow's-feet wrinkles
  - Raised cheeks
  - Deepened nasolabial folds: inverted U
  - Nose wrinkling
  - Raised upper and lower lips
  - Slightly protruding lower lips
  - Asymmetry: contempt
- Surprise and fear
  - Raised and drawn together eyebrows
  - Raised upper eyelids
  - Tensed lower eyelids: fear
  - Horizontally stretched lips toward ears: fear
  - Jaw dropped down: surprise
  - Pulled back chin
- Sadness
  - Angling upward of the inner corners of the eyebrows (triangulation of inner brows): the sad brows
  - Vertical wrinkle between the brows
  - Drooping of upper eyelids
  - Tensing of lower eyelids
  - Downward gaze
  - Raised cheeks, sometimes causing a false grin
  - Horizontal stretching of lips
  - Pushing up of lower lips
  - Pulling down of lip corners
  - Opening of mouth
  - Chin pouting

- Happiness
    - Raised lip corners: smile
    - Raised cheeks
- Accuracy of facial emotional recognition
    - Happiness   100%
    - Sadness   80%
    - Anger   80%
    - Fear   80%
    - Disgust   80%

Emotional recognition from bodily expression (Darwin 1965)

- Anger
    - Head erect
    - Shoulders squared
    - Arms rigidly suspended by the sides
    - Elbows squared
    - Fist clenched and shaking
    - Intends to push or strike
    - Purposeless or frantic gestures
    - Chest well expanded
    - Whole body trembles
    - Feet planted firmly on the grounded
    - Pacing up and down
- Disgust and contempt
    - Spitting
    - Shoulders raised as when horror is experienced
    - Arms pressed close to the sides
    - Gestures as if to push away or to guard oneself
    - Turning away of the whole body: contempt
    - Snapping one's fingers: contempt

- Fear
    - Head sinks between shoulders
    - Shoulders raised
    - Arms bent and pressed closely against sides or chest
    - Arms thrown wildly over the head
    - Arms violently protruded as if to push away
    - Hands clenched and opened alternately with twitching
    - Whole body often turned away or shrinks
    - Motionless or crouches down
- Sadness
    - Head hangs on contracted chest
    - Motionless
    - Passive
- Shame
    - Turning away the whole body
    - Face averted, bent down
    - Ackward
    - Nervous movement
- Joy
    - Head upright
    - Head nods to and fro while laughing
    - Various purposeless movement
    - Clapping of hands
    - Body held erect
    - Whole body is thrown backward and shakes or almost convulsed during excessive laughter
    - Stamping
    - Jumping
    - Dancing for joy
- Pride
    - Head and body held erect

Listening

- Language
  - Expression of physical complaints
  - Expression of thoughts
    - Ideas
    - Concerns
    - Hope and expectation
  - Expression of emotions
  - Expression of relationships and social interactions
  - Expression of spirituality
- Paralanguage (paralinguistics)
  - Non-verbal elements of speech
  - Not related to content or verbal message
  - Pitch: the degree of highness or lowness of a tone
  - Rate: the speed of speaking
  - Volume: the loudness of a voice
  - Prosody: the rhythm, stress and intonation of a speech
    - Rhythm: the flow of speech produced from the variation of pitch, rate and volume
    - Stress: making a syllable prominent
    - Intonation: pitch variation not to distinguish words
    - Inflection: pitch variation to distinguish words
    - Pause: a break while speaking
  - Articulation: the act of speaking clearly
  - Pronunciation: the act of speaking a word correctly
  - Quality: the unique vocal characteristics of every person
  - Tone of voice: the feelings added while speaking
  - Paralinguistic respirations
    - Gasp: sudden sharp inhalation through mouth
    - Sigh: deep, audible exhalation through mouth/nose
  - Side sounds
    - Laughter, cry, scream, cough

Speech emotional recognition: (Juslin & Laukka 2003)

- Anger: higher mean pitch, higher pitch variation, upward pitch inflection, faster voice onsets, faster speech rate, higher volume, higher volume variation, more high frequency spectral energy, higher first formant, higher precision of articulation, less pauses
- Disgust: lower mean pitch, downward pitch inflection, faster voice onsets, more high frequency spectral energy, higher first formant
- Fear: higher mean pitch, lower pitch variation, upward pitch inflection, faster speech rate, higher volume, higher volume variation, lesser high frequency spectral energy than anger, lower first formant, variable precision of articulation, less pauses
- Anxiety: higher mean pitch, lower pitch variation, lesser high frequency spectral energy than anger
- Sadness: lower mean pitch, lower pitch variation, downward pitch inflection, slower speech rate, lower volume, lower volume variation, longer voicing duration, least high frequency spectral energy, lower first formant, lower precision of articulation, more pauses
- Happiness: higher mean pitch, higher pitch variation, upward pitch inflection, faster speech rate, higher volume, higher volume variation, more high frequency spectral energy, higher precision of articulation, less pauses
- Accuracy of speech emotional recognition (Scherer 1991)
    - Sadness   72%
    - Anger   68%
    - Joy   59%
    - Fear   52%
    - Disgust   28%

Empathy

- Diagnostic empathy
    - A state of being conscious or aware of another person's feeling or perspective through observing the person and the body language, listening to the voice and experiences, and imagining oneself in his or her position
- Therapeutic empathy
    - A caring response to another's mental state, verbally or non-verbally, that causes the person to feel better

Therapeutic non-verbal empathy

- Oculesics
    - Maintain good eye contact
    - Maintain a kind look
    - Sit down at same eye level
- Facial kinesics
    - Face the person
    - Smile if appropriate
- Body kinesics
    - Kind first impression
    - Open posture: no crossed arms or legs
    - Leaning forward to show genuine interest
    - Mirror the body language during rapport building
    - Minimize unintentional body movements or gestures
- Paralanguage
    - Speak with a gentle voice
    - Articulate clearly to show confidence
    - Match the vocal cues of the person
    - Follow their pitch, volume, rate and rhythm if appropriate
    - Adjust your pitch, volume, rate and rhythm if appropriate
        - Higher pitch, higher volume, faster rate: motivating
        - Lower pitch, lower volume, slower rate: calming

- Haptics
  - Be aware of cultural or gender sensitivity to touch
  - Touch shoulder or elbow if appropriate
- Proxemics
  - Be aware of a comfortable distance
  - Be aware of arrangement of sitting position
  - No barrier: medical notes, side rails
- Chronemics
  - Proper communication of appointment time
  - Punctuality
  - Avoid rushing
  - State time limitation politely if time is a constraint

Smile in palliative care

- Smile is a very important facial expression
- Smile releases the following "feel good" neurotransmitters:
  - Endorphins
  - Serotonin
  - Dopamine
- Smile is contagious
- Smile lifts our mood as well as the mood of those around us
- A calm and genuine smile is appropriate in most situations
- A barely noticeable, calm and genuine smile can be appropriate even in the setting of angry or sad atmosphere

12 Muscles of smiling	11 Muscles of frowning
- Orbicularis oculi (2) - Zygomaticus major (2) - Zygomaticus minor (2) - Levator labii superioris (2) - Levator anguli oris (2) - Risorius (2)	- Corrugator supercilii (2) - Orbicularis oculi (2) - Procerus (1) - Orbicularis oris (1) - Depressor anguli oris (2) - Mentalis (1) - Platysma (2)

Types of smile

- True smile (Duchenne smile)
    - Involves eyes and lips
    - Orbicularis oculi muscles narrow eyes
    - Zygomatic major muscles raise lip corners
    - Timing matches with stimulus
    - Slow onset
    - Short apex duration, usually <5s
    - Smooth offset
    - Symmetrical
- Social smile (fake smile, botox smile, Pan American smile)
    - Involves lips only
    - Zygomatic major muscles raise lip corners
    - Timing too early or too late compared to stimulus
    - Abrupt onset
    - Long apex duration
    - Abrupt offset
    - Slightly asymmetrical

Therapeutic verbal empathy

- The key expression of empathy is to "ALLOW"
- Allow patients or family to talk about their experiences
- Allow patients or family members to express their thoughts
- Allow patients or family to express their emotions
- The primary obstacle of expressing empathy is to "BLOCK"
- Do not block the expression of thoughts and emotions:
    - Interrupting the conversation
    - Deviating away from the topic
    - Giving explanation prematurely
    - Giving advice prematurely
    - Focusing on the biomedical aspect of the person
    - Giving tissues as a signal for patient to stop crying

- Express empathy verbally once the catharsis is complete:
    - Acknowledging the emotion: talk about the emotion
    - Validating the emotion: tell patient it is ok or normal
    - Normalizing the emotion: tell patient you or others would feel the same too given the same situation

---

Little experience

Once I was standing at the bedside of a breast cancer patient. She was accompanied by her family on the other side of the bed. Her pain had been well controlled. I asked her, "Is there anything else you would like me to do for you?" She said, "Can you give me a hug?" I was completely unprepared and her family hugged her instead. The next day she passed away. I felt sorry about that. Then I started to accept hugging from patients and families. I was quite stiff in the beginning but now I have improved a lot. Hugging is often a sign of gratitude in palliative care. So next time if your patient wants to hug you, go for it and hug him or her with all your body, heart and spirit.

Breaking Bad News

Introduction

Breaking bad news, done poorly, can cause devastating effects on patients, family members as well as health care providers. There is no one simple way to break bad news. The aim of this chapter is to provide a short introduction to what is bad news and describe how to apply the SPIKES strategy in delivering bad news.

Definition (Buckman 1984)

- Bad news can be defined as any information that seriously and adversely changes a person's view of his future

Cleopatra's syndrome

- The bearer of the bad news is blamed for the bad news itself

  No one loves the messenger who brings bad news. Sophocles

SPIKES (Walter 2000)

- S = Setting
    - Set up the interview
    - Get all the facts ready before the discussion
    - Switch your handphone to silent or vibration mode
    - Arrange for a quiet room if possible
    - Sit down with the patient or family
- P = Perception
    - Assess patient's perception
    - Find out what is known or suspected
    - Examples
        - How much do you know about your situation?
        - What have you been told by the other doctors?

- What do you think is going on?
- Have you been suspecting anything serious?
- I = Invitation
  - Obtain permission to share the information
  - Examples
    - Would you like me to tell you about your results?
    - How much would you like to know?
    - Are you the kind of person who would like to know everything in details?
- K = Knowledge
  - Consider giving a warning shot
  - Example: I am afraid the news is not good
  - Give information following patient's pace
  - Give information in small pieces
  - Avoid medical jargons
  - Be honest but sensitive
  - Be mindful of emotional cues
- E = Emotions
  - Address patient's emotions with empathy
    - Pick up emotional cues
    - Allow patient to express emotion
    - Be comfortable with silence
    - Do not block emotional expression
      - Continuing to talk about medical facts
      - Diverting from the conversation
      - Asking patient to stop crying
      - Explaining away patient's anger
  - Acknowledge the emotion
  - Validate the emotion
  - Normalize the emotion
  - Imagine yourself in the situation and see whether you can find out what patient wants you to say or do

- Never say "there is nothing more can be done"
- Never say "there is no more hope"
- S = Strategy
  - Summarize the discussion when patient is ready
  - Give a plan when patient is ready
  - Give hope: refer to the "Hope" chapter

Little opinion

Strictly speaking, all news is neutral in its own sense. There is no such thing as bad news. It is the perception of the patient that makes it good or bad. This is why some patients are hardly affected by the so-called "bad" news but some can be devastated by it. So, as physicians, we have to be mindful of our own perception too.

Communicating Prognosis

Introduction

Foreseeing is the science of formulating a prognosis. Foretelling is the art of communicating it. Majority of patients want to know about their prognosis, but how we communicate it to them may affect how they live the rest of their lives.

Doctor, how much time do I have?

- Be mindful of what you are going to say when you hear this
- This is a common question in palliative care
- Great sensitivity is needed in answering it
- How we answer may give a long-lasting impact on patients

What is the reason patient asks this question?

- Find out the reason behind the question
- Is there anything that the patient wants to do?
- Is patient expecting some important event?
- Knowing this can help us a lot

Does the patient have the answer?

- Find out how much time does the patient think he or she has
- Patient may have been told about their prognosis by others
- Patient may know deep inside how much time is left

How long does the patient want to live?

- It is prudent to find out patient's expectation
- This gives us a clue how ready they are to know their prognosis
- This can help us on how to answer

Is it appropriate to answer without answering?

- For some patients, they are aware of their prognosis
- We may not need to answer their question about prognosis

Is it appropriate to answer without giving the prognosis?

- For some patients, they don't really want to know if it is short
- We may say doctors do not know the actual prognosis

Is it appropriate to answer without giving the duration?

- For some patients, they are asking because they want to know whether they have enough time to complete certain unfinished business or celebrate certain important event
- If it is a yes, we may tell them the likehood of being able to do it or celebrate the event
- If it is a no, think of what the patient wants us to say when the likelihood is low

Is it appropriate to answer without giving the time range?

- For some patients, they just want to know whether it is short
- If it is long, we can tell them that they still have time
- We can tell them that time is running short only when they are completely bed-ridden and no longer conscious
- If it is short, we may tell them: I am afraid time could be short

Is it appropriate to answer based on functional decline?

- If one is getting weaker and weaker every month, then the time could be in months
- If one is getting weaker and weaker every weeks, then the time could be in weeks
- If one is getting weaker and weaker every days, then the time could be in days

Is it appropriate to give the estimated time range?

- If nothing happens suddenly, the time could be:
    - Months to years
    - Weeks to months
    - Days to weeks
    - Hours to days

Is it appropriate to give an exact number?

- No
- Do not give exact number
    - You have 3 months to live
    - You have 2 weeks to live
- These are death sentences
- Don't be a judge; be a doctor

What is next after communicating prognosis?

- Communicate empathy: refer to the "Communication" chapter
- Communicate hope: refer to the "Hope" chapter

End-of-life Discussion

Introduction

End-of-life discussion is one of the most important conversations in the care of the dying. A skilled physician can help patients to slowly come to terms to what is happening so that they can make the most out of their remaining time.

Insight and acceptance

- Assess patient's insight into his or her illness and prognosis
- Assess patient's acceptance towards illness and prognosis

Goals of care

- Assess patient's goals of care
    - Survival: to live as long as possible
    - Function: to live as independent as possible
    - Comfort: to live as comfortable as possible

Readiness

- Ready: discuss end of life and preferences
- Not ready: discuss advance care planning (ACP)
- Not ready to discuss ACP: give time

Preferred information

- Assess what patient wants to know
- Assess how much patient wants to know

Communicating information

- Communicate information according to patient's wish
- Communicate information according to patient's pace

- Illness
- Prognosis
- Realistic goals
- Disease trajectories
- Clinical features of dying if appropriate
- Potential medical problems during dying if appropriate

Hope and preferences

- Assess hope
  - Hope regarding their illness
  - Hope regarding their life
    - Things to complete
    - Things to do
    - Things to see
    - Things to say
      - Ask for forgiveness from someone
      - Express forgiveness to someone
      - Express love to someone
      - Express thank you to someone
      - Express farewell to someone
  - Hope after death if appropriate
  - Consider helping patients to fulfil their hope if possible
- Preferences
  - Place of care
  - Place of dying if appropriate
  - Ritual and ceremonies if appropriate

Suffering of Palliative Care Patients

Introduction

The importance of suffering has been highlighted in the 2002 WHO definition of palliative care: Palliative care is an approach that improves the quality of life of patients and their families facing the problem associated with life-threatening illness, through the prevention and relief of **_SUFFERING_** by means of early identification and impeccable assessment and treatment of pain and other problems, physical, psychosocial and spiritual.

Definitions of suffering

- A state of severe distress associated with actual or perceived threat to the intactness of a person (Eric Cassell 1982)
    - A simplified description of a person
        - A person cannot be reduced to their parts
        - A person has a past
        - A person has a family
        - A person has a cultural background
        - A person has roles
        - A person has a relationship with himself or herself
        - A person is a political being
        - A person does things
        - A person has an unconscious component
        - A person has regular behaviour
        - A person has a body
        - A person has a secret life
        - A person has a perceived future
        - A person has a transcendent dimension
    - Suffering is experienced by person, not bodies (Cassell 1991)

- A perceived threat to the integrity of the self, helplessness in the face of the threat, and exhaustion of psychosocial and personal resources of coping (Chapman 1993)
- An aversive emotional experience characterized by the perception of personal distress that is generated by adverse factors that undermine the quality of life (Cherny 1994)
- An experience of distress and disharmony caused by loss or threatened loss of what we most cherish (Coulehan 2012)

The biopsychosocial-spiritual model of suffering

- Based on the concept of total pain (Saunders 1983)
- Suffering has four dimensions
- Physical suffering, such as
  - Pain
  - Breathlessness
  - Nausea and vomiting
  - Constipation
- Psychological suffering, such as
  - Anxiety
  - Depression
  - Delirium
  - Insomnia
- Social suffering, such as
  - Loss of employment and income
  - Loss of social connections or roles
  - Concerns about family
  - Distress related to healthcare services
- Spiritual suffering, such as
  - Hopelessness
  - Meaninglessness
  - Fear of death
  - Why me?

The existential-experiential model of suffering (Tan 2014)

- Suffering is an unpleasant existential experience
- Suffering can be seen from two perspectives
  - Existential suffering: the view of suffering from the perspective of the events that make one suffer
  - Experiential suffering: the view of suffering from the perspective of the inner experiences of the person
- Existential suffering
  - Loss-related events
    - Loss and change
      - Loss of function
      - Loss of independence
      - Loss of freedom
      - Loss of sense of control
      - Loss of job and income
      - Loss of role
      - Loss of normality
      - Loss of quality of life
      - Loss of future
      - Loss of hope
      - Loss of confidence
      - Loss of fighting spirit
      - Anticipated loss
    - Dependence on others
      - Dependence on family
      - Dependence on friends
      - Dependence on healthcare providers
      - Perceived burdening of others
      - Perceived uselessness
      - Embarrassment of dependence
      - Loss of self-image due to dependence
      - Anticipated dependence

- Witnessing family suffering
  - Witnessing physical exhaustion of family
  - Witnessing emotional exhaustion
  - Witnessing helplessness
  - Witnessing family grief
  - Lack of self-concern in family
  - Concerns about family future
- Gain-related events
  - Facing terminal disease and death
    - Diagnosis of a terminal illness
    - Disease progression
    - Multiple recurrences
    - Multiple complications
    - Fear of dying
    - Fear of suffering
    - Fear of the unknown
    - Near-death experiences
    - Short estimated life span
    - Dying young
    - Unfinished business
  - Unpleasant healthcare encounter
    - Lack of full attention
    - Lack of immediate attention
    - Lack of listening
    - Lack of empathy
    - Lack of information
    - Different information from different teams
    - Poor communication
    - Hearing "nothing more can be done"
    - Perceived lack of competency
    - Lack of efficiency
    - Lack of coordination of different teams

- Unpleasant hospital stay
    - Hospital confinement
    - Mobility restriction from tubes and lines
    - Boredom in hospital
    - Loneliness in hospital
    - Noisy hospital environment
    - Unpalatable hospital food
    - Witnessing suffering of other patients
    - Witnessing death in the hospital
- Experiential suffering
    - Physical experience
        - Various physical symptoms
        - Impact of symptoms
            - Physical functions
            - Mental functions
            - Routines
            - Social activities
            - Employment
            - Sleep
            - Family
        - Sense of impending death due to intense symptoms
        - Desire to die due to refractory symptoms
    - Emotional experience
        - Shock
        - Surprise
        - Worry
        - Fear
        - Anger
        - Frustration
        - Boredom
        - Sadness
        - Loneliness

- Regret
- Cognitive experience
  - Hope-hopelessness spectrum
    - Hope for cure
    - Hope for survival
    - Hope for function
    - Hope for comfort
    - Hope for peace
    - Hope for sooner death
    - Hopelessness
  - Denial-acceptance spectrum
    - Complete denial
    - Partial acceptance
    - Choiceless acceptance
- Spiritual experience
  - Unanswered questions
    - Reason of having the disease
    - Reason of having to suffer
    - Reason of having to die
    - Contribution of past actions
    - Time of death
    - The unknown after death
  - Loss of faith
  - Religious doubts
  - Spiritual loneliness

Psychological processes of suffering (Tan 2016)

- Although patients have unique suffering experiences at their end of life, the psychological processes follow 5 set patterns
  - Perceptions: becoming aware of the sources of suffering through the senses

- Cognitive appraisals: interpretation of the sources of suffering
- Hope and the struggles with acceptance: the cognitive processes that occur when patients are relating with the sources of suffering
- Emotions: the subjective experiences of perceptions, cognitive appraisals, hope and acceptance that move patients to fight with or run away from the sources of suffering
- Clinging: the fixation on the suffering experiences and the difficulty to move forward

Perceptions (seeing, hearing, feeling, knowing)

- Experiencing loss of function
- Experiencing loss of ability to do things
- Experiencing loss of ability to walk far
- Experiencing loss of ability to go out
- Experiencing loss bit by bit
- Experiencing loss of confidence
- Experiencing loss of faith while in pain
- Experiencing loss of social engagement
- Experiencing dependence on others
- Experiencing pain
- Experiencing pain all of a sudden
- Experiencing pain all the time
- Experiencing pain everywhere
- Experiencing pain for the whole day
- Experiencing pain from injections
- Experiencing worst pain in life
- Experiencing sleeplessness
- Experiencing other symptoms
- Experiencing side effects of treatment

- Experiencing impoliteness of medical staff
- Experiencing hospital confinement
- Seeing family crying
- Seeing family feeling scared
- Seeing family getting stressed
- Seeing family not getting enough sleep
- Seeing the corpse trolley
- Seeing death in the hospital
- Hearing 'I have seen worse cases than you' from the doctors
- Knowing that the disease is incurable
- Knowing that death is imminent
- Knowing that death is inevitable
- Knowing that death is unpredictable
- Knowing that no one else can die for you
- Knowing that one is troubling the family
- Knowing that family is stressed

Cognitive appraisals

Interpreting

- Interpreting loss of ability to do many things as worst suffering
- Interpreting loss of ability to do enjoyable things as no life
- Interpreting lying on bed all the time as the same as a corpse
- Interpreting that one is no longer the same as before
- Interpreting that it is not easy to live with the changes
- Interpreting that the reminder of being sick is always there
- Interpreting that one is depending on others for everything
- Interpreting that one is burdening others
- Interpreting accepting help from others as a form of stress
- Interpreting depending on others as a sign of uselessness
- Interpreting that the children are not independent enough
- Interpreting that the waiting time to see doctors is very long
- Interpreting that the services of nurses are slow

- Interpreting that receiving chemotherapy is suffering
- Interpreting that medical students are inconsiderate
- Interpreting that the hospital food is not nutritious
- Interpreting that being sick is full of pain and suffering
- Interpreting the pain experience as a terrible experience
- Interpreting a life full of pain as a life of suffering
- Interpreting feelings as the most difficult thing about being sick
- Interpreting that God has abandoned oneself
- Interpreting that life is unfair
- Interpreting that life is not worth living

Comparing

- Comparing current disability with past ability
- Comparing current disability with past enjoyment
- Comparing current suffering with past happiness
- Comparing current quality of life with past quality of life
- Comparing the impact of bad news as the stab of a knife

Imagining

- Imagining oneself as a living corpse
- Imagining oneself like being trapped in the hospital
- Imagining oneself like being treated as an experiment
- Imagining oneself like being attacked by pain one after another

Believing

- Believing that one is giving extra work to others
- Believing that the children cannot live without oneself
- Believing that one is socially out
- Believing that nobody is ready to die at a young age
- Believing that nobody can tell how long one can live
- Believing that nobody can understand the suffering
- Believing that suffering is due to actions of past life

- Believing that what other people says of retribution is true
- Believing that one has to answer to God after death
- Believing that there is no reason to live if one cannot recover
- Believing that it is impossible not to worry

Filtering

- Focusing on loss
- Focusing on loss of function
- Focusing on loss of a happy life
- Focusing on burdening of others
- Focusing on worrying about family
- Focusing on pain
- Focusing on side effects of treatment
- Focusing on dying
- Focusing intensively on fear
- Zooming in pain and suffering
- Emphasizing loss of ability to walk
- Emphasizing side effects of treatment
- Mentioning fear repetitively
- Not focusing on what one still can do
- Not focusing on how to live until death

Magnifying

- Magnifying frequent episodes of pain to a life full of suffering
- Magnifying inability to do many things to everything
- Magnifying partial mobility restriction to complete immobility

Catastrophizing

- Catastrophizing current loss to loss of everything in the future
- Catastrophizing that bad things are going to happen one by one

Generalizing

- Generalizing that all doctors are busy
- Generalizing that everybody is scared to die
- Generalizing that nobody can remain fearless at the end of life
- Generalizing that nobody can help

Blaming

- Blaming the disease for poor quality of life
- Blaming the disease for hastening death
- Blaming God for abandoning oneself
- Blaming the devil for causing the disease

Dichotomous thinking

- Either to improve or die
- Either to remain functionally independent or die
- Either to have no pain or die
- Life is either happy or suffering

'Should' thinking

- One should depend on oneself rather than others
- One should take care of family rather than the other way round
- One should work, get married and bear children before dying
- One should do many things in life before dying

Hope and the struggles with acceptance

Hope

- Hoping for cure
- Hoping for life prolongation
- Hoping to live one day at a time
- Hoping for physical independence
- Hoping to be able to take care of oneself

- Hoping to be able to walk around freely
- Hoping for quality of life
- Hoping for a normal life
- Hoping to do many normal things in life
- Hoping to try many things in life
- Hoping to see more people
- Hoping to see the world more
- Hoping that family won't feel so sad
- Hoping to face dying later
- Hoping for hastening of death
- Hoping for death if burdening others
- Wanting to do many things but breathless
- Wanting to have own family before dying
- Wanting to know the entire picture
- Wanting to see the same doctor
- Wanting empathy from the doctor
- Intending to die if not improving
- Intending to die if suffering
- Bargaining to live longer
- Bargaining to live one extra day at a time
- Bargaining to delay death
- Expecting a cure but not possible
- Expecting life prolongation with quality
- Preferring to die if suffering
- Having no hope for recovery

Hope not

- Not wanting the disease
- Not wanting to have cancer
- Not wanting to suffer
- Not wanting to suffer anymore
- Not wanting to depend on others

- Not wanting to be disturbed
- Not wanting family to get sick from caring
- Not wanting family to suffer together
- Not wanting tubes and lines
- Not wanting to lie on hospital bed
- Not wanting to take medications
- Not wanting to wait in the clinic
- Not wanting to be treated like experiment
- Not wanting to eat hospital food
- Not wanting to die with pain
- Not wanting to die by losing bit by bit
- Having to depend on others
- Having to go through side effects of chemotherapy
- Having to wake up because of pain
- Having to walk slowly because of the pain
- Having difficulty in passing time
- Not able to do anything about the pain
- Not able to forget that one is sick
- Not able to sit still for minutes
- Not able to walk for ten minutes

The struggles with acceptance

- Not accepting the disease
- Not accepting the terminality of the disease
- Not accepting pain
- Not accepting the dependence on others
- Not accepting but no choice
- Finding it hard to accept the prognosis
- Feeling unprepared to die
- Completely unprepared to die
- Not scared of dying but not ready to die
- Not believing the told prognosis

- Arguing with the doctor for disparaging one's experience
- Complaining about lack of communication
- Complaining about lack of empathy
- Complaining about lack of care continuity
- Not satisfied with slow nursing service
- Not satisfied with hospital food
- Asking family to go home to rest

Emotions

- Feeling shocked with the diagnosis
- Feeling shocked with the prognosis
- Feeling frustrated with the disease
- Feeling angry and unfair
- Feeling bored with nothing to do
- Fear of no carer
- Fear of burdening others
- Fear of getting infection from friends
- Fear of needles
- Fear of dying
- Fear of suffering
- Fear of suffering but not dying
- Feeling fearful knowing what is cancer
- Feeling scared about many things
- Feeling scared to answer God
- Feeling scared not knowing the prognosis
- Feeling anxious
- Feeling hopeless
- Feeling lonely
- Feeling lonely in the experiencing of pain
- Feeling lonely not knowing where God is
- Feeling unhappy connected to lines
- Feeling sorry to see family having stress

- Feeling sad when diagnosed with cancer
- Feeling sad because of incurability
- Feeling sad for the family
- Feeling sad when thinking about dying
- Feeling depressed
- Feeling devastated to see family sadness
- Feeling terrible because of pain
- Feeling useless

Clinging

Ruminating

- Ruminating about the disease
- Ruminating about the pain
- Ruminating about the changes
- Ruminating about troubling family
- Ruminating about the impact on children
- Ruminating about dying
- Ruminating about dying all the time
- Ruminating about not wanting to die
- Ruminating about not the right time to die
- Ruminating about unfairness of life
- Chain of fearful thoughts
- Chain of worrying thoughts

Worrying

- Worrying about the future of oneself
- Worrying about losing the ability to walk
- Worrying about coping
- Worrying about depending on others
- Worrying about the future of family
- Worrying about the well-being of family

- Worrying about small children
- Worrying about the risk of getting infection

Wondering

- Wondering why there is no forewarning
- Wondering why this is happening
- Wondering how it is possible
- Wondering why me
- Wondering what one has done wrong
- Wondering what to do if one cannot walk
- Wondering how long one has to suffer
- Wondering where God is while in pain
- Not knowing how to describe suffering
- Not knowing what to do
- Not knowing what one is doing
- Not knowing who to turn to
- Not knowing how long one can live

Diagnosing suffering

- Screening question: Are you suffering? (Cassell 1999)

General questions for suffering assessment

- Can you tell me a little about your experience?
- How has this illness affected you physically?
- What about your emotions?
- How have your family been throughout your illness?
- What about your friends?
- How do you find the doctors and nurses here?
- How is it like staying in the hospital?
- What things do you believe in that are important to you now?
- Is there anything else that you would like to share with me about your experience?

Specific questions for suffering assessment

- Existential questions
    - Loss and change
        - Can you tell me a little about the changes in your life because of the sickness?
        - How has your routine changed?
        - Are there specific things that you are planning to do?
    - Dependence on others
        - Tell me a little about your family support
        - How about the support from your friends?
        - How do you feel about their care?
    - Witnessing family suffering
        - What are your concerns for your family?
        - What are their routines now?
        - How is your family coping?
    - Facing terminal disease and death
        - What are your concerns regarding your sickness?
        - What about your treatment?
        - What are your concerns about the future?
    - Healthcare encounter
        - How do you find the communication from doctors and nurses?
        - How would you comment on the level of care you have received?
        - What are your opinions regarding the knowledge and skills of doctors and nurses?
    - Hospital stay
        - How do you find the hospital environment?
        - How do you find the hospital food?
        - What about the hospital facilities?

- Experiential questions
    - Physical experience
        - Tell me about your physical symptoms
        - How have your symptoms affected you?
        - What are your concerns about the symptoms?
    - Emotional experience
        - Tell me a little about your mood when you go through the sickness
        - How are you affected by your emotions?
        - How do you deal with your emotions?
    - Cognitive experience
        - What are your beliefs regarding the sickness?
        - What are your hopes and expectations?
        - How do you come to terms with your sickness?
    - Spiritual experience
        - Are there things that you can't make sense when you experience the sickness?
        - How has your faith affected by the sickness?
        - What support do you look for when life is difficult?

Measuring suffering

- PRISM
    - Pictorial Representation of Illness and Self Measure
    - Measurement of self-illness-separation (SIS)
    - Red disc = illness
    - Yellow disc = self
    - Place red disc on the plate in such as way that it shows which place the illness occupies in one's life
    - SIS = distance between center of "self" and "illness" in cm
    - Range: 0-27cm

- SISC
  - Structured Interview for Symptoms and Concerns
  - 13 items
    - Pain
    - Drowsiness
    - Nausea
    - Weakness
    - Dyspnoea
    - Loss of control
    - Loss of dignity
    - Sense of burden
    - Anxiety
    - Depression
    - Loss of interest
    - Hopelessness
    - Desire for death
- Distress thermometer
  - Measures distress
  - 0 = no distress
  - 10 = extreme distress
- Suffering pictogram
  - Measures overall suffering score
    - Write at center of pictogram
    - 0 = no suffering
    - 10 = worst possible suffering
  - Also measures 8 suffering experiences
    - 0 = none
    - 1 = a little bit
    - 2 = somewhat
    - 3 = quite a bit
    - 4 = a lot

Suffering pictogram

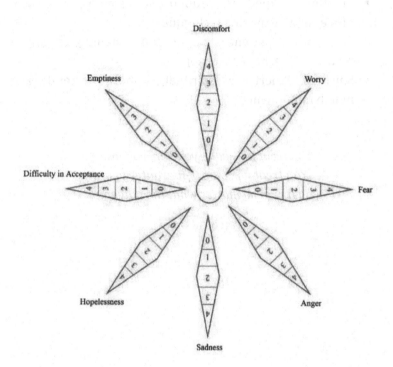

The relief of suffering

- Existential approaches (targeting events)
    - Loss and change: rehabilitation
    - Dependence on others: mobilizing support and resources
    - Witnessing family suffering: care of family caregivers
    - Terminal disease and death: disease-modifying treatment
    - Healthcare encounter: communication training
    - Hospital stay: patient-centered hospital design

- Experiential approaches (targeting experiences)
  - Physical experience: symptom control
  - Emotional experience: supportive listening, emotional processing, relaxation techniques
  - Cognitive experience: supportive listening, cognitive restructuring, hope fostering
  - Spiritual experience: spiritual support, pastoral care, nonabandonment

You treat a disease, you win, you lose.
You treat a person, I guarantee you,
you'll win, no matter what the outcome.

Patch Adams

Psychological Stages of Dying

Introduction

Elisabeth Kübler-Ross described five stages of dying in her 1969 masterpiece – On Death and Dying: What the dying have to teach doctors, nurses, clergy, and their own families.

The five stages

- Denial
- Anger
- Bargaining
- Depression
- Acceptance

Denial

- First reaction may be a temporary state of shock
- Followed by "No, not me, it cannot be true."
- A healthy way of dealing with a painful situation
- Usually a temporary defense
- Will soon be replaced by partial acceptance
- Maintained denial until the end is a rarity
- We should listen, acknowledge and allow them their defenses

Anger

- When the first stage of denial cannot be maintained any longer
- Replaced by feelings of anger, rage, envy and resentment
- The next question becomes: "Why me?"
- "Well, why couldn't it have been him?"
- The anger can be displaced in all directions
- We should not take it personally

Bargaining

- Entering into some sort of an agreement which may postpone the inevitable happening
- "If God has decided to take us from this earth and he did not respond to my angry pleas, he may be more favourable if I ask nicely."
- Wish to be rewarded for good behaviour
- Bargaining for extension of life
- Most bargains are made with God and are usually kept a secret
- The promises may be associated with quiet guilt
- We should not brush aside their remarks
- We should explore any sense of guilt and reasons behind

Depression

- Patient cannot smile it off anymore
- Numbness and stoicism, anger and rage will soon be replaced with a sense of great loss
- Reactive depression
    - A reaction to the disease and loss
    - Address the disease and symptoms
    - Address the loss
    - Encourage patient to look at the bright side
- Preparatory depression
    - A preparatory grief
    - Preparation for final separation from the world
    - Not a result of past loss but impending losses
    - Encouragements and reassurances are not meaningful
    - Allow patient to express his or her sorrow
    - Sit with patient silently
    - No or little need for words
    - Non-verbal: a touch of a hand, a stroking of the hair

Acceptance

- Patient is no longer angry nor depressed
- Has expressed feelings
- Has mourned the impending loss
- Contemplating the coming end with a certain degree of quiet expectation
- Not a happy stage
- Almost void of feelings
- It is as if the pain has gone, the struggle is over
- "The final rest before the long journey"
- Patient wishes to be left alone
- Visitors are often not desired
- Television is off
- We should focus more on non-verbal communication
- Sit in silence
- May reassure that it is alright to say nothing
- May reassure that he or she is not left alone
- Family needs more help during this stage
- A visit in the evening may lend itself best
- It is comforting for the patient to know that he or she is not forgotten

Hope

- The one thing that persists through all the stages
- Even the most accepting patients leave the possibility open for some cure, for the discovery of a new drug or the "last-minute success in a research project"
- This glimpse of hope maintains patients through their suffering
- The feeling that all this must have some meaning, will pay off eventually if they endure it for a little longer
- We should allow them to hope – realistic or unrealistic

Little sharing

My colleague said, "There is no such thing as a difficult patient or a difficult family member. They are just in a difficult situation." It is important not to judge others based on their reactions to a difficult situation because given the same situation, we may react the same too.

Hope in Palliative Care

Introduction

Many doctors think that being terminally ill means hopelessness. This is not true. Hope is present at all times.

What is hope?

> *"Hope" is the thing with feathers*
> *That perches in the soul*
> *And sings the tune without the words*
> *And never stops at all*

> Emily Dickinson

- A desire for a particular thing to happen (Oxford 2010)
- A psychological function of a person that involves the desiring of a particular outcome (Tan 2014)
- A positive motivational state that is based on an interactively derived sense of successful agency [goal-directed energy] and pathways [planning to meet goals] (Snyder 1991)

The theory of hope (Snyder 2000)

- Where there is a will, there is a way
- Will power (agency thinking)
  - The will to shape the future
- Way power (pathway thinking)
  - The ability to see ways to shape the future
- Goals: provide direction and endpoint for hopeful thinking
- Barriers: things that block attainment of goals

Hope assessment

- Will power assessment (agency)
    - Could you tell me a little about your hope?
- Way power assessment (pathway)
    - What are the ways you see that can achieve your hope?

Herth Hope Index

- 12 items
    - I have a positive outlook toward life
    - I have short or long range goals
    - I feel all alone
    - I can see possibilities in the midst of difficulties
    - I have a faith that gives me comfort
    - I feel scared about my future
    - I can recall happy times
    - I have deep inner strength
    - I am able to give and receive love
    - I have a sense of direction
    - I believe that each day has potential
    - I feel my life has value and worth
- The higher the score the higher the level of hope

Types of hope of palliative care patients (Tan 2014)

- Regarding suffering
    - Hope to recover
    - Hope to live longer
    - Hope to stay independent
    - Hope to be discharged
    - Hope to be normal
    - Hope to be pain-free
    - Hope to die peacefully

- Regarding quality of life
    - Hope to do
        - Take care of family
        - Do housework
        - Go for holiday
        - Just sit and relax
        - Be a better person
        - Do charity
    - Hope to see
        - Children grow up, enter university, graduate, get married, bear children
        - Grandchildren grow up, enter university, graduate, get married, bear children
        - Harmony in the family

Hope and well-being

- Hope is a coping mechanism
- It is a positive thought that can fill the gap of a stream of negative thoughts

The change of hope in terminally ill patients

- Initial hope
    - Hope that the news is not true
    - Hope that there is treatment
    - Hope that treatment is effective
    - Hope that treatment is not causing any side effects
- Feeling hopeless when treatment is ineffective
- Subsequent hope
    - Hope for family
    - Hope for symptom control
    - Hope for meaningful time
    - Hope for a peaceful death
    - Hope after death
- Denial and hope (Runbold 1986)
    - First order denial
        - Denial of symptoms
        - Denying the significance of symptoms
        - Ignoring worrying symptoms
        - Enables patient to continue functioning
        - Can delay the seeking or accepting of treatment
        - Do not confront this denial prematurely
        - Give patient some time to sink in
        - First order denial breaks down
            → Hope for recovery (first order hope)
    - Second order denial
        - Denial of non-recovery
        - Often encouraged by doctors
        - Gives medical access to symptoms
        - Enables the suppression of fear of death
        - Can result in resignation and despair later
        - Give patient honest information gently
        - Continue support

- Second order denial breaks down
  → Despair if collusion or lack of support
  → Hope beyond recovery
  (second order hope)
    - Hope to die with dignity
    - Hope for the continuing success of children
    - Hope that partner will find the needed support
    - Hope that life's contribution will continue
- Third order denial
  - Denying the possibility that death will be the end
  - Third order denial breaks down
    → Hope that accepts the existential possibility of extinction at death, but that nevertheless finds a sense of ultimate meaning in the life that has been lived (third order hope)

Sources of hope (Herth 1990)

- Family
- Friends
- Healthcare professionals
- God or higher spiritual being

Obstacles of hope (Herth 1990)

- Abandonment and isolation
- Uncontrolled pain
- Devaluation of personhood

The Zeigarnik effect

- Nagging from the unconscious mind to fulfil a hope
- Stops when a hope is fulfilled or a plan is made
- Recommendations:fulfil patient's hope or give patient a plan

Interventions that engender hope (Herth 1990, Storey 1997)

- Adequate control of symptoms
- Fostering interpersonal connectedness and relationship
- Assistance in attaining practical goals
- Exploring spiritual beliefs
- Supporting and identifying personal attributes, such as determination, courage, and serenity
- Encouraging light-heartedness when appropriate
- Affirming worth by treating the patient as a valued individual
- Recalling uplifting memories with life review

Communicating hope

- It is important NOT to take away patient's hope by
  - Saying "there is no more hope"
  - Saying "there is nothing more can be done"
- Always give hope by saying:
  - I will never leave you in pain
  - I will never abandon you
  - I will never give up hope on you

Realistic and unrealistic hope

- Realistic hope
  - Always provide realistic hope
  - Relieve pain
  - Non-abandonment
  - Fulfil patient's wish
- Unrealistic hope
  - Never give false hope
  - Never destroy patient's hope, realistic or unrealistic
  - Communicate sensitively
  - Give patient time to sink in
  - Hope is never unrealistic from a patient's perspective

Hope from a family perspective (Catherine 2015)

- Hope is a form of strength that is always there and can be passed on from one person to another
- Giving and receiving hope can lead to a positive reaction
- It is important to realize and respect that each individual has their own perception of hope
- Communication and trust will align hopes and expectations

Hope continues to bloom

My mother, the queen of my heart,

Before... any portrait is just in that moment in time

She hopes to do her best and to give everything
So her family is happy and her kids are successful

She hopes to be healthy and active
To be able to enjoy the little things in life

She wants to live as long as possible to see my brother and I get married and have kids

I hope my 'best friend' will never leave my side
So I can always be her little girl

She was diagnosed with lung cancer stage 1
And the prognosis was grim

She hopes to be healthy and recover soon
So she gives her best and is willing to do anything

I hope my 'daughter' will be healthy again
So she can do what she loves like before

She hopes that we will not be worried or unhappy
So she continues smiling

Four months later, after radio and chemotherapy
She is already in stage 4

She hopes to be home with her loved ones
Because she does not know how long she has

I hope I can take her pain and suffering away
For I am so helpless my 'daughter' is suffering

She hopes we will be happy always and taken care of
And wish that someday she would come back as my daughter

We hope that you are happy
and having a wonderful journey wherever you are

For you have given us unconditional LOVE, JOY and HOPE

By Catherine Yee Chiew Huei

Spirituality in Palliative Care

Introduction

Spirituality is one of the most important areas in palliative care. Stricty speaking, palliative care is a form of spiritual care because treating patients as whole persons is spiritual care.

What is spirituality?

- Spirit in Latin: spiritus – breath, life, soul
- Of, or pertaining to, affecting or concerning the spirit or higher moral questions. (Oxford 1988)
- That which is deepest and most genuine in us, the ground of our being, and what we, and others, refer to as spiritual pain is the experience of alienation from this depth. (Saunders 1988)
- Whomever or whatever gives one a transcendent meaning in life. (Puchalski 1999)
- Concerned with an aspect of human nature that is rooted in our experience of relatedness to both an inner and outer world. (Cobb 2003)
- Spirituality is a fundamental element of human experience. It encompasses the individual's search for meaning and purpose in life and the experience of the transcendent. (Puchalski 2009)
- Spirituality is the aspect of humanity that refers to the way individuals seek and express meaning and purpose, and the way they experience their connectedness to the moment, to self, to others, to nature, and to the significant or sacred. (Puchalski 2009)

The meaning of life is to find your gift.
The purpose of life is to give it away.

Pablo Picasso

What is religion?

- The structured and communal aspects of belief related to one's ultimate concern (Hoffman 2008)
- Religion is a formal structure through which a person expresses spirituality within a community
- A religious community is then organized around common beliefs, attitudes, practices, traditions, and relationships

Spirituality and religion

- Not interchangeable
- The spirit is a dimension of personhood
- Religion is a construct of human making that, for some, enables conceptualization and expression of spirituality (Hill 2003)
- Spirituality explains what is important to the life of a person
- Religion is one of the many explanations
- The hand and glove analogue of Jean Radley
  - Hand
    - Spirituality
    - An integral part of human being
  - Glove
    - Religion
    - Some people find a glove that their hand can fit in
    - Some people choose to forgo the glove
- A religious person may still experience spiritual pain
- A spiritual person may have strengths even without a religion

Spiritual components

Existential component (Yalom 1980)

- 4 ultimate concerns:
- Existential freedom
    - The absence of inherent design in the universe
    - We are absolutely responsible for how we live our life
    - We are absolutely responsible for our choices
    - Causes: awareness of this terrifying responsibility, fear of this groundlessness, erecting defences to suppress the fear, passing the responsibility to others in an attempt to escape from the freedom
- Existential isolation
    - The unbridgeable gap between self and others
    - Deeper than loneliness, which is bridgeable
    - Our aloneness in the universe
    - We enter and leave the world alone
    - Causes: recognizing this basic isolation, recognizing that one's death is always solitary, recognizing the terror of feeling that there may be moments when no one in the world is thinking of us, connecting with others to buffer against the experience of existential isolation
    - A deep sense of connection does not solve the problem of existential isolation, but it provides solace
    - An important milestone in therapy is the patient's realization that, "there is a point beyond which the therapist can offer nothing more."
- Meaning
    - Finding meaning in life, although none is absolute and none is given to us
    - We create our own world and have to answer for ourselves why we live and how we shall live

- Causes: searching for meaning and purpose in life, the crisis of meaning seeking, feeling empty, passionless or pointless in life
- The big questions
  - Why me?
  - Why now?
  - Why am I living?
- If all purpose is self-authored, then one must confront the ultimate groundlessness of existence
- We create our own meaning and purpose in life
- Death
  - Existential obliteration
  - Causes: the awareness of our inevitable demise, death anxiety, fear of death, denial of death to suppress fear, projecting ourselves into the future through our children, trying to grow rich and famous, developing compulsive behaviours, or fostering an impregnable belief in an ultimate rescuer
  - Confronting death allows us to live fuller, richer, and more compassionate lives

Connectedness component (Puchalski 2009)

- The sense and experience of connectedness
  - Connectedness to the moment
  - Connectedness to self
  - Connectedness to others
  - Connectedness to nature
  - Connectedness to the significant or sacred

Religious component

- Faith
- Beliefs
- Rituals and practices
- Relationship with God
- Relationship with the ultimate

Spiritual needs (Flannelly 2005)

- Need for meaning and purpose
- Need for love and a sense of belonging
- Need for appreciation of nature and beauty
- Need for positivity, gratitude and peace
- Need for spiritual or religious practices
- Need for resolution of issues involving life and death

Spiritual assessment

- Acronym FICA (Christina Puchalski 1999)

F = Faith

- What do you believe in that gives meaning to your life?

I = Importance

- How important is your faith, religion or spirituality to you?

C = Community

- Are you part of a spiritual or religious community?

A = Address

- How would you like me to address these issues?

- Acronym SPIRIT (Maugans 1997)
  - S = spiritual belief system
  - P = personal spirituality
  - I = integration with a spiritual community
  - R = ritualized practices and restrictions
  - I = implications for medical practices
  - T = terminal events planning
- Acronym HOPE (Anandarajah 2001)
  - H = sources of hope, meaning, comfort, strength, peace, love and compassion
  - O = organized religion
  - P = personal spirituality or practices
  - E = effects on medical care and end-of-life issues
- FACIT-Sp-12 (Version 4)
  - Assess spiritual well-being
  - 12 items
  - I feel peaceful
  - I have a reason for living
  - My life has been productive
  - I have trouble feeling peace of mind
  - I feel a sense of purpose in my life
  - I am able to reach down deep into myself for comfort
  - I feel a sense of harmony within myself
  - My life lacks meaning and purpose
  - I find comfort in my faith or spiritual beliefs
  - I find strength in my faith or spiritual beliefs
  - My illness has strengthened my faith or spiritual beliefs
  - I know that whatever happens with my illness, things will be ok

Spiritual suffering

- Pain deep in your being that is not physical (Mako 2006)
    - Three domains of expression
        - An intrapsychic conflict
        - An interpersonal loss or conflict
        - In relation to the divine
- Pain caused by extinction of the being and the meaning of the self (Murata 2003)
    - Three dimensions
        - A being founded on temporality
        - A being in relationship
        - A being with autonomy
- Arises when there is a gap between a person's innermost sense of value and meaning and the external reality

Types of spiritual suffering

- Existential suffering
    - Existential groundlessness
        - The key existential dynamic is the clash between our confrontation with groundlessness and our wish for ground and structure
        - Experience (Bruce 2011)
            - Being shaken to the core
            - Recognizing life is ending
            - Profound sense of hopelessness
            - Unable to reconcile experience with their faith
            - Not understanding why God is doing this
            - Having one's belief system shattered
            - Experiencing extreme dissonance
            - Feeling of deep despair and unmalleable grief

- Existential loneliness
  - The existential conflict is the tension between the awareness of our isolation and our wish for contact, for protection, our wish to be part of a larger whole
  - Experience
    - The feeling of fundamental aloneness as human
    - Feeling "separated" from the rest of the world
    - Loneliness unrelieved by presence of others
    - Feeling nobody can understand one's feeling
    - Feeling nobody cares
- Meaninglessness
  - Conflict arising from the issue of meaning, stems from the dilemma of a meaning-seeking creature who is thrown into a universe that has no meaning
  - Experience
    - Feeling the lack of meaning and purpose in life
    - Cannot make sense of the suffering
    - Cannot make sense of what is happening
    - Feeling meaningless, hopeless and helpless
    - Feeling empty and futile: existential vacuum
    - Desire to die
- Death anxiety
  - The core existential conflict is the tension between the awareness of the inevitability of death and the wish to continue to be
  - Definitions of death anxiety
    - A negative emotional reaction provoked by the anticipation of a state in which the self does not exist (Tomer 1996)
    - Feeling of dread, apprehension and solicitude (anxiety) when one thinks of the process of dying, or ceasing to be (Farley 2010)

- Experience
  - Fear of death
  - Fear of a painful death
  - Fear of suffering
  - Fear of loss
  - Fear of separation
  - Fear of the unknown
  - Paradoxical desire to hasten death
- Connectedness-related suffering
  - Failure to live in the moment
    - Ruminating excessively about the past
    - Worrying excessively about the future
  - Disrupted self integrity
    - Hopelessness and despair
    - Grief
    - Guilt and shame
  - Impaired sense of belonging
    - Abandonment
    - Loneliness
    - Reconciliation issues
    - Dispute
  - Disconnected from nature
    - Hospital confinement
  - Disrupted spiritual practices
    - Inability to practice spirituality
- Religion-specific
  - Loss of ability to practice religion
    - Inability to pray
    - Inability to meditate
    - Inability to attend religious activities
    - Inability to observe religious ethics
    - Inability to perform rituals

- Loss of faith
  - Feeling unfair
  - Feeling being abandoned by God
  - Feeling angry at God
  - Feeling angry at religious community
  - Challenged belief system
- Religious-specific fear
  - Fear of retribution
  - Fear of punishment
  - Fear of God
- Religious-specific guilt
  - Failure to practice religion
  - Failure to progress
  - Failure to do good
  - Failure to live a moral life
- Interfaith distress
  - Lack of understanding from people of other faiths
  - Distress due to preaching from others
  - Fear of being evangelized
  - Concerns regarding different rituals and ceremonies
  - Dispute due to different faiths in the family

Spiritual care

- Spiritual care is defined as interventions, individual or communal, that facilitate the ability to express the integration of the body, mind, and spirit to achieve wholeness, health, and a sense of connection to self, others, and/or a higher power (Health Minitries Association 2005)
- Spiritual care is care that encourages and supports reflection on experience, the search for meaning and the development of inner resources for the journey

- Responding to spiritual suffering (Kearney 1997)
    - Surface-work
        - Interventions aimed at easing distress at the surface, the conscious and concrete level of an individual's experience
        - Not "superficial", but the way to the deep
        - For many, caring, effective surface-work is also depth-work and all that is needed to bring individuals into depth
    - Depth-work
        - Approach or intervention that brings individual inward and downward toward the deeper layers of the psyche
        - Helping patient to reconnect with those very simple and ordinary aspects of life that have, in the past, brought them a sense of depth or significance
        - This may involve encouraging patients
            - To share memories
            - To spend time with their loved ones
            - To visit a place of special importance to them
            - To return home from the hospital if possible
            - To bring 'home' to the hospital if cannot return
                - Photographs
                - A particular treasured object
    - Depth skills
        - Image work
        - Dream work
        - Art therapy
        - Music therapy
        - Reminiscence and biography therapy
        - Body work (including massage)
        - Meditations

- Control of physical symptoms
- Existential approaches
    - Explore fear of death
    - Explore the meaning of illness and suffering
    - Explore the sources of meaning in patient's life
    - Encourage the search for meaning and purpose
    - Fostering hope
    - Reframing goals and redefining hope
- Connectedness approaches
    - Establish a therapeutic relationship
        - Being presence
        - Supportive listening
        - Understanding suffering
        - Working with love
    - Practice non-abandonment
    - Encourage life review
    - Explore guilt, shame, remorse and regret
    - Explore the need for reconciliation
    - Encourage mindful practices to connect to the moment
    - Encourage engagement in art and music if appropriate
- Religious approaches
    - Facilitate religious expression
    - Facilitate ritual practices
    - Encourage prayers that assist healing
    - Encourage meditative practices that focus on healing
    - Involve chaplain or spiritual care workers

Specific therapy for spiritual suffering

- Existential therapy (Yalom 1980)
- Meaning-centered group therapy (Breitbart 2010)
- Dignity therapy (Chochinov 2005)
- Mindfulness-based supportive therapy (Tan 2015)

UNIPAC's acronym for spiritual care: LET GO (Storey 1997)

- Listen to the patient's story
- Encourage the search for meaning
- Tell of your concern and acknowledge the pain of loss
- Generate hope whenever possible
- Own your limitation and refer when appropriate

Life Review

Introduction

Life review is a structured evaluation of one's life with the intention to derive a sense of meaning and purpose from the recalled memories.

Life review and reminiscence (Butler 1963)

- Life review
  - Structured
  - Involves one or more life themes
  - Evaluative process
    - To derive a sense of meaning and purpose
    - To come to terms with difficult memories
- Reminiscence
  - Unstructured
  - Involves spontaneous recall of memories
  - Passive process
  - May be part of life review but not synonymous

Everybody is a story. When I was a child, people sat around kitchen tables and told their stories. We don't do that so much anymore. Sitting around the table telling stories is not just a way of passing time. It is the way the wisdom gets passed along. The stuff that helps us to live a life worth remembering.

Rachel Naomi Remen

Techniques (Butler 1963)

- Patients are asked to describe important life events
    - Time periods
        - Childhood
        - Adolescence
        - Adulthood
        - Present situation
    - Life events
        - Schooling
        - Working
        - Marriage
        - Parenting
        - Illness
- Use of mementos to enhance life review
    - Music
    - Scrapbooks
    - Photos
    - Letters
    - Cherished possessions
    - Family trees
- Create a legacy from life review
    - Audio
    - Video
    - Notebooks
    - Album with pictures
- Review the creation with patient and family
- Facilitate
    - Expression of emotions
    - Finding meaning from recalled memories
    - Coming to terms with difficult memories
    - Closure

Existential Therapy

Introduction

Existential therapy is a way of thinking about human experience. It is a philosophical approach to therapy that assumes we are free to choose and are responsible for our choices.

Basic concepts (Yalom 1980)

- Based on principles of humanistic and existential psychology
  - Humanism: emphasizes the whole person
  - Existentialism: emphasizes the four ultimate concerns of human existence
    - Existential freedom
    - Existential isolation
    - Meaninglessness
    - Death
- Assists patient
  - In confronting the ultimate concerns
    - Freedom and responsibility
    - Loneliness and loss
    - Meaninglessness and suffering
    - Death and finitude
  - To live more fully in each moment
- Focuses on
  - The person as the center of the therapeutic process
  - The subjective experience of self
  - The will and intentionality
  - The therapeutic encounter
  - The here-and-now

Existential maturity (Spira 2000)

- Hermeneutic basis of the self
  - The "self" arises from social interpretations formed from a lifetime of social conditioning
- Inauthentic assumptions of our self and our world
  - Our assumptions of our "self" and our "world" are merely mental constructions
  - We assume our "self" as fixed, stable entity
  - We assume our "world" as fixed, predictable world
  - These are inauthentic assumptions
- Breakdown of inauthentic assumptions
  - External crisis can lead to the breakdown of assumptions
  - Breakdown of our habitual assumptions leads to either covering up of the breakdown by fleeing into conveniently provided alternative social conventions and returning to inauthentic assumptions; or to existential anxiety (Angst) and feeling of a sense of dissociated depersonalization (Unheimlicheit)
- Moment of vision
  - Becoming aware of the inauthentic assumptions one has been making unconsciously in one's life
  - One may realize that they have done nothing that is truly rewarding but only things that the society or others expect of them
- Authentic commitment
  - Reevaluation of how one wants to live more fully in the remaining time
  - Choosing life acivities that will bring greatest meaning, purpose and value to one's life

- The severity of the external disruption corresponds to the extent to which assumptions breakdown (live as it has been lived), corresponds to the extent which one will recognize prior assumptions (habitual, nonchosen activities), which in turn corresponds to the extent to which new activities can be authentically chosen for greatest meaning, purpose and value in one's life

Methods of existential therapy (Spira 2000)

- Establish an authentic relationship
    - Establish rapport
        - The therapeutic stance
            - "The fellow traveller"
            - Not doctor and patient
            - Not therapist and client
            - We are all in this together
        - Sharing the essence of human conditions
        - Treat encounter as a learning experience for both
        - Active listening
        - Non-judgmental acceptance of the patient
            - Acknowledge beliefs
            - Acknowledge emotions
            - Acknowledge existential concerns
            - Acknowledge potential for existential maturity
    - Ask questions that encourage exploration of existential issues and development of existential maturity
        - What is important to you in the time you have left?
        - Are there things you would like to do for yourself that are not what others expect from you?

- Ask questions that encourage open intimacy with self and others that lead to existential process
  - Cognitive openness
    - Acceptance versus denial
    - Question: Can you give me a specific example of how that affects you personally?
  - Affective openness
    - Integrated feeling versus repression
    - Question: How does that make you feel?
  - Interpersonal
    - Open expression versus isolation
    - Question: Can you tell your family your fears about losing control?
  - Active coping
    - Explore ways to deal with what one can control and let go of what one cannot control
    - Question: What can you do to lessen your pain?
- Facilitate the breakdown
  - Acknowledge patient's suffering and explore the basis of such suffering rather than helping to cover up patient's distress
  - Assist in making unconscious assumptions conscious
    - Facilitate the development of "lateral perspective"
      - How do family members view what is going on?
      - How do friends view what is going on?
      - How do doctors view what is going on?
      - How do other patients view what is going on?
    - Facilitate appreciation of the idea that any view is personally created over a lifetime, rather than mirroring a "realistic" view of the world
    - Facilitate suspension of patient's fixed view of self and life to explore ways that allow adjustment

- Another way to facilitate the breakdown is to discuss death and dying openly

Exercise 1: Living in the face of dying

- If you have one year (month, week) to live and you want to make it the most meaningful year of your life
  - What personal characteristics (self-image, personality, assumptions about life) would you want to let go of?
  - What activities would you let go of that you find more of a burden than a joy?
  - What personal characteristics would you want to have to help you make this year a valuable one for you?
  - What activities would you want to engage in that would bring greatest meaning and value to your life?
  - What is stopping you from having these qualities and doing these activities now?
  - What can you do to overcome these barriers to live more fully?

Exercise 2: Identifying beliefs that limit ability to live fully

- When was this belief developed? Under what circumstances did you form this belief?
  - How did this belief help you at that time? How does this belief still help you now?
  - How has this belief limited you in the past? How does this belief limit you at this time?
  - What is an alternative belief that would help you at this time, and would keep the habit belief in check?
  - In what situations will the old belief influence you, and what will help you recall the alternative belief?

Exercise 3: Being in the moment

- Can you describe the present state?
- Can you discuss what you feel in your body?
- What do you see in the room?
- What sounds come to your ears?
- How do you feel in the relationship with the therapist?
- Patients can practice this each day for one minute and then use this "presencing" method to become calm whenever they start "thinking too much"

- Support a "moment of vision"
    - A moment of vision occurs when patients realize they are more than their limited view of themselves
    - They also come to appreciate that they contain all the resources they have from their entire lives, releasing their full potential for acting
    - Must allow full grieving to occur, supporting the state of despair, until such time as the patient can fully accept his or her condition without attempting to flee it
    - Must be kept in mind that different patients will have different capacities for existential maturation
    - Must be flexible enough to support patients in the way that works best for them
- Encourage the pragmatic development of commitment
    - Promote active strategies to develop meaningful actions in the patient's life
    - Assist patients in reprioritizing life activities

Exercise 4: reprioritizing life activities

- Make a list of activities you spend your time doing during a typical week

- Prioritize this list, with the activities you spend most time with at the top and those you spend less time on toward the bottom
- Prioritize these activities again, but this time list at the top the activities that bring more meaning and personal value to your life, with progressively less meaningful activities toward the bottom. To the list can also be added any activities you wish you were doing, even though you have not gotten around to them
- Examine the last two columns. If the lists are ordered differently, then it is important to ask what you can do to spend more time engaged in those activities that bring more meaning and value to your life and less in activities that you do out of habit

Principles of existential psychotherapy (Spira 2000)

- Development of an authentic relationship between therapist and patient, and between patient and others
- The valuing of patient experience, resources, and capacity for development at any point in life
- The importance of facilitating the breakdown of conditioned habitual assumptions about life
- Assisting patients to accept their suffering and potential for death without attempting to cover up
- Helping patients to trust in the present moment as the fullest experience possible in life
- Engaging in activities that bring greatest meaning, purpose, and value to one's life

Meaning-centered Therapy

Introduction

Meaning-centered therapy or logotherapy was developed by Viktor Frankl, an Austrian neurologist, psychiatrist as well as a Holocaust survivor. A short introduction to the therapy was given in his famous book, Man's Search for Meaning.

Basic concepts

- Logos = "meaning" in Greek
- Less retrospective compared to psychoanalysis
- Less introspective compared to psychoanalysis
- Focuses on the meaning to be fulfilled by patient in the future
- Primary motivational force in human
    - Freudian psychoanalysis: will to pleasure
    - Adlerian psychotherapy: will to power
    - Logotherapy: will to meaning
- Human's will to meaning can lead to existential frustration
    - Existential frustration = an existential distress
    - Not pathological
    - Not pathogenic
    - Not a mental disease
    - Can result in noögenic neurosis (vs psychogenic neurosis)
- Logotherapy assists patient to find meaning in his or her life

He who has a why to live for can bear almost any how

Nietzsche

Logodrama

- A technique based on logotherapy for discovering meaning and responding meaningfully to a life situation
- Dramatization of an imagined experience in the here-and-now
- Stages
    - Present-moment awareness
        - Awareness of bodily sensations
        - Awareness of thoughts
        - Awareness of emotions
    - Engagement
        - Counters the instinct to run away from emotions
        - Counters the instinct to run away from a person
        - Counters the instinct to run away from a situation
    - Stepping back
        - Allows one to see the situation subjectively
        - To find the choice between stimulus and response
    - Expectant presence
        - To look for meaning of what the situation is about in terms of values
        - To respond in a way that makes life worth living

Meaning-centered group psychotherapy (Breitbart 2010)

- A psychoeducational model
- Developed from logotherapy
- Designed for patients with life-threatening illness
- 6-8 weekly sessions
- 90min sessions
- Includes
    - Teachings on the philosophy of meaning
    - Discussion of topic such as "good death"
    - Engagement in experiential exercises
    - Home exercises that reinforce similar themes

- Themes
  - Summary of concepts and sources of meaning
  - Cancer and meaning
  - Meaning derived from historical context in life
  - Meaning derived from attitudinal values
  - Meaning derived from creative values and responsibility
  - Meaning derived through experiential values
  - Termination and feedback

Dignity Therapy

Introduction

Dignity therapy is a brief, individualized psychotherapeutic intervention designed to address psychosocial and existential distress among terminally ill patients.

Three major domains of dignity (Chochinov 2002)

- Illness-related concerns that influence dignity
  - Physical distress
  - Psychological distress
  - Cognitive acuity
  - Functional capacity
  - Medical uncertainty
  - Death anxiety
- Dignity conserving repertoire
  - Dignity conserving perspectives
    - Continuity of self
    - Role preservation
    - Generativity
    - Maintenance of pride
    - Hopefulness
    - Autonomy and control
    - Acceptance
    - Resilience and fighting spirit
  - Dignity conserving practices
    - Living in the moment
    - Maintaining normalcy
    - Seeking spiritual comfort

- Social dignity inventory
  - Privacy boundaries
  - Social support
  - Care tenor
  - Burden to others
  - Aftermath concerns

Dignity themes (Chochinov 2005)

- Generativity
  - The notion that, for some patients, dignity is intertwined with a sense that one's life has stood for something or has some influence transcendent of death
  - Implication: sessions are tape-recorded and transcribed, with an edited transcript or "generativity document" being returned to patient to bequeath to a friend or family member
- Continuity of self
  - Being able to maintain a feeling that one's essence is intact despite advancing illness
  - Implication: patients are invited to speak to issues that are foundational to their sense of personhood or self
- Role preservation
  - Being able to maintain a sense of identification with one or more previously held roles
  - Implication: patients are questioned about previous or currently held roles that may contribute to their core identity
- Maintenance of pride
  - An ability to sustain a sense of positive self-regard
  - Implication: providing opportunities to speak about previous accomplishments or achievements that engender a sense of pride

- Hopefulness
  - Hopefulness relates to the ability to find or maintain a sense of meaning or purpose
  - Implication: patients are invited to engage in a therapeutic process intended to instill a sense of meaning and purpose
- Aftermath concerns
  - Worries or fears concerning the burden or challenges that their death will impose on others
  - Implication: inviting the patient to speak to issues that might prepare their loved ones for a future without them
- Care tenor
  - Refers to the attitude and manner with which others interact with the patient that may or may not promote dignity
  - The tenor of dignity therapy is empathic, nonjudgmental, encouraging and respectful

Dignity psychotherapy question protocol (Chochinov 2005)

- Tell me a little about your life history; particularly the parts that you either remember most or think are the most important? When did you feel most alive?
- Are there specific things that you would want your family to know about you, and are there particular things you would want them to remember?
- What are the most important roles you have played in life (family roles, vocational roles, community-service roles, etc)? Why were they so important to you, and what do you think you accomplished in those roles?
- What are your most important accomplishments, and what do you feel most proud of?

- Are there particular things that you feel still need to be said to your loved ones or things that you would want to take your time to say once again?
- What are your hopes and dreams for your loved ones?
- What have you learned about life that you would want to pass along to others? What advices or words of guidance would you wish to pass along to your (son, daughter, husband, wife, parents, others)?
- Are there words or perhaps even instructions that you would like to offer your family to help prepare them for the future?
- In creating this permanent record, are there other things that you woud like to include?

Well-being of Palliative Care Patients

Introduction

Relieving suffering and increasing well-being are interrelated but not equal. We may be very good in relieving suffering of patients but not very good in making them happy.

Types of well-being

- Hedonic well-being
  - Advocates maximizing pleasure and minimizing pain
  - Model of subjective well-being (Diener 1984)
    - Subjective well-being (SWB) = high level of positive affect (maximizing pleasure) + low level of negative affect (minimizing pain) + high degree of life satisfaction
- Eudaimonic well-being
  - Single-minded pursuit of sensory pleasure and avoidance of pain does not lead to a lasting form of well-being
  - True well-being is found by living a virtuous life
  - Multiple models
    - Psychological well-being (Ryff 1995)
      - Self-acceptance
      - Personal growth
      - Positive relationships
      - Autonomy
      - Purpose in life
      - Environmental mastery
    - Self-determination theory (Deci 2000)
      - Competence
      - Relatedness

- Autonomy
- The theory of flow (Csikszentmihalyi 1975)
  - Flow denotes the holistis sensation present when we act with total involvement
  - Characteristics of flow (Nakamura 2002)
    - Intense and focused concentration
    - Merging of action and awareness
    - Loss of self-consciousness
    - A sense of control
    - Distortion of temporal experience
    - Experience of the activity as intrinsically rewarding (autotelic experience)
- The authentic happiness model (Seligman 2011)
  - Positive emotions
  - Engagement
  - Meaningful life
  - Positive relationships
  - Positive accomplishments

Types of well-being of palliative care patients (Tan 2014)

- Attitudinal well-being
  - Positive attitude: the psychological tendency of a person to think, feel, or act in a particular way that is conducive to his or her own well-being
    - Acceptance: an attitude that allows things to happen as it is without any denial or resistance
    - Kindness: an attitude characterized by the concern for others
    - Resilience: the universal capacity which allows a person to overcome the damaging effects of adversity (Newman 2004)

- Volitional well-being
    - Positive volitional activities
        - Positive cognitions: thoughts that contribute to one's own well-being
            - Hope: a psychological function of a person that involves the desiring of a specific outcome
            - Optimism: the positive view of a person that enables him or her to interpret events with the best possible explanation that is conducive to his or her own well-being
            - Faith: the confident belief in something that gives the person energy to move forward irrespective of the direness of the situations
            - Wisdom: the awareness of a person regarding the truth of a situation or an experience and the ways to deal with it
        - Positive emotions: emotions that contribute to one's own well-being
            - Happiness: a pleasant emotion that occurs when one is involved in a relationship, activity, or thought that is perceived by him or her as pleasurable or meaningful
            - Calmness: an emotion that occurs when one is completely or partially free from negative thoughts or emotions
        - Positive engagement: the active participation of a person in activities that promote well-being
            - Routine activities: customary activities
            - Leisure activities: enjoyable activities
        - Positive relationships: supportive relationships
            - Practical support
            - Psychological support

- Perceptual well-being
  - Positive circumstances: situations that contribute to the well-being of a person
    - Symptom-free
    - Functional

Six approaches to enhance well-being (Tan 2014)

- Attitudinal interventions
  - Facilitate acceptance
  - Foster kindness
  - Promote resilience
- Cognitive interventions
  - Foster hope
  - Support optimism
  - Strengthen faith
  - Acknowledge wisdom
- Emotional interventions
  - Conduct practices that promote happiness
  - Conduct practices that promote calmness
- Behavioural interventions
  - Encourage engagement in meaningful routines
  - Encourage engagement in enjoyable activities
- Interpersonal interventions
  - Mobilize practical support
  - Mobilize psychological support
- Circumstantial interventions
  - Symptom control
  - Support making full use of remaining functions

Caregiver Suffering

Introduction

Suffering affects both patients and family caregivers reciprocally. However, family caregivers are often left out by healthcare professionals, to the degree that we can label their suffering as "disenfranchised suffering". Family caregivers are "second-order patients" with their own care needs requiring medical attention.

The model of compassion suffering (Tan 2013)

- Compassion is the perception of another's suffering, coupled with the intention and action to relieve it
- Compassion suffering is a state of severe distress associated with caring of another person
  - Perception component
  - Intention component
  - Action component
- Perception component
  - Empathic suffering
    - Empathic suffering from seeing
      - Seeing suffering of patient
        - Physical suffering
        - Functional decline
        - Emotional suffering
        - Treatment-related suffering
        - Death and dying
      - Seeing family stress
        - Tiredness in the family
        - Sadness in the family
        - Denial in the family

- Seeing suffering of other patients
    - Abandonment by family
- Empathic suffering from hearing
    - Hearing bad news from doctors
        - Terminal diagnosis
        - Abnormal blood results
        - Disease progression
        - Additional chemotherapy
        - Coma
        - Short prognosis
    - Hearing expression of suffering from patient
        - Expression of unbearable suffering
        - Expression of the desire to give up
        - Expression of death and dying
- Empathic suffering from worrying
    - Worrying about patient
        - Pain and suffering
        - Nutritional status
        - Complications
        - Side effects of treatment
        - Prognosis
    - Worrying about other family members
        - Grief in the family
- Anticipatory grief
    - Perceived impending death of patient
        - Perceptions
            - Recognizing dying
                - Knowing the incurability of sickness
                - Hearing treatment discontinuation
            - Witnessing dying
                - Seeing patient deteriorate
                - Seeing patient eat less

- Seeing patient talk less
- Seeing patient sleep most of the time
- Seeing patient unresponsive
- Cognitions
  - Hopes for patient
    - Hope for cure
    - Hope for survival
    - Hope for function
    - Hope for quality of life
    - Hope for a good after-life
    - Hopelessness
  - Hopes for oneself
    - Hope to return to a normal life
    - Hope to be with patient
  - Beliefs
    - Belief in staying positive
    - Belief in decision of God
  - Denial
    - Complete denial
    - Partial denial
- Emotions
  - Shock
  - Fear
  - Anxiety
  - Sadness
  - Frustration
  - A mixture of emotions
- Perceived impending absence of patient
  - Current absence
    - Absence of company for daily activities
    - Absence of company at home
    - Absence of company for talking

- Absence of company for support
- Role substitution
- Perceived absence when patient can't talk
- Future absence
  - Anticipated loneliness
  - Anticipated quietness
  - Anticipated sadness
  - Anticipated aimlessness
  - Anticipated supportlessness
  - Anticipated life changes
  - Concerns about new life without patient
- Intention component
  - Obsessive-compulsive suffering
    - Compassion obsession
      - Obsession with giving the best care
      - Obsession with giving 24-hour company
      - Obsession with pleasing patient
      - Obsession with motivating patient
      - Ignoring career
      - Ignoring job and income
      - Ignoring own social life
      - Ignoring own health
      - Concealing own grief
      - Concealing own exhaustion
      - Avoidance of discussing sickness with patient
      - Avoidance of discussing death with patient
    - Existential obsession
      - Obsession with keeping patient alive
        - Seeking multiple medical opinions
        - Seeking alternative medicine
        - Seeking various nutritional supplements
        - Pressurizing medical team to treat

- Promising to do good
- Performing life-prolonging rituals
- Praying for miracle
- Willingness to sacrifice own life
- Doing compulsion
  - Compulsion to do something for patient
    - Not comfortable in doing nothing
    - Not comfortable in sitting down and cry
    - Doing something without knowing benefit
    - Doing something despite own exhaustion
- Helpless-powerless suffering
  - Lack of information
    - Not knowing what to do
      - When patient is getting weaker
      - When patient is dying
      - When patient is not eating
      - When patient is not talking
      - When patient is restless
      - When patient is in pain
      - When patient insists to go home
    - Not knowing what to say
      - When patient expresses
        - Unberable suffering
        - Burdening of family
        - Knowledge about impending death
        - Desire to give up
        - Desire to die
        - Unwillingness to die
    - Not knowing what to expect
    - Not knowing how long patient can live

- Lack of support
  - Lack of support
    - Assisting patient functionally
    - Temporary relief
    - Overnight relief
    - Home medical support
    - Home nursing support
  - Difficulty to get support
    - Everyone has own commitment
    - Lack of leave during year end
    - Dispute in scheduling care
    - Fear of troubling others
    - Belief that help should be voluntary
  - Dissatisfaction with support
    - Nonsupportive family
    - Family is not doing enough
      - Not talking to patient
      - Not motivating patient
      - Not cheering patient up
  - Criticism from family and friends
    - Criticism in the way of caring
    - Criticism in sacrificing own job for caring
- Action component
  - Obligatory suffering
    - Companionship burden
      - 24-hour company
      - Overnight company
      - Final days company
      - Final moments presence
    - Functional burden
      - Functional assistance
        - Activities of daily living

- - Instrumental activities
  - Unfinished business
  - Decision input
- Financial burden
  - Expenses
    - Treatment
    - Hospitalization
    - Medical equipment
    - Traditional medicine
    - Daily necessities like milk and diapers
- Cheer-making burden
  - Making patient happy
    - Family gatherings
    - Outdoor activities
- Impedimental suffering
  - Patient-related obstacles
    - Difficult circumstances
      - Excessive dependence
      - Bad temper
      - Conflict in opinion
      - Desire to die
      - Confusion state
      - Withdrawal from external world
    - Lack of appreciation from patient
    - Complaints from patient
  - Family-related obstacles
    - Family conflict
      - Continuation vs stopping treatment
      - Conventional vs alternative treatment
      - Different alternative medicine options
      - Different levels of acceptance in the family
      - Different levels of involvement

- Different ways of caring
- Healthcare-related obstacles
  - Information issues
    - Lack of medical information
      - Disease
      - Complications
      - Side effects of treatment
      - Updates on progress of patient
    - Lack of opportunity to meet doctors
  - Interaction issues
    - Poor communication
      - Lack of listening
      - Lack of sensitivity
      - Lack of hope-giving
      - Lack of nonabandonment statement
      - Told "nothing much can be done"
      - Paternalistic communication
    - Lack of empathy
    - Lack of compassion
    - Poor attitude
  - Institution issues
    - Long waiting time
    - Noisy hospital environment
    - Witnessing suffering of other patients
    - Witnessing death of other patients
- Repercussion suffering
  - Personal life repercussion
    - Physical exhaustion
    - Psychological exhaustion
      - Sadness
      - Worry
      - Rumination

- Guilt
- Regret
- Fear
- Countertransferences
    - Fear of getting cancer
    - Fear of dying
    - Fear of burdening family in the future
- Sleep disturbances
- Loss of freedom
- Loss of personal time
- Spiritual suffering
    - Questioning "Why me?"
    - Questioning God
- Social life repercussion
    - Loss of family life
    - Loss of socialization with friends
    - Loss of recreational activities
    - Loss of promotion
    - Loss of job

The relief of caregiver suffering

- Perception approaches
    - Empathic suffering
        - Palliation of patient's suffering
    - Anticipatory grief
        - Supportive listening
- Intention approaches
    - Obsessive-compulsive suffering
        - Self-care emphasis
        - Supportive listening
        - Shift of curing to caring duties

- Helpless-powerless suffering
  - Information giving
  - Mobilizing support
- Action approaches
  - Obligatory suffering
    - Mobilizing support
    - Respite care
  - Impedimental suffering
    - Conflict resolution
    - Family meeting
    - Communication training of healthcare providers
  - Repercussion suffering
    - Self-care emphasis
    - Social connection encouragement

Little advices

- Pay attention to family caregivers
- Explore caregiver suffering
- Remind caregivers to take care of themselves too
- Remind caregivers to **EAT**, **SLEEP** and **RELAX**
- Teach caregivers to practice mindful caregiving as opposed to automatic caregiving

Mindful caregiving:

Paying attention to caregiving on purpose
Paying attention in the present moment
Paying attention nonjudgmentally

Grief and Bereavement

Introduction

Most bereaved family members require no specific intervention. They recover with the support of family and friends, and time. Only 10-20% of family members who remain stuck in their grief require further assistance.

Terms

- Grief: the distressing emotional response to any loss, including related feelings, cognitions and behaviours (Genevro 2004)
- Bereavement: the state of having experienced a loss resulting from death (Genevro 2004)
- Mourning: the process of adaptation to a loss, which includes expression of grief and behaviours influenced by culture, religion, and social evens, such as grieving rituals (Raphael 1983)
- Anticipated grief: the distress and related emotions, cognitions, and behaviours that occur before an expected loss (Raphael 1983)
- Pathological grief: a severely distressing and disabling abnormal emotional response to loss that involves mental and physical dysfunction (Jacobs 1993)
- Disenfranchised grief: grief that occurs with losses that are not recognized by society, resulting in less social permission to express one's grief (Doka 1989)

Theories of grief and bereavement

- The four phases of grief (Bowlby 1973, Parkes 1998)
    - Phase 1: shock and numbness
        - Feeling that the loss is not real
        - Feeling impossible to accept
        - Somatic symptoms
        - Emotional shut-down if stuck
    - Phase 2: yearning and searching
        - Acutely aware of the void left from the loss
        - The imagined future is no longer possible
        - Searching for comfort one used to have together
        - Trying to fill the void
        - Preoccupied with the person
        - Looking for reminders of the person
        - Looking for ways to be close to the person
        - Remain preoccupied with the person if stuck
    - Phase 3: despair and disorganization
        - Accepted the irreversible loss
        - Hopelessness and despair
        - Anger and questioning
        - Feeling meaningless without the person
        - Remain negative and hopeless if stuck
    - Phase 4: reorganization and recovery
        - Faith in life restored
        - New goals and patterns of day-to-day life established
        - Realizing that life can still be positive
        - Grief continues to influence oneself but no longer at the forefront of the mind

- The five phases of grief (Lindemann 1994)
    - Somatic disturbances
    - Preoccupation with the image of the deceased
    - Guilt, reviewing behaviour that occurred before the death for evidence of negligence or failure
    - Feeling of hostility or anger
    - Difficulty in carrying out everyday routines
- The five stages of grief (Kübler-Ross 1969)
    - Denial
    - Anger
    - Bargaining
    - Depression
    - Acceptance
- The four tasks of mourning (Worden 1991)
    - Task 1: to accept the reality of loss
    - Task 2: to work through and experience the pain of grief
    - Task 3: to adjust to an environment without the deceased
    - Task 4: to withdraw emotionally from or relocate the deceased and move on
- The dual process model of coping with bereavement (Stroebe and Schut 1999)
    - Loss-orientated processes
        - Grief work
        - Intrusion of grief
        - Denial or avoidance of restoration changes
        - Breaking bonds or ties
    - Restoration-orientated processes
        - Attending to life changes
        - Distraction from grief
        - Doing new things
        - Establishing new roles/identities/relationships

Prolonged grief disorder (Prigerson 2009)

- Bereavement: loss of a significant other
- Separation distress: yearning daily or to a disabling degree
- ≥ 5 symptoms
    - Confusion about one's role in life or diminished sense of self (feeling that a part of oneself has died)
    - Difficulty accepting the loss
    - Avoidance of reminders of the reality of the loss
    - Inability to trust others since the loss
    - Bitterness or anger related to the loss
    - Difficulty moving on with life
    - Numbness
    - Feeling that life is unfulfilling, empty, and meaningless
    - Feeling stunned, dazed, or shocked by the loss
- > 6 months since the death
- Social impairment
- No Major Depressive Disorder, Generalized Anxiety Disorder or Posttraumatic Stress Disorder

Addressing grief and bereavement

- Before death
    - Communicate prognosis timely and sensitively
    - Prepare family
    - Allow family to grieve
    - Facilitate expression of grief if suppressed
- At the time of death
    - Allow family to see the deceased before last office
    - Allow family time to grieve before last office
    - Give practical information on procedures after death
- After death
    - Follow up contact
        - Condolences phone call

- Sympathy card
- Home visits
- Attending funeral if appropriate
- Annual commemoration services
- Grief and bereavement counseling
  - Bereaved individuals who request help
  - High risk bereaved individuals
  - Prolonged grief disorders

Self-care

Introduction

Caring of oneself and caring of others are inseparable. If we cannot take good care of ourselves, we cannot take good care of others. If we ourselves are unhappy, it will be hard for us to make others happy, more so in terminally ill patients.

Stress

- Definitions of stress
    - The non-specific response of the body to any demand for change (Selye 1956)
    - Non-specific: different noxious stimuli → similar response
    - A constellation of physiological, cognitive, emotional and behavioural reactions as a person is confronted with perceived threat and challenges (Harrington 2013)
- Stressor: an event that provokes stress
- Acute stress reaction: fight-or-flight response (Cannon 1932)
- Chronic stress reaction (Selye 1956)
    - General adaptation syndrome
        - Alarm stage
        - Resistance stage
        - Exhaustion stage
- Types of stress
    - Eustress: positive stress
    - Distress: negative stress
- Sources of stress
    - Major life events or daily hassles
    - Internal or self-generated

The transactional model of stress and coping

- By Lazarus and Folkman 1984
- Stress is a transaction (two-way process) between a person and the situation in the form of cognitive appraisals
- Primary appraisal
  - The relevant significance of the situation as a threat
    - Motivational relevance: relevance of the situation to the person own well-being
    - Motivation congruence: congruence of the situation with the person's goals
  - Stress is the perceived discrepancy between what one has in a given situation and what one wants in that situation
- Secondary appraisal: the capacity of the person to cope
  - Problem-focused coping: the capacity to improve the situation so that it is more congruent with one's goals
  - Emotion-focused coping: the capacity to adapt to the situation when the situation remains incongruent with one's goals

Types of stressors in palliative care (Vachon 1995)

- Personal factors
  - Age
  - Sex
  - Ethnicity
  - Family status
  - Financial status
  - Work experiences
  - Qualifications
  - Personal values
  - Coping styles
  - Social support

- Work factors
  - Work environment problems
    - Communication problems within the organization
    - Inadequate resources
    - Unrealistic expectations of the system
  - Role problems
    - Role strain
    - Role ambiguity
    - Role conflict
  - Patient-family problems
    - Dealing and communicating with dying patients
    - Dealing and communicating with young patients
    - Dealing and communicating with non-coping family

Cognitive appraisals of palliative care providers

- Primary appraisals
  - Perceived mismatch between the person and the working environment
  - Perceived imbalance between job demands, job resources and workplace support
- Secondary appraisals
  - Problem-focused coping
    - Good communication with patients
    - Good communication with family members
    - Good communication with colleagues
    - Being connected with patients
    - Practice of exquisite empathy
    - Optimism
    - Self-efficacy
    - Receiving social support
  - Emotion-focused coping
    - Positive reinterpretation

- Meaning making
- Humour
- Practice of mindfulness
- Healthy lifestyle engagement
- Turning to religion
- Praying
- Taking a break

The Total Care Model of Palliative Care Stress (Tan 2013)

- Stress of palliative care providers
    - Problems in caring for others (healthcare)
    - Problems in interacting with others (interpersonal care)
    - Problems in caring for oneself (self-care)
- Healthcare
    - Organizational challenges
        - Team dysfunction
            - Lack of shared team philosophy
            - Lack of caring attitude in team members
            - Lack of team cooperation
            - Lack of competence in team members
            - Lack of team communication
            - Lack of team support
            - Inter-team dispute
        - Resources, staffing and working environment
            - Lack of hospital resources
            - Lack of staffing
            - Lack of understanding of the complex system
    - Care overload
        - Heavy workloads
            - Incapacity to attend to all distressed patients
            - Multiple calls from patients and family
            - Time-consuming nature of the work of caring

- - Too many orders from the superior
  - Difficult encounters
    - Uncontrolled pain
    - Repetitive requests for more analgesia
    - Difficult branula insertions
    - Unrealistic expectations from patients or family
    - Request for hastening of death
    - Pressure from family to monitor closely
    - Pressure from family to do everything possible
    - Pressure from family to give futile treatment
    - Family interfering with treatment decisions
    - Family giving instructions for doctors to follow
    - Family's impatience
    - Family's inability to accept patient's death
    - Family's begging to hasten patient's death
    - Too many visiting family members
- Interpersonal care
  - Communication challenges
    - With patients
      - Communicating prognosis
      - Dealing with strong emotions
      - Dealing with strong denial
      - Dealing with difficult questions
      - Lack of time to build rapport
      - Repetitive listening to patient's suffering
      - Language barrier
      - Attending to non-communicative patients
    - With family members
      - Being asked too many questions
      - Different relatives asking same questions
      - Dealing with big family
      - Difficult to please all family members

- Dealing with fussy family members
- Dealing with non-disclosure
- Dealing with intense grief
  - With colleagues
    - Lack of communication
    - Lack of consideration
    - Lack of listening
    - Lack of empathy
- Differences in opinion
  - With patients and family members
    - Disagreement in prognosis
    - Disagreement in treatment option
    - Disagreement in treatment futility
    - Disagreement in goals of care
    - Disagreement in end-of-life discussion
    - Conflicting views among different relatives
  - With colleagues
    - Disagreement in prognosis
    - Disagreement in treatment option
    - Disagreement in treatment futility
    - Disagreement in goals of care
    - Disagreement among different specialists
- Misperceptions and misconceptions
  - From patients and family members
    - Regarding palliative care referral
      - A sign of giving up
      - A sign of nothing more can be done
      - A sign of not doing anything
    - Regarding morphine and sedatives
      - Rejecting use of morphine
      - Rejecting dose titration
      - Requesting for discontinuation of sedative

- Regarding cancer
  - Cancer means suffering
  - Cancer means death
- Regarding disclosure of cancer diagnosis
  - Disclosure generates depression
  - Disclosure causes giving up
  - Disclosure expedites death
- Self-care
  - Personal expectations
    - Perception of having not done enough
      - Lack of time to see patients
      - Lack fo time to see patients regularly
      - Lack of time to attend to patients immediately
      - Feeling upset for the incapacity to fulfil request
      - Feeling guilty for not doing enough
      - Being criticized for not doing anything
    - Perceived failure
      - Failure to prevent young deaths
      - Failure to extend life of patients
      - Failure to relieve suffering
      - Failure to fulfil patient's wish
      - Failure to change misperceptions
      - Failure to help patients in strong denial
    - Perceived helplessness
      - Feeling helpless when young patients die
      - Feeling helpless when patients die alone
      - Feeling helpless when nothing can be done
      - Feeling helpless when patients gasp for breath
      - Feeling powerless when patients desire death

- Emotional involvement
  - Emotional vulnerability
    - In seeing pain and suffering
      - Patient devastated by bad news
      - Patient develops multiple problems
      - Patient confused by different information
      - Patient stuck at emergency
      - Patient has unnecessary investigations
      - Patient asked to fast for investigations
      - Patient cries
      - Patient gives up
      - Relative grieves
    - In seeing death and dying
      - Seeing patient deteriorates
      - Seeing patient dies
      - Harder to see certain patients die
        - Close patients
        - Children
        - Young patients
        - Young patients with children
        - Patients who are breadwinners
        - Elderly patients for some
      - Circumstantial vulnerability
        - Sudden death
        - Sudden absences in ward
        - Multiple deaths in short time
  - Emotional reactivity
    - Feeling sad when patient dies
    - Feeling angry with demanding family
    - Feeling frustrated when patient presents late
    - Feeling guilty when patient dies post-treatment
    - Feeling helpless when not knowing what to do

- Feeling puzzled why patient has to die
- Difficulty controlling emotions before patient
- Grieving after patient's death
  - Death and dying thoughts
    - Worrying about own death
    - Worrying about how one will die in the future
    - Worrying about getting cancer
    - Worrying about dying with pain and suffering
    - Fear of death
    - Fear of suffering
    - Fear of separation with family
    - Fear of death of other family members
    - Fear of suffering of family members

Countertransference

- A result of the patient's influence on the physician's unconscious feelings (Freud 1910)
- The reactions that arise in the therapist as a result of the patient's influence on the therapist's unconscious feelings and have their origins in the therapist's identification and projection (Noyes 1963)
- The totality of feelings experienced by the clinician towards the patient – whether conscious or unconscious or whether prompted by the client's dynamics or by issues or events in the clinician's own life (Katz 2006)

Vicarious traumatization

- The negative transformation in the therapist's inner experience resulting from empathic engagement with clients' trauma material (Pearlman 1995)

Compassion fatigue

- The natural consequent behaviors and emotions resulting from knowing about a traumatizing event experienced by a significant other – the stress resulting from helping or wanting to help a traumatized or suffering person (Figley 1995)

Moral distress

- Moral distress occurs when one knows the right thing to do, but institutional constraints make it nearly impossible to pursue the right course of action (Jameton 1984)
- Moral distress is the painful psychological disequilibrium that results from recognizing the ethically appropriate action, yet not taking it, because of such obstacles as lack of time, supervisory reluctance, an inhibiting medical power structure, institution policy, or legal considerations (Corley 2001)
- Moral distress is the physical or emotional suffering that is experienced when constraints (internal or external) prevent one from following the course of action that one believes is right

Burnout

- A psychological syndrome in response to chronic interpersonal stressors on the job (Maslach 1982)
- A state of mental and physical exhaustion caused by excessive and prolonged stress (Girdin 1996)
- Dimensions of burnout
    - Emotional exhaustion
        - The basic individual stress dimension of burnout
        - The feelings of being overextended and depleted of one's emotional and physical resources
    - Depersonalization (cynicism)
        - The interpersonal context dimension of burnout

- A negative, callous, or excessively detached response to various aspects of the job
  - Personal accomplishment
    - The self-evaluation dimension of burnout
    - Feelings of incompetence and lack of achievement and productivity at work
- The 12 phases of burnout cycle (Freudenberger 2006)
  - A compulsion to prove oneself
  - Working harder
  - Neglecting own needs
  - Displacement of conflicts
  - Revision of values
  - Denial of emerging problems
  - Withdrawal
  - Obvious behavioural changes
  - Depersonalization
  - Inner emptiness
  - Depression
  - Burnout syndrome

Coping

- Coping comprises both behavioral and cognitive strategies aimed at managing the internal and external demands of stressful transactions (Lazarus 1984)
- Defence mechanism: an unconscious psychological mechanism that reduces anxiety arising from unacceptable or potentially harmful stimuli (Schacter 2011)
- Defence mechanisms are not to be confused with conscious coping strategies

- Maladaptive defence mechanisms
  - Acting out: direct expression of an unconscious wish or impulse in action, without conscious awareness of the emotion that drives that expressive behaviour
  - Blocking: temporary or transiently inhibiting thinking
  - Controlling: attempting to manage or regulate events or objects in the environment to minimize anxiety and to resolve inner conflicts
  - Delusional projection: grossly frank delusions about external reality, usually of a persecutory nature
  - Denial: refusal to accept external reality because it is too threatening
  - Displacement: redirection of an intense emotion toward someone or something that is less offensive or threatening in order to avoid dealing directly with what is frightening or threatening
  - Dissociation: temporary drastic modification of one's personal identity or character to avoid emotional distress
  - Distortion: a gross reshaping of external reality to meet internal needs
  - Externalization: tending to perceive in the external world and in external objects elements of one's own personality, including instinctual impulses, conflicts, moods, attitudes, and styles of thinking
  - Fantasy: tendency to retreat into fantasy in order to resolve inner and outer conflicts
  - Hypochondriasis: an excessive preoccupation or worry about having a serious illness
  - Idealization: unconsciously choosing to perceive another individual as having more positive qualities than he or she may actually have

- Identification: the unconscious modelling of one's self upon another person's character and behaviour
- Inhibition: consciously limiting or renouncing some ego functions, alone or in combinations, to evade anxiety arising out of conflict with instinctual impulses, the superego, or environmental forces or figures
- Intellectualization: concentrating on the intellectual components of a situation so as to distance oneself from the associated anxiety-provoking emotions
- Introjection: identifying with some idea or object so deeply that it becomes a part of that person
- Isolation: separation of feelings from ideas and events
- Passive aggression: aggression towards others expressed indirectly or passively such as using procrastination
- Projection: shifting one's unacceptable thoughts, feelings and impulses within oneself onto someone else, such that those same thoughts, feelings, beliefs and motivations are perceived as being possessed by the other
- Projective identification: the object of projection invokes in that person precisely the thoughts, feelings or behaviours projected
- Rationalization (making excuses): offering rational explanations in an attempt to justify attitudes, beliefs or behaviour that may otherwise be unacceptable
- Reaction formation: transforming an unacceptable impulse into its opposite
- Regression: temporary reversion of the ego to an earlier stage of development rather than handling unacceptable impulses in a more adult way
- Repression: expelling or withholding from consciousness an idea or feeling

- Somatization: converting psychic derivatives into bodily symptoms and tending to react with somatic manifestations, rather than psychic manifestations
- Splitting: segregating experiences into all-good and all-bad categories, with no room for ambiguity
- Undoing: trying to 'undo' an unhealthy, destructive or threatening thought by engaging in contrary behaviour
- Upward and downward social comparisons: looking to another individual or group who is considered to be worse off in order to dissociate oneself from perceived similarities and to make oneself feel better
- Wishful thinking: making decisions according to what might be pleasing to imagine instead of by appealing to evidence, rationality or reality
- Adaptive defence mechanisms
  - Altruism: constructive service to others that brings pleasure and personal satisfaction
  - Anticipation: realistic planning for future discomfort
  - Humour: overt expression of ideas and feelings (especially those that are unpleasant to focus on or too terrible to talk about) that gives pleasure to others
  - Sublimation: transformation of negative emotions or instincts into positive actions, behaviour, or emotion
  - Thought suppression: consciously or semiconsciously postponing attention to a conscious impulse or conflict
- Cognitive distortions: irrational thinking patterns
  - All-or-none thinking, dichotomous reasoning, polarized thinking, splitting: seeing things in absolute, black-and-white categories
  - Always being right: actively trying to prove one's actions or thoughts to be correct

- Blaming: holding other people responsible for the harm they cause
- Catastrophizing: an extreme form of magnification, giving greater weight to the worst possible outcome, however unlikely
- Control fallacies: feeling oneself as a victim of fate (external control) or assuming responsibility for the well-being of others (internal control)
- Disqualifying the positive: discounting positive events
- Emotional reasoning: thinking something is true, solely based on a feeling
- Fallacy of change: expecting others to change to suit oneself if one just pressures or cajoles them enough
- Fallacy of fairness: believing that life is fair according to your definition
- Filtering: picking out a single negative detail and dwelling on it exclusively
- Heaven's reward fallacy: expecting one's sacrifice to pay off, as if someone is keeping score
- Jumping to conclusions: making a negative interpretation though there are no definite facts that convincingly support conclusion
- Labeling: attaching a negative label to oneself or others
- Magical thinking: attributing causal relationships between actions and events which seemingly cannot be justified by reason and observation
- Magnification: exaggerating the importance of things
- Mind reading: a form of jumping to conclusion, concluding arbitrarily that someone is reacting negatively to oneself
- Minimization: shrinking things inappropriately until they appear tiny

- Overgeneralization: seeing a single negative event as a never-ending pattern of defeat
- Oversimplification: looking for incorrect mental shortcuts
- Personalization: seeing oneself as the cause of some negative external event which in fact one was not primarily responsible for
- Should statements: criticizing oneself or others with "Shoulds" or "Shouldn'ts". "Musts", "Oughts" and "Have tos" are similar offenders
- The Fortune Teller Error: a form of jumping to conclusion, anticipating that things will turn out badly
- Conscious coping strategies (Lazarus and Folkman 1984)
  - Problem-focused coping
    - To change or eliminate stressors
      - Taking control
      - Information seeking
      - Evaluating the pros and cons
  - Emotion-focused coping
    - To alleviate distress triggered by stressors
      - Disclaiming
      - Escape-avoidance
      - Accepting responsibility or blame
      - Exercising self-control
      - Positive reappraisal

Coping strategies in palliative care (Tan 2013)

Healthcare

- Organizational challenges
  - Team dysfunction
    - Adopt similar team philosophy
    - Define role clearly
    - Encourage team cooperation and commitment

490

- Open team communication
- Regular team meeting
  - Resources, staffing and working environment
    - Mobilize resources
    - Increase staffing
    - Improve working environment
- Care overload
  - Heavy workload
    - Prioritize visits based on needs
    - Help patients bit by bit
    - Practice teamworking
  - Difficult encounter
    - Try to understand patient's perspective
    - Try to understand family's perspective
    - Cognitive reappraisal of the situation
    - Facilitate shifting of expectation
    - Facilitate grieving
    - Debriefing sessions

Interpersonal care

- Communication challenges
  - Learn and practice good communication skills
  - Practice empathy
  - Explore hope and preferences
  - Give hope
- Differences in opinion
  - Learn to agree to disagree
  - Respect differences in opinion
  - Allow time for change
- Misperceptions and misconceptions
  - Give adequate information
  - Acknowledge misperceptions and misconceptions

- Respect preferences
- Allow time for change

Self-care

- Personal expectation
    - Debriefing sessions
    - Cognitive reappraisal
    - Practice mindfulness
        - Non-appraisal
        - Non-attachment to outcome
- Emotional involvement
    - Improve emotional competence
    - Debriefing sessions
    - Practice mindfulness
        - Non-reactive
        - Letting go
    - Work-life balance
        - Eat well
        - Sleep well
        - Exercise
        - Socialize
        - Hobbies
        - Relaxation
        - Meditation
        - Taking a break
- Death and dying thought
    - Spirituality
        - Having a personal philosophy of life and death
        - Finding meaning in work
        - Finding meaning in life
        - Reflection on personal mortality
        - Imagine the deceased going to a better place

- Connect with family, friends, nature, art, music
- Connect with the significance and the sacred
- Prayer
- Meditate
- Rituals

The 3 essential practices of self-care

1. Practice mindfulness
2. Practice happiness
3. Practice kindness

Mindfulness

Introduction

While science is an excellent method to study the natural world, mindfulness is a universal human capacity to study the inner world, or the mind. The former focuses on looking "outside" and the latter focuses on "looking inside". Looking inside is crucial in the pursuit of an enduring happiness.

The three stages in practicing mindfulness

- Understanding mindfulness
- Experiencing mindfulness
- Living mindfully

What is mindfulness?

- Mindfulness = sati in Pali = bare attention
- Paying attention in a particular way: on purpose, in the present moment, nonjudgmentally (Kabat-Zinn 1994)
- When you first become aware of something, there is a fleeting instant of pure awareness just before you conceptualize the thing, before you identify it. That is a state of awareness. Ordinarily, this state is short-lived. It is that flashing split second just as you focus your eyes on the thing, just as you focus your mind on the thing, just before you objectify it, clamp down on it mentally, and segregate it from the rest of existence. It takes place just before you start thinking about it – before your mind says, "Oh, it's a dog." That flowing, soft-focused moment of pure awareness is mindfulness. (Gunaratana 2011)

Characteristics of mindfulness (Gunaratana 2011)

- Mindfulness is mirror-thought: it reflects only what is happening and in exactly the way it is happening
- Mindfulness is nonjudgmental observation: it is that ability of the mind to observe without criticism
- Mindfulness accepts whatever experience we may be having
- Mindfulness is impartial watchfulness: it does not take sides
- Mindfulness is nonconceptual awareness: it does not get involved with thoughts or concepts. It just looks.
- Mindfulness is present-moment awareness: it takes place in the here and now
- Mindfulness is nonegotistic alertness: it takes place without reference to self
- Mindfulness is awareness of change: it is observing the passing flow of experience
- Mindfulness is participatory observation: the meditator is both participant and observer at one and the same time
- Mindfulness is extremely difficult to define in words: not because it is complex, but because it is too simple and open
- Mindfulness is a presymbolic function: we can never fully express what it is

Three core elements of mindfulness (Shapiro 2006)

- Intention
  - Self-regulation
  - Self-exploration
  - Self-liberation
  - Selfless service
- Attention
  - Temporal: moment-to-moment attention
  - Quality: deep attention that "sinks" into its object

- Attitude
  - Acronym COAL (Siegel 2007)
    - Curiosity
    - Openness
    - Acceptance
    - Love
  - Nonjudging
  - Nonstriving
  - Nonattachment
  - Nonreactivity
  - Gentleness
  - Patience
  - Trust
  - Letting go

Benefits of mindfulness

- Improves pain acceptance
- Improves sleep
- Reduces stress
- Reduces anxiety and depression
- Integrates emotions
- Calms the body
- Increases cortical thickness (Lazar 2005)
- Increases telomerases and decelerates aging (Lengacher 2014)
- Improves immune function (Witek-Janusek 2008)

Mechanisms of mindfulness in stress reduction

- Paying attention on purpose
  - Attention regulation
- Paying attention in the present moment
  - Reduces rumination of the past
  - Reduces worry of the future

- Paying attention nonreactively
    - Metacognitive awareness: the ability to see one's thoughts and feelings as mental events, rather than the self
    - Decentering: the ability to observe one's thoughts and feelings as temporary, objective mental events
    - Defusion: the ability to be aware of one's thoughts, feelings and memories as passing events rather than "things" that are valid or invalid
    - Reperception: the ability to disidentify from the contents of consciousness, such as one's thoughts, feelings, and judgments and view one's moment-to-moment experience with greater clarity and objectivity

Measuring mindfulness

- Freiburg Mindfulness Inventory (Buchheld 2001)
    - 30 items
    - Nonjudgmental present-moment observation
    - Openness to negative experience
    - Designed for experienced meditators
- Mindful Attention Awareness Scale (Brown 2003)
    - 15 items
    - Awareness of present-moment experience in daily life
- Kentucky Inventory of Mindfulness Skills (Baer 2004)
    - 39 items
    - Observing present-moment experience
    - Describing: applying verbal labels
    - Acting with awareness
    - Accepting present-moment experience without judgment
- The Toronto Mindfulness Scale (Lau 2006)
    - 13 items
    - Curiosity
    - Decentering

- The Five Facet Mindfulness Questionnaire (Baer 2006)
  - 39 items
  - Observing
  - Describing
  - Acting with awareness
  - Non-judging of inner experience
  - Non-reactivity to inner experience
- The Cognitive and Affective Mindfulness Scale (Feldman 2007)
  - 12 items
  - Attention
  - Awareness
  - Present-focus
  - Acceptance
  - Non-judgment of thoughts and feelings
- The Southampton Mindfulness Questionnaire (Chadwick 2008)
  - 16 items
  - Mindful observation
  - Letting go
  - Non-aversion
  - Non-judgment
- The Philadelphia Mindfulness Scale (Cardaciotto 2008)
  - 20 items
  - Awareness
  - Acceptance

Slowing down

Slowing down is a prerequisite for the practice of mindfulness. With the current pace of our modern society, we rush a lot. We seldom have time for ourselves. The first step in establishing mindfulness is to slow down and to stop rushing. Then, it is easier for us to pay full attention to whatever we are doing. Try not to multi-task. Do one thing at a time, with our full attention.

The four foundation practices to establish mindfulness

- From <u>The Discourse on the Foundations of Mindfulness</u>
- Or <u>Satipatthana Sutta</u> in Pali
    - Mindfulness of the body
    - Mindfulness of feelings
    - Mindfulness of mind
    - Mindfulness of reality

Mindfulness of the body

- The first way to establish mindfulness
- The simplest and most direct way to reduce stress
- The basis of all other practices

Mindfulness of the breath

Exercise 1: conscious breathing

- Go to a quiet place
- Sit down comfortably
- Fold or cross legs; or sit on a chair
- Sit upright
- Observe the breath at the nose area
- Breathing in, I know I am breathing in
- Breathing out, I know I am breathing out
- Do not control the breath in any way
- Breathe naturally
- Do not be distracted by other thoughts
- Come back to the breath once we are distracted
- Practice for our own welfare , others and even the whole world
- Just be aware of the breath
- Breathe with full awareness of each breath

Exercise 2: following the breath

- Follow the breath closely
- Follow the entire length of the breath: "the breath body"
- Do not allow any distracting thought to enter
- Breathing in a long breath,
  I know I am breathing in a long breath
- Breathing out a long breath,
  I know I am breathing out a long breath
- Breathing in a short breath,
  I know I am breathing in a short breath
- Breathing out a short breath,
  I know I am breathing out a short breath
- Do not force ourselves to take long or short breath
- Breathe naturally
- Just be aware of the entire length of the breath
- Breathe with full awareness of the entire length of the breath
- As we follow the breath, the breath will calm naturally
- The breath will become smooth, regular and harmonious
- The flow of air will change from turbulent to laminar

Exercise 3: bringing our mind home to the body

- Use our breathing to bring our mind home to our body
- Stop ruminating about the past
- Stop worrying about the future
- Bring our mind back to the present moment
- Bring our mind and body together as one
- Breathing in, I am aware of my whole body
- Breathing out, I am aware of my whole body
- Feel the different parts of our body, from the top to the bottom
- Feel the body as a whole, fully united with the mind
- Feel the wholeness of ourselves with each breath

Exercise 4: calming the body

- Once our breath is harmonious, it will calm our body naturally
- Breathing in, I calm my body
- Breathing out, I calm my body
- Notice whether there is any tension in any part of our body
- Breathe and relax the tension one by one, from top to bottom
- Then relax the whole body all at once
- Feel the breath entering our body and calming all parts of body
- Feel the breath leaving our body and taking away our tiredness
- Feel the breath and the body calm down together

Mindfulness of postures

Exercise 5: awareness of postures

- Be aware of our bodily postures
- When sitting, I know I am sitting
- When sitting, just sit
- When standing, I know I am standing
- When standing, just stand
- When walking, I know I am walking
- When walking, just walk
- When lying down, I know I am lying down
- When lying down, just lie down
- The benefits of mindfulness of postures
    - It helps to maintain the continuity of mindfulness
    - It reveals our states of mind
    - It reveals the three universal characteristics of reality
        - The reality of impermanence (time)
        - The reality of selflessness (space)
        - The reality of suffering (mind)

- The reality of impermanence (anicca in Pali)
    - Notice the big changes from one posture to another
    - Notice the minute changes of sensation during movement
    - Slow down to notice the minute sensations
- The reality of selflessness (anatta in Pali)
    - Notice the different body parts during different postures
    - Notice the contact between the body and any support
    - Observe "who" is sitting, standing, walking or lying down
    - Observe the intention that initiates each action
    - Find out what and where is the "I" during each posture
- The reality of suffering (dukkha in Pali)
    - Notice the discomfort that causes us to change posture
    - Notice the temporary relief of discomfort with movement

Mindfulness of activities

Exercise 6: awareness of activities

- Practice full awareness of every activity
    - Waking up and falling asleep
    - Eating and drinking
    - Urinating and defecating
    - Sitting, standing and walking
    - Talking and keeping silent
- Full awareness (sampajanna)
    - Awareness of the purpose of an activity
        - Notice the purpose of an activity
        - Is the purpose wholesome or unwholesome?
        - Is the activity beneficial to us and others?
        - Notice the possibility to choose
        - Choose a wholesome activity
    - Awareness of the appropriateness of an activity
        - Notice the appropriateness of a wholesome activity
        - Is it the right time and place to perform the activity?

- Awareness of the four fields of practice
  - Knowing which field we are practicing
    - Mindfulness of the body
    - Mindfulness of feelings
    - Mindfulness of mind
    - Mindfulness of reality
  - Knowing when we are distracted
- Awareness of the three universal characteristics of reality
  - Notice the impermanent nature of each activity
    - The big change of an activity
    - The small change of an activity
  - Notice the selfless nature of each activity
    - The "self" is just a mental construction
    - The "self" is just a combination of:
      - The physical body
      - Sensations
      - Perceptions
      - Mental activities: cognitions and emotions
      - Consciousness
    - The "doing" without a "doer"
  - Notice the unsatisfactory nature of each activity

Mindfulness of the physical body

Exercise 7: bodily awareness

- Scan our body bottom-up from the soles of our feet
- Scan our body top-down from the top of the hair
- Scan the different parts of the body
  - Superficial somatic: head hair, body hair, nails, teeth, skin
  - Deep somatic: fat, muscles, tendon, ligament, bones, bone marrow, diaphragm
  - Solid visceral: brain, heart, lungs, liver, kidneys, spleen
  - Hollow visceral: stomach, small bowel, large bowel, feces

- Excretion fluid: tears, saliva, phlegm, mucus, sweat, urine
- Body fluid: bile, blood, lymph, pus, synovial fluid
- Notice the attractive and unattractive aspects of the body parts
- The benefits of mindfulness of the physical body
  - To decondition our strong identification with the body
    - Liking the superficial parts
    - Disliking the deeper parts
  - To lessen suffering that results from that identification
  - To deepen understanding of the three characteristics
    - Notice the impermanent nature of the body
      - The changes of the body
    - Notice the selfless nature of the body
      - The interdependent nature of the body
    - Notice the unsatisfactory nature of the body
      - The changes that we cannot accept

Exercise 8: awareness of body composition

- Be aware of the presence of earth elements in our body
  - Earth element: the solid nature of matter
- Be aware of the presence of water elements in our body
  - Water element: the liquid nature of matter
- Be aware of the presence of fire elements in our body
  - Fire element: the heat nature of matter
- Be aware of the presence of air elements in our body
  - Air element: the movement nature of matter
- Notice similar elements that constitute the earth and universe
- Notice the interrelated nature of our body and the earth
- Notice the interrelated nature of our body and the universe
- See our lives outside our bodies
- Transcend the boundary between self and nature
- Go beyond the limiting concepts of life and death

Exercise 9: contemplation of decomposition of a corpse

- The benefits of this exercise
    - Helps us to understand the decaying nature of our body
    - Helps us to become less attached to our body
    - Helps us to use and care for the body without attachment
    - Helps us to see the preciousness of life
    - Helps us to see the preciousness of time
- Visualize a corpse in various stages of decay
    - The body is bloated, discolored, festered and stinky
    - The body is crawling with insects and worms
    - The body is eaten by animals
    - The body is left with skeleton with little flesh and blood
    - The body is left with skeleton with no flesh but little blood
    - The body is left with skeleton with no more blood
    - The body is left with scattered bones
    - The body is left with bleached bones
    - The body is left with dried bones
    - The bones are reduced to a pile of dust
    - The dust disappears with a gust of wind
- It is not a pleasant exercise
- It is meant for someone with good physical and mental health
- The effect of this exercise can be liberating

Mindfulness of feelings

- Feeling is the English translation of the Pali word *vedana*
- Feeling in English can be a sensation, an emotion or an opinion
- Vedana carries a more specific meaning
    - It refers to the feeling tone
    - The quality of pleasantness, unpleasantness or neutrality
    - Key factor to free us from our deepest conditioning
    - Key factor to eliminate stress permanently

- The conditioning of reaction and action by *vedana*
    - Pleasant feeling
        - Reaction: craving, attachment
        - Action: addictive behaviour
    - Unpleasant feeling
        - Reaction: hate, aversion
        - Action: avoidance behaviour
    - Neutral feeling
        - Reaction: indifference, delusion
        - Action: couldn't-care-less behaviour
- The benefits of mindfulness of feelings
    - To recognize the transitory nature of feelings
    - To recognize our ingrained habitual reactions to feelings
    - To recognize our reactions to feelings, and not the object
    - To become less identified with feelings
        - Less attached to pleasant feeling
        - Less resistant to unpleasant feeling
        - Less unaware of neutral feeling
    - To become less judgmental and reactive
    - To foster calmness and equanimity

Exercise 10: identifying the feeling tone

- When a feeling arises, notice its feeling tone
- Watch the arising, maintaining and disappearing of the tone
- Do not attempt to control or change the feeling tone
- Just observe and return our attention to the breath
- Feeling a pleasant feeling,
  I know I am feeling a pleasant feeling
- Feeling an unpleasant feeling,
  I know I am feeling an unpleasant feeling
- Feeling a neutral feeling,
  I know I am feeling a neutral feeling

- Abandon the tendency to crave for pleasant feeling
- Abandon the tendency to hate unpleasant feeling
- Abandon the tendency to ignore neutral feeling
- Practice nonreactivity towards feeling
- Notice the moment-to-moment changes of feelings
- Notice the suffering that arises from resisting painful feeling
- Notice the suffering that arises from craving pleasant feeling
- Whether the feeling is pleasant, unpleasant or neutral
  - Contemplate impermanence in those feelings
  - Watch the feelings come, stay and fade away
  - Let the feelings come when they come
  - Let the feelings stay when they stay
  - Let the feelings fade away when they fade away
  - Do not cling to any feeling
- When we do not cling to anything, we are not agitated
- When we are not agitated, we experience stresslessness

Exercise 11: identifying the source of the feeling tone

- Notice the source of the feeling tone
- Is it from the body or from the mind?
- Feeling a pleasant feeling from the body,
  I know I am feeling a pleasant feeling from the body
- Feeling a pleasant feeling from the mind,
  I know I am feeling a pleasant feeling from the mind
- Feeling an unpleasant feeling from the body,
  I know I am feeling an unpleasant feeling from the body
- Feeling an unpleasant feeling from the mind,
  I know I am feeling an unpleasant feeling from the mind
- Feeling a neutral feeling from the body,
  I know I am feeling a neutral feeling from the body
- Feeling a neutral feeling from the mind,
  I know I am feeling a neutral feeling from the mind

- Notice the source of the feeling tone
    - From sight?
    - From hearing?
    - From smell?
    - From taste?
    - From touch?
    - From thoughts?
- Notice the source of the feeling tone
    - Is it a physical sensation?
    - Is it an internally generated emotion?
- Notice how the sensation or emotion changes

Exercise 12: identifying worldly and unworldly feelings

- Notice whether it is a worldly or unworldly feeling
    - Worldly pleasant feeling
        - Sensory pleasure
        - Psychological pleasure
    - Worldly unpleasant feeling
        - Sensory pain
        - Psychological pain
    - Worldly neutral feeling
        - Sensory indifference
        - Psychological indifference
    - Unworldly pleasant and unpleasant feeling
        - Spiritual pleasure and pain
            - Practicing generosity without expectation
            - Practicing love without attachment
            - Practicing compassion without attachment
            - Practicing renunciation
            - Practicing mindfulness and meditation
    - Unworldly neutral feeling
        - Equanimity in mindfulness and meditation

- Both kinds of feelings will arise naturally in our lives
- Recognize the tendencies of the worldly feelings
    - Chasing worldly pleasant feeling
    - Running away from worldly painful feeling
    - Ignoring worldly neutral feeling
- Abandon these tendencies
- Appreciate and cultivate the unworldly feelings

Mindfulness of mind

- Two mental states
    - Unwholesome mental states
        - The mental state of craving (attachment)
        - The mental state of hating (aversion)
        - The mental state of indifference (delusion)
    - Wholesome mental states
        - The mental state of non-craving (non-attachment)
        - The mental state of non-hating (non-aversion)
        - The mental state of awareness (non-delusion)

Exercise 13: identifying unwholesome/wholesome mental states

- Notice our mental state
- The mental state of craving
    - Notice the arising of craving thoughts
    - Observe the craving thoughts without following them
    - Observe until the craving thoughts fade away
    - Recognize that the craving thoughts have gone
    - Reflect on the nature of a craving-free mind
    - It is free, happy, generous, loving and compassionate
- The mental state of hating
    - Notice the arising of hateful thoughts
    - Observe the hateful thoughts without following them
    - Observe until the hateful thoughts fade away

- Recognize that the hateful thoughts have gone
- Reflect on the nature of a hate-free mind
- It is free, happy, relaxed, peaceful and friendly
- The mental state of awareness
    - The mind is clear and aware before delusion arises
    - Notice the arising of delusion
    - Once we pay attention, the clouds of delusion fade away
    - Recognize the re-appearance of the clear mind
    - Recognize the nature of a delusion-free mind
    - It is clear, aware, sky-like and luminous
- Delusion
    - A false belief based on incorrect inference about external reality that is firmly sustained despite what almost everyone else believes and despite what constitutes the inconvertible and obvious proof or evidence to the contrary (DSM IV)
    - Delusion in the context of mindfulness
        - Is not similar to DSM IV definition
        - Is *moha* in Pali
        - Is the unawareness of the reality
            - The reality of impermanence (time)
                - That things change from time to time
            - The reality of selflessness (space)
                - That things are conditioned
            - The reality of suffering (mind)
                - That suffering arises when we cannot accept things as they are
    - Delusion of permanence: the false belief that things remain unchanged all the time (reality: nothing lasts)
    - Delusion of self: the false belief that the self is an independent entity (reality: the self is just a mental construction)

510

- Delusion of happiness: the false belief that true happiness is achieved through avoiding pain and the pursuit of sensory pleasure (reality: pain is inevitable in life, pleasure is transient, true happiness is achieved through abandoning the root causes of suffering and practicing the eight noble paths – please refer to mindfulness of reality)

Exercise 14: the removal of distracting thoughts

- This exercise combines mindfulness of thoughts and cognitive methods to remove distracting thoughts
- From <u>The Discourse on The Removal of Distracting Thoughts</u>
- Or <u>Vitakkasanthana Sutta</u> in Pali
- 5 cognitive methods in the removal of distracting thoughts
  - Replacing the thoughts
    - Identify unwholesome thoughts
    - Notice the arising of craving, hate or delusion
    - Replace the thoughts with wholesome thoughts
    - Metaphor: like a carpenter striking hard at, pushing out, and getting rid of a coarse peg to replace it with a fine one
  - Reflecting on the negative effects of the thoughts
    - When unwholesome thoughts remain
    - Examine the danger of the unwholesome thoughts
    - Reflect on the negative effects of the thoughts
    - Metaphor: like a well-dressed young man or woman feeling disgusted with the carcass of a snake hung around his or her neck
  - Ignoring the thoughts
    - When unwholesome thoughts remain
    - Pay no attention to the unwholesome thoughts
    - Metaphor: like a man shutting his eyes or looking away from a visible object

- Removing the source of the negative thoughts
  - When unwholesome thoughts remain
  - Reflect on the removal of the source
  - Metaphor: like a man slowing down because he found no reason to walk fast
- Suppressing unwholesome thoughts
  - When unwholesome thoughts remain
  - Use all our energy to suppress the thoughts
  - With teeth clenched and tongue pressed on palate
  - Metaphor: like a strong man holding a weaker man by the head or shoulders, restraining, subduing and beating him down

Exercise 15: identifying the eight pairs of mental states

- Pause and look at our mind
- Recognize whether the mind is:
  - Greedy or not greedy
    - Greedy: burning with the fire of craving
    - Not greedy: calm, cool, peaceful and relaxed
  - Angry or not angry
    - Angry: gripped by anger or hate
    - Not angry: calm, cool, peaceful and relaxed
  - Deluded or not deluded
    - Deluded: being trapped in the net of cognitive errors
    - Not deluded: calm, cool, peaceful, clear and free
  - Contracted/distracted or not contracted/distracted
    - Contracted: dull and heavy, collapsing inward
    - Distracted: agitated and restless, expanding outward
  - Narrow or wide
    - Narrow: our day-to-day ordinary consciousness
    - Wide: altered consciousness in meditation, the mind is calm, peaceful, tranquil, harmonious, relaxed

- Not supreme or supreme
    - Not supreme: not in the highest state of meditation
    - Supreme: in the highest state of meditation
- Not concentrated or concentrated
    - Not concentrated: not in meditative states
    - Concentrated: in meditative states
- Not liberated or liberated
    - Not liberated: bound by problems; greedy, angry or deluded; narrow, not supreme or not concentrated
    - Liberated: free of all problems; not greedy, not angry and not deluded; wide, supreme, concentrated

Mindfulness of reality

- The three universal characteristics of reality
    - Temporal reality: the reality of impermanence
    - Spatial reality: the reality of selflessness
    - Psychological reality: the reality of suffering

Exercise 16: recognizing impermanence

- Be mindful of impermanence
- Watch the arising, maintaining, dissolving and disappearing of:
    - The breath and other bodily experiences
    - Feelings: pleasantness, unpleasantness, neutrality
    - The ordinary mind: mental states, thoughts and emotions
    - The meditative mind: altered mental states
- Recognize the impermanence of impermanence awareness
    - Drifting of mind from unawareness of impermanence to awareness of impermanence
    - Drifting of mind from awareness of impermanence back to unawareness of impermanence again
- Recognize the freedom when we reduce our clinging to the idea of permanence (the wish for pleasant things to stay the same)

Exercise 17: recognizing selflessness

- Recognize that the sense of "self":
    - Is a faulty mental construction
    - Is not an independent entity
    - Is dependent on various causes and conditions
    - Arises as we think about our body, feelings, perceptions, mental formations and consciousness
    - Is impermanent
- Recognizing selflessness (conditionality)
    - That conditioned things change
    - That things arise, maintain, dissolve and disappear based on causes and conditions
    - The body: birth, aging, sickness and death
    - Feelings: come and go based on causes and conditions
    - Mental states: change from time to time based on causes and conditions
- Recognize the freedom when we reduce our clinging to the idea of self (the wish for things the way "I" want, not as they are)

Time Magazine 2002

After more than a century looking for it, brain researchers have long since concluded that there is no conceivable place for a self to be located in the physical brain, and that it simply does not exist.

Exercise 18: recognizing suffering

- Suffering is not inherent in the phenomena of the world
- It exists only in the way the ordinary mind experiences it
- It arises when we are unable to accept changes
- It arises when we cannot accept the reality of impermanence and conditionality
- The 4 noble truths
    - The truth of suffering
    - The truth of causes of suffering
    - The truth of cessation of suffering
    - The truth of paths leading to cessation of suffering
- The truth of suffering (dukkha in Pali)
    - Notice the arising of suffering when it arises
    - Notice the suffering as it is
    - Notice the unsatisfactory nature of suffering
    - Contemplate on the 8 types of suffering associated with:
        - Birth
        - Aging
        - Sickness
        - Death
        - Separating from what or who we love
        - Not getting what we want
        - Getting what we do not want
        - Clinging to our body and mind
    - Contemplate on the 3 types of suffering
        - Suffering due to unpleasant experiences
            - The obvious biopsychosocial-spiritual suffering
        - Suffering due to impermanence
            - The potential suffering hidden in all changes
        - Suffering due to conditionality
            - The potential suffering hidden in conditioned things

- The truth of causes of suffering (samudaya in Pali)
    - Notice the arising of the causes of suffering
        - Delusion: the mistaken belief of the reality
            - The belief that things are permanent
            - The belief that things are independent
            - The belief that long-lasting happiness can be achieved by indulging in things we crave
            - The belief that suffering can be removed totally by resisting or avoiding things we hate
        - Attachment: the craving of things that one likes
        - Aversion: the hating of things that one dislikes
    - When delusion arises, I know this is delusion
    - Notice delusion as it is without sustaining it
    - When attachment arises, I know this is attachment
    - Notice attachment as it is without sustaining it
    - When aversion arises, I know this is aversion
    - Notice aversion as it is without sustaining it
    - Watch how suffering arises based on causes & conditions
        - Notice the arising of feeling tone
            - Pleasant
            - Unpleasant
            - Neutral
        - Notice the conditioned reactions to feeling tones
            - Pleasant feeling → attachment
            - Unpleasant feeling → aversion
            - Neutral feeling → delusion
        - Notice the reaction to attachment/aversion
            - Clinging
                - Holding on to attachment
                - Holding on to aversion
                - Holding on to delusion

- Notice the arising of suffering
    - From feelings to attachment/aversion
    - From attachment/aversion to clinging
- The truth of cessation of suffering (nirodha in Pali)
    - Suffering arises, maintains, dissolves and disappears due to impermanence and conditionality
    - Observe the mind when it is free of suffering
    - Delusion, craving and hate arise, maintain, dissolve and disappear due to impermanence and conditionality
    - Observe the mind when it is free of the causes of suffering
        - Free of delusion
        - Free of craving
        - Free of hate
    - Observe the mind when it is free of clinging
    - Feel the radical freedom that is independent of favourable or unfavourable conditions
    - Feel the extinction of negative mental states
- The truth of paths (magga in Pali)
    - Notice the paths/factors leading to cessation of suffering
    - The 8 noble paths
        - Right understanding
            - Understanding the reality as it is
            - Understanding the 4 noble truths
        - Right intention
            - The intention to do no harm
            - The intention to do good
        - Right speech
            - Communicating truthfully
            - Communicating meaningfully
            - Communicating sensitively
            - Communicating timely

- Right action
    - To protect life
    - To give
    - To preserve dignity
    - To listen deeply and speak with love
    - To promote health
- Right livelihood
    - Not engaging in profession that may do harm
    - Engaging in profession that may do good
- Right progress
    - Prevent negative thoughts from arising
    - Abandon negative thoughts that have arisen
    - Invite positive thoughts that have not arisen
    - Sustain positive thoughts that have arisen
- Right mindfulness
    - Mindfulness of the body
    - Mindfulness of feelings
    - Mindfulness of mind
    - Mindfulness of reality
- Right meditation
    - Meditation to calm down our mind
    - Meditation to look inside our mind
        - Insight into reality of impermanence
        - Insight into reality of selflessness
        - Insight into reality of suffering
- Notice the arising of these factors from time to time
- Notice the cessation of suffering with these factors
- Practice the 8 noble paths continuously

Mindfulness in Palliative Care

Introduction

Although mindfulness has great potential in reducing suffering, the practice of mindfulness in palliative care has many challenges.

Challenges of practicing mindfulness in palliative care

- Patients/families may not have the intention to practice
- Patients/families may be too tired to pay attention
- Patients/families may be too overwhelmed with suffering
- Patients may experience rapid change in suffering
- Patients may experience rapid change in physical strength
- Patients may experience rapid change in conscious level
- Healthcare staff may be too busy with work

Mini-mindfulness meditation (MMM)

- Designed for palliative care patients since most patients do not have the time or energy to attend formal mindfulness practices
- Recommended duration: at least 5 minutes a day
- Flexibility
  - Can choose from any of the following practices
  - Can practice for 5min, 15min, 30min, or more
  - Can practice for any number of sessions
  - Can practice at any setting
  - Can stop at any time
  - Can be a practice for family members
  - Can be a practice for healthcare providers
  - Can be a guided practice except mindful bathing
  - Can be a self-practice

Instructions for mindful breathing

- Make yourself comfortable
- Relax your body
- Close your eyes gently
- Take two deep breaths slowly
- Then, breathe naturally
- Notice the flow of air through your nose
- Rest your attention gently on your breath
- If you are distracted by any sounds, body sensations, thoughts or feelings, gently come back to your breath
- Be aware of the breath for the next five minutes

Instructions for mindful eating

- Enjoy your breathing while waiting for the food
- Feel grateful when the food arrives
- Be there fully for the food
- Put your food gently into your mouth
- Chew slowly
- Feel the taste, texture and temperature of the food
- Feel every nook and corner of the food
- Feel the movement of the food as you chew and swallow

- Follow the food down to the foodpipe and stomach
- Take the next portion or sip a drink when you are ready
- If you are lost in thinking, gently come back to your meal

Instructions for mindful movement

- Breathe in and out to center yourself
- Stop rushing
- Move slowly
- It can be any exercise or walking
- Feel the joint movement
- Feel the muscles contraction and relaxation
- Feel the skin and the gentle wind caused by the movement
- Synchronize you breathing with your movement
- As you stop moving, rest your attention on your posture
- If you are distracted, gently come back to yourself
- Rest your attention on movement for the next five minutes

Instructions for mindful bathing

- Breathe in and out
- Lock the door
- Take off your clothes slowly
- Turn on the shower
- Bathe slowly
- Feel the contact and flow of the running water
- Feel the temperature of the water
- Wipe your body with soap
- Feel the soap and the foam
- Focus on the skin sensation
- Do not get lost in thoughts
- If your mind wanders, come back to your skin sensation
- Wash away all your worries and stress
- Rest your attention on the water showering all over your body

Instructions for mindful smiling

- Breathe in and out to center yourself
- Imagine your face as a flower bud
- Choose your favourite flower
- Visualize the flower blooming as you start to smile
- Smile very slowly until your smile is blooming fully
- Rest your mind in the feeling of happiness
- Let the feeling spread to your whole body as you breathe
- Do not let other feelings, thoughts or sensations distract you
- Stay with this feeling of happiness for the next five minutes

Instructions for mindful chanting

- Breathe in and out to center yourself
- Choose a positive phrase
- Phrases: may I be happy, may I be calm, may I be peaceful
- Rest your mind on this phrase
- Chant it slowly and silently in your mind
- Use it as an anchor to stabilize your mind
- If you are distracted, come back to it again and again
- Rest your mind on it for the next five minutes

Instructions for mindfulness of love

- Love is an intention to bring happiness to someone
- Breathe in and out naturally
- Imagine your loved one in front of you
- Imagine sending love to the person
- Visualize him or her getting happier and happier
- Let go of any distraction
- Rest your attention on your love to the person
- Then, imagine receiving love from the person too
- See yourself getting happier and happier with the love
- Stay with the feeling of love for the next five minutes

Instructions for mindfulness of nature

- Choose a leaf, a flower, a tree, the sky or a picture of nature
- Breathe in and out naturally
- If you have chosen a leaf, look at it deeply
- Appreciate the general characteristics of the leaf
- Then, appreciate its details
- See the beauty of the leaf
- See until you can picture the leaf completely in your mind
- Let go of any distraction
- Rest your attention on the leaf and be one with it

Instructions for mindfulness of pain

- Seek help from your doctor for analgesia
- Breathe in and out to center yourself
- Breathe until you feel you are calmer
- Bring your attention to the pain
- Try to keep a curious mind to see what pain is
- Notice the sensations, emotions and thoughts of pain
- Pay particular attention to the unpleasantness of pain
- Notice how the mind resists pain
- Relax the resistance
- Smile to your pain

Instructions for mindful suffering

- Relax your body
- Take two deep breaths slowly
- Then, breathe naturally
- Allow your mind to settle down
- When you feel calmer, bring your attention to your suffering
- Observe the sensations, emotions and thoughts of suffering
- Watch suffering like an observer rather than an experiencer
- Notice how your suffering arises and disappears naturally

- Do not increase your suffering by overthinking about it
- Do not reject your suffering
- Embrace your suffering with kindness
- Imagine breathing in kindness to dissolve your suffering
- Imagine breathing out the remnants of suffering
- Continue breathing in and out for the next five minutes

Instructions for mindfulness of death

- Recommended for advanced mindfulness practitioners
- May cause considerable distress for those who are not
- Death is a natural process in life
- It can happen to us at anytime and anywhere
- Breathe in and out to center yourself
- Openly acknowledge that death can happen to you at anytime
- Imagine you are dying and lying on a bed surrounded by family
- Imagine the sensations caused by failure of many organs
- Imagine the negative thoughts and emotions that can arise
- Watch them and let them be as they are without rejecting them
- If fear arises, just breathe and let go
- If anger arises, just breathe and let go
- If worry arises, just breathe and let go
- If sadness arises, just breathe and let go
- Breathing in, I see dying as falling leaves
- Breathing out, I smile in peace
- Breathing in, I embrace my journey of living and dying
- Breathing out, mindfulness is my lead
- Rest your mind on the imagined scene for the next 5 minutes

Mindfulness-based supportive therapy (MBST)(Tan 2015)

- Designed for healthcare providers (HCP)
- Allow HCP to practice mindfulness during patient care
- Recommended duration: limited by available time of HCP
- Flexibility
    - No restriction in time
    - No restriction in number of sessions
    - Can be delivered by any HCP
    - Can be delivered to patients, family members or both
    - Can be delivered at hospital, home or hospice
    - Can be terminated at any time
    - Can be a bridge to other psychotherapies
- Reciprocity
    - May alleviate suffering of patients and family members
    - May reduce stress of HCP
- Simultaneity
    - Allow HCP to practice mindfulness at work
    - No need to change any schedule

The foundations of MBST (refer to chapter of suffering)

- Based on the theory of suffering in palliative care
    - Patients: the existential-experiential model of suffering
    - Families: the model of compassion suffering
- Open-ended questions for assessment of suffering
    - General questions
    - Specific questions
- Types of suffering as a guide in the diagnosis of suffering
    - Suffering of patients
    - Suffering of family caregivers

The framework of MBST

- Mindful presence
- Mindful listening
- Mindful empathy
- Mindful compassion
- Mindfulness of boundaries

The application techniques of MBST

- Directing attention (paying attention on purpose)
- Sustaining attention (paying attention on purpose)
- Distraction monitoring
    - Temporal distraction
      (paying attention in the present moment)
    - Reactive distraction
      (paying attention nonreactively)

Instructions for mindful presence

- Practice mindful breathing
    - Breathe consciously
    - Follow the entire length of the breath
    - Feel your whole body while you are breathing
    - Calm your body
- Give patient 100% of your attention
- Treat patient as if he or she is the only person in the world
- Maintain good eye contact from moment to moment
- See patient as a whole
- Observe his or her facial expression and body movement
- If you find yourself judging patient, feeling anxious or rushing, breathe and relax your body and mind again
- Be there fully for the patient during the entire encounter

Instructions for mindful listening

- Continue with mindful breathing
- Listen to patient with 100% of your attention
- Do not interrupt unnecessarily
- Do not judge patient
- Do not give your opinion prematurely
- Listen to the speech
- Listen to the rate, rhythm, pitch and volume
- Be comfortable with the speech and the silence in between
- Listen with an open and curious heart to understand patient
- Create a safe space for patient to express his or her suffering
- Try to understand what is being expressed
- Try to understand what is behind the expression
- If you are distracted by your judgment, just breathe and relax
- Let the barrier between you and patient dissolves
- Listen with all of yourself during the entire encounter

Instructions for mindful empathy

- Continue with mindful breathing
- Imagine "entering into" the feelings and perspectives of patient
- Imagine experiencing the emotions and thoughts of patient
- Imagine yourself going through the same experience
- If you notice any overimagination, just breathe and relax
- Try to understand what are the hopes, expectations and wishes
- Allow patient to express everything, thoughts and emotions
- Allow silence
- Abandon your impulse to block any form of expression
- Acknowledge, validate or normalize the expression if necessary
- Continue to put yourself in patient's shoes from time to time

Instructions for mindful compassion

- Continue with mindful breathing to anchor your attention
- Compassion is the motivation to relieve suffering
- Cultivate the sincere motivation to alleviate patient's suffering
- Repeat silently: May you be free from suffering
- Focus on the thoughts and feelings of compassion
- Let compassion manifest in your speech and action
- Speak consciously in consistent with the hopes, expectations, wishes and preferences of patient
- Act consciously in consistent with the hopes, expectations, wishes and preferences of patient
- Be mindful not to speak or act unwisely
- If you are excessively concerned in fixing the suffering, breathe
- If you are excessively attached to any expectation, breathe
- Breathe, relax and come back to compassion

Instructions for mindfulness of boundaries

- Mindfulness of boundaries is a practice of self-awareness
- Continue to practice mindful breathing
- Consciously monitor boundary issues that arise during your practices of presence, listening, empathy and compassion
- Be aware when boundaries are approached
- Cross boundaries consciously only if you are convinced that crossing boundary in that particular situation is beneficial to patient and the therapeutic relationship, without violating your professional conduct or compromising the equity of care
- Mindfulness of boundaries protects you from burnout due to:
  - Time constraint (presence)
  - Countertransferences (listening)
  - Vicarious traumatization (empathy)
  - Compassion fatigue (compassion)
- Maintain self-awareness throughout the encounter

The Neuroscience of Mindfulness

Introduction

With regular practice, mindfulness can change the brain areas involved in attention regulation, emotional regulation and self-awareness.

Default mode network (DMN)

- The wandering mind
- Active when we are not engaged in performing a task
- Active when we are not processing external events
  - Daydreaming or mind wandering
  - Thinking about ourselves or others
  - Thinking about the past or future
- Comprises 3 midline regions and inferior parietal lobule
  - Ventromedial prefrontal cortex (vmPFC)
    - Emotion processing
  - Dorsomedial prefrontal cortex (dmPFC)
    - Self-referential processing
  - Posterior cingulate cortex (PCC) + adjacent precuneus
    - Recollection of prior experiences
  - Inferior parietal lobule (IPL)
    - Perspective taking
- Mindfulness practices
  - Reduce activation of DMN (mPFC and PCC)
    - Less mind wandering
  - Increase connectivity between PCC, dACC and dlPFC
    - More self-monitoring and cognitive control
  - Increase DMN functional connectivity
    - More communication within DMN

The habit loop

- 3Rs
    - Reminder: cue, stimulus
    - Routine: triggered behaviour
    - Reward: the benefit that makes us repeat the loop
- Habit learning
    - Basal ganglia (the habit center)
        - Dorsal striatum: caudate, putamen
        - Ventral striatum: nucleus accumbens
        - Globus pallidus
    - Basal-ganglia-thalamocortical loops
        - Cortex → striatum
            - Caudate nucleus and vmPFC
                - Initial learning
                - Flexible goal-directed behaviour
            - Putamen
                - Later
                - Stimulus-driven habitual behaviour
        - Striatum → globus pallidus
        - Globus pallidus → thalamus
        - Thalamus → cortex
- Neurotransmitter
    - Dopamine: released in response to reward
        - Food
        - Sex
        - Money
        - Praise
- Mindfulness practices
    - Increase functional connectivity
        - Caudate nucleus
        - Basal-ganglia-thalamocortical loops
            - Mindfulness becomes more spontaneous

Shifting from DMN to mindfulness

- Mind wandering
    - Activation of vmPFC, dmPFC, PCC
- Awareness of mind wandering
    - Activation of dorsal anterior cingulate cortex (dACC)
        - Salience network
        - Conflict monitoring and error detection
- Shifting and sustaining attention to the breath
    - Activation of dorsolateral prefrontal cortex (dlPFC)
        - Central executive network
        - Cognitive and emotional regulation

Summary of brain regions involved in mindfulness

- Anterior cingulate cortex (ACC)
    - Salience network
        - Attention regulation
        - Cognitive regulation
        - Emotional regulation
        - Self-regulation
- Dorsolateral prefrontal cortex (dlPFC)
    - Central executive network
        - Cognitive regulation
        - Emotional regulation
        - Meta-awareness: consciously aware of awareness
- Insular cortex
    - Body awareness
- Striatum
    - Habit formation
- Amygdala
    - Shrinks after 8 weeks of mindfulness practices
    - Fight-or-flight center
        - Emotional learning

Happiness

Introduction

If we are not happy, it is difficult for us to make patients happy. To be happy, we have to study and practice happiness.

Terms

- Positive psychology: the study of happiness
- Hedonism
    - Living a pleasant life
    - Pursuing pleasure and avoiding pain
        - Sensory pleasures are short-lived
        - Constant pursuit is needed
        - Tendency to adapt: hedonic treadmill or adaptation
        - May not lead to personal growth
        - Pain is inevitable in life
    - Model of subjective well-being (Diener 1984)
        - Subjective well-being
            - High level of positive affect
            - Low level of negative affect
            - High degree of life satisfaction
    - The happiness pie chart (Lyubomirsky 2005)
        - Happiness set point 50%
        - Intentional activities 40%
        - Life circumstances 10%
    - Happiness set point
        - An average level of happiness after temporary highs and lows in emotionality
        - Attributed to genetic predeterminism
        - Assumed to be fixed and stable over time

- Eudaimonia
    - Living a good life
    - Pursuing virtues and strengths
        - Happiness from living a virtuous life is more stable
        - Promotes personal growth
    - The authentic happiness model (Seligman 2011)
        - Positive emotions
        - Engagement
        - Meaningful life
        - Positive relationships
        - Positive accomplishments
    - Flourishing (Fredrickson 2005)
        - Living within an optimal range of human functioning
        - One that connotes goodness, generativity, growth and resilience
    - Mental health functioning (Keyes 2002)
        - Flourishing: high well-being, low mental illness
        - Struggling: high well-being, high mental illness
        - Floundering: low well-being, high mental illness
        - Languishing: low well-being, low mental illness
    - Resilience (Newman 2004)
        - A universal capacity which allows a person, group or community, to prevent, minimize or overcome damaging effects of adversity
    - Flow (Csikszentmihalyi 1975)
        - The holistic sensation present when we act with total involvement

Savouring: the pursuit of pleasure

- Noticing and appreciating the positive aspects of life
- Positive counterpart of coping
- Involves mindfulness and conscious attention to pleasure

- Types of savouring (Bryant 2005, 2007)
    - Anticipation: enjoying future pleasure
    - Being in the moment: enjoying present pleasure
        - Luxuriating: indulging in sensory pleasure
        - Marveling: feeling wonderful
        - Basking: receiving praise
        - Thanksgiving: expressing gratitude
    - Reminiscing: enjoying past pleasure

Flow: the pursuit of optimal experience

- The psychology of optimal experience
- The process of total involvement in life
- The elements of enjoyment
    - Involved in a challenging activity that requires skills
    - The merging of action and awareness
    - Clear goals, immediate feedback and sense of reward
    - Concentration on the task at hand
    - The paradox of control
    - The loss of self-consciousness
    - The transformation of time

The pursuit of love (Sternberg 1986)

- Passion: an intense emotional response to another person
- Intimacy: warmth, closeness, sharing of self in a relationship
- Commitment: decision to maintain the relationship
- Infatuation: passion alone
- Liking: intimacy alone
- Empty love: commitment alone
- Romantic love: passion + intimacy
- Fatuous love: passion + commitment
- Companionate love: intimacy + commitment
- Consummate love: passion + intimacy + commitment

The pursuit of excellence

- Excellence: the acquisition of extraordinary skill in a specific area of expertise (Ericsson 1994)
- Elements of excellence
    - Cognitive: large knowledge base in one's specific domain
    - Motivational: passion and commitment
    - Action: consistent deliberate practice, persistence
- Grit (Duckworth 2007)
    - Passion + persistence
- Ten-year rule
    - It takes at least a decade of dedicated, consistent practice before one can attain a high level of excellence

Aesthetics: the pursuit of beauty

- Aesthetics: an appreciation of the beautiful and the sublime
- Four attributes of the aesthetic experience
    - Pleasure
    - Absorption
    - Intrinsic interest
    - Challenge

The pursuit of creativity

- Creativity: adaptive originality (Simonton 2009)
    - Adaptive: provides a useful solution to a real-life problem
    - Originality: original, novel, surprising or unexpected
- The creative process
    - Preparation: gathering information
    - Incubation: subconscious processing of information
    - Illumination: rapid emerging of a creative solution
    - Verification: turning an insight into real-world solution

The pursuit of virtues and strengths (Martin Seligman 2002)

- Virtue: good character or moral excellence
- Strength: route in achieving virtue
- The six virtues and twenty four strengths
  - Wisdom
    - Curiosity
    - Love of learning
    - Open-mindedness
    - Creativity
    - Emotional intelligence
    - Perspective
  - Courage
    - Bravery
    - Perseverance
    - Integrity
  - Love
    - Kindness
    - Loving and loved
  - Justice
    - Responsibility
    - Fairness
    - Leadership
  - Temperance
    - Self-control
    - Prudence
    - Humility
  - Spirituality
    - Appreciation of beauty
    - Gratitude
    - Hope and optimism
    - Sense of purpose
    - Forgiveness

- Humour
- Passion

The reward system

- Reward: the attractive and motivational property of a stimulus that induces approach behaviour (Schultz 2015)
- Reward system: a group of neural structures responsible for:
    - Liking or pleasure
    - Wanting or desire (incentive salience)
    - Learning or positive reinforcement
- Intrinsic rewards
    - Unconditioned rewards that are attractive and motivate behaviour because they are inherently pleasurable
- Extrinsic rewards
    - Conditioned rewards that are attractive and motivate behaviour, but are not pleasurable
- Neuroscience of the reward system
    - Primarily within cortico-basal ganglia-thalamic loop
    - Pleasure centers or hedonic hotspots
        - Mediate pleasure or "liking"
            - Subcortical
                - Nucleus accumbens shell
                - Ventral pallidum
                - Parabrachial nucleus of pons
            - Cortical:
                - Orbitofrontal cortex
                - Insular cortex
                - Medial prefrontal cortex
                - Anterior cingulate cortex
    - Mesolimbic dopamine pathway
        - Ventral tegmental area (VTA) to nucleus accumbens
        - Mediates motivational processes or "wanting"

- Medial forebrain bundle (MFB)
  - Fibers from basal olfactory regions
  - Fibers from periamygdaloid region
  - Fibers from the septal nuclei
  - Fibers from ventral tegmentum area (VTA)
  - Integration of reward and pleasure
- Basal ganglia
  - Mediates learning and drives activities
    - Dorsal striatum: caudate and putamen
    - Substantia nigra
    - Globus pallidus
- Possible neural correlates of eudaimonic happiness
  - Link between cortical and hedonic brain circuits
  - Cortical regions
    - Orbitofrontal cortex
    - Medial prefrontal cortex
    - Anterior cingulate cortex
    - Dorsolateral prefrontal cortex
    - Insular cortex

Happiness activities (Sonja Lyubomirsky 2008)

- Expressing gratitude
- Cultivating optimism
- Avoiding overthinking
- Practicing acts of kindness
- Nurturing social relationships
- Develop strategies for coping with stress
- Learning to forgive
- Increasing flow experiences
- Savouring life's joys
- Committing to our goals
- Practicing spirituality or religion

- Practicing mindfulness or meditation
- Exercise
- Smile

Little quote

If you want others to be happy, practice compassion.
If you want to be happy, practice compassion.

Dalai Lama

Kindness

Introduction

Kindness is the most important quality of a human being. If we cultivate kindness every day, it will grow every day and embrace everyone. We will become happier. Everyone around us will become happier.

Kindness

- The quality of being friendly, generous and considerate
- Synonyms of kindness
    - Altruism
    - Benevolence
    - Big-heartedness
    - Care
    - Compassion
    - Concern
    - Charitableness
    - Friendliness
    - Generosity
    - Gentleness
    - Goodwill
    - Helpfulness
    - Humaneness
    - Kind-heartedness
    - Love
    - Selflessness
    - Thoughtfulness
    - Understanding
    - Warm-heartedness

The four mental states of kindness

Love

- The intention and capacity to bring happiness
- Requires
    - Attentive looking and listening
    - Empathy and understanding
        - Knowing what to think and what not to think
        - Knowing what to say and what not to say
        - Knowing what to do and what not to do
- Love with understanding brings happiness
- Love without understanding causes suffering
- Love starts with ourselves
- If we cannot love ourselves, it can be hard to love others

Compassion

- The intention and capacity to relieve suffering
- Roots: passion (suffer) and com (with)
- We do not need to 'suffer with' to relieve another's suffering
- Requires
    - Attentive looking and listening
    - Empathy and understanding
    - Deep concern
    - Calmness, clarity and strength
- Calmness, clarity and strength are needed in relieving suffering
- Otherwise we will be overwhelmed by suffering

If your compassion does not include yourself, it is incomplete.

Jack Kornfield

Joy

- The intention and capacity to abide in a state of joy
- Requires
    - Feeling blessed for many things in life
    - Feeling grateful to many persons in life
    - Rejoicing in our own happiness
    - Rejoicing in others' happiness
- A joy that is filled with peace and contentment

Equanimity

- The intention and capacity to abide in a state of freedom
- The state of freedom
    - Freedom from judgment and conditions
    - Freedom from attachment to outcome
    - Freedom from discrimination
- The practices of love, compassion and joy are incomplete without the practice of freedom
    - Practice love without judgment and conditions
    - Practice compassion without attachment to outcome
    - Practice joy without discrimination
- Associated with the cognition of clarity
- Associated with the emotion of calmness

Guided meditations on the four mental states of kindness

Love meditation (metta meditation)

- Sit comfortably and relax your body
- Breathe in and breathe out naturally
- Make a wish from the depth of your heart: I am going to train myself in developing love for the sake of all beings
- Imagine someone you love in front of you
- Imagine receiving unconditional love from the person

- Feel the love from the bottom of your heart
- Rest in this love for a few moments
- Make a sincere wish for this person to be happy
- "May he or she be happy"
- Imagine sending unconditional love toward the person
- Rest in this love for the next few moments
- Now imagine extending unconditional love to:
    - All family members
    - All friends
    - All strangers
    - All enemeies
    - All beings
- Take time to deepen your unconditional love to each group
- End by imagining the whole universe filled with boundless love

Compassion meditation (karuna meditation)

- Sit comfortably and relax your body
- Breathe in and breathe out naturally
- Make a wish from the depth of your heart: I am going to train myself in developing compassion for the sake of all beings
- Imagine someone you love suffering in front of you
- Open your heart to feel the suffering of the person
- Feel the suffering from the bottom of your heart
- Rest in this suffering for a few moments
- Make a sincere wish for this person to be free from suffering
- "May he or she be free from all suffering"
- Imagine directing your compassion toward the person
- Rest in this compassion for the next few moments
- Now imagine extending compassion to:
    - All family members
    - All friends
    - All strangers

- All enemies
- All beings
- Take time to deepen your compassion to each group
- Imagine the whole universe filled with boundless compassion

Joy meditation (mudita meditation)

- Sit comfortably and relax your body
- Breathe in and out naturally
- Make a wish from the depth of your heart: I am going to train myself in developing joy for the sake of all beings
- Imagine you are with a very joyful person
- Feel the lightness and joy that this person brings to others
- Rejoice in his or her joy
- Feel his or her joy flowing into every part of your body
- Rest in this joy for a few moments
- Make a sincere wish for everyone to be full of joy
- "May everyone be full of joy"
- Imagine radiating this joy to:
    - Everyone in the northern direction
    - Everyone in the southern direction
    - Everyone in the eastern direction
    - Everyone in the western direction
    - All living beings above
    - All living beings below
- Take time to radiate joy to each direction
- Imagine the whole universe filled with boundless joy

Equanimity meditation (upekkha meditation)

- Sit comfortably and relax your body
- Breathe in and out naturally
- Make a wish from the depth of your heart: I am going to train myself in developing equanimity for the sake of all beings

- Imagine you are with a very calm and peaceful person
- Feel the calmness and peace of this person
- Imagine the peace of this person entering your body
- Feel the peace flowing into every part of your body
- Rest in this feeling of peace for a few moments
- Let go of everything in your mind
    - Your body
    - Your feelings
    - Your perceptions
    - Your thoughts and emotions
    - Your consciousness
- Just let them be as they are
- Do not try to change or manipulate any of them
- Just let them be as they are
- Feel the freedom and peace when you have let go of everything
- Rest in this freedom of your mind for the next few moments
- Make a sincere wish for everyone to be full of peace
- "May everyone be calm and peaceful"
- Imagine radiating this peace to:
    - Everyone in the northern direction
    - Everyone in the southern direction
    - Everyone in the eastern direction
    - Everyone in the western direction
    - All living beings above
    - All living beings below
- Take time to radiate peace to each direction
- Imagine the whole universe filled with boundless peace

18 qualities of kindness (Piero Ferrucci 2006)

- Honesty: everything becomes easier
- Warmth: the temperature of happiness
- Forgiveness: live in the present

- Contact: to touch and be touched
- Sense of belonging: I belong, therefore I am
- Trust: are you willing to risk?
- Mindfulness: the only time is now
- Empathy: expansion of consciousness
- Humility: you are not the only one around
- Patience: have you left your soul behind?
- Generosity: redefining boundaries
- Respect: look and listen
- Flexibility: adapt or perish
- Memory: have you forgotten anyone?
- Loyalty: don't lose your thread
- Gratitude: the easiest way to be happy
- Service: a wonderful opportunity
- Joy: our natural state

Cultivating the qualities of kindness

Generosity

- Sit down and listen to a patient
- Help a patient to pour water
- Help a patient to eat or drink
- Help a patient to adjust the bed linen
- Help a patient to comb hair
- Help a patient to adjust shoes or slippers
- Give a hand for a patient to sit up
- Bring flowers to a patient
- Buy a handheld fan for a patient with breathlessness
- Arrange a hairstylist to cut hair for a long-staying patient
- Arrange a musician to play music for a patient
- Hand out balloons for paediatric patients
- Make a patient smile
- Call and visit a dying patient

- Sit beside a dying patient
- Ask a family member "How are you doing?"
- Give a lazy chair to a family member
- Serve a drink to a family member
- Say something nice to a family member
- Bring a colleague out for lunch
- Write a small note of appreciation to a colleague
- Bring a small gift for a colleague
- Be a friend to a new colleague
- Buy a copy of book on kindness and give to a colleague
- Give a compliment to a colleague
- Allow staff to go home a bit earlier
- Write a thank you note to boss
- Take a picture with staff
- Offer to help the nurses during bed-making
- Give some cookies to a medical attendant
- Create a kindness board for daily kindness quote
- Plant some indoor flowers in the hospital
- Give our loved ones 100% of our attention
- Give our loved ones little surprises
- Listen with our heart
- Give a big hug to a friend
- Make a new friend
- Smile to a stranger
- Say something nice to everyone we meet
- Crack a joke
- Press the lift button for a stranger
- Say hello to a stranger
- Make some kindness bookmark and distribute it
- Play with a children
- Pick up a rubbish
- Plant a tree

Patience

- Slow down
- Stop rushing
- Listen to a patient without interrupting
- Give a patient time to come to terms with illness
- Give a patient time to come to terms with dying
- Allow a talkative patient to talk a bit more
- Allow an angry patient to express anger
- Allow an anxious patient to ask question
- Continue to review an unappreciative patient
- Continue to review a withdrawn patient
- Acknowledge differences in opinion with family member
- Acknowledge request for futile treatment from family member
- Respect the mistaken belief of family member
- Agree to disagree with a colleague
- Accept criticism of a colleague and respond thoughtfully
- Respect the impatience of a colleague
- Give a colleague time to change
- Listen attentively to a nagging spouse
- Keep calm and respond thoughtfully to a negative remark
- Keep calm and respond thoughtfully to a noisy neighbour
- Remain mindful during a queue
- Let someone cut in front of us in line
- Be a courteous driver
- Let someone merge into our lane in traffic
- Enjoy a traffic jam
- Leave nice comments on social media
- Complain less
- Say a timely apology
- Respect politicians
- Clean the toilet
- Keep calm and smile

Humility

- Avoid seeing a patient with a huge team
- See a patient in small group if necessary
- See a patient one-to-one if possible
- Sit down at the same level as patient
- Remove our sense of superiority over patient
- Spend more time listening than talking
- Learn from the experiences of a patient
- Speak without medical jargon
- Speak at the same level as patient
- Accept our limitations
- Accept credit when credit is due
- Give other people credit when it is due
- Avoid showing off
- Ask for help when appropriate
- Work as a team
- Recognize the contribution of each team member
- Acknowledge the importance of each team member
- Stop identifying ourselves as the center of the universe
- Stop identifying ourselves as someone very important
- Stop identifying ourselves as someone special
- Stop identifying our stress as something very overwhelming
- Stop identifying our contributions as highly important
- Learn to develop concern for others
- Learn to see others as very important person
- Learn to see others as very special person
- Learn to understand others' pain and suffering
- Learn to appreciate the contribution of others
- Adopt the beginner mind
- Keep an open mind
- Accept kindness from others
- Show gratitude to others

Forgiveness

- Forgive ourselves
- Write down our past mistake
- Feel the burden we are carrying: pain, guilt, fear, regret
- Make a confession
- Say sorry for any wrongs
- Ask for forgiveness
- Let go of our past misconduct
- Do not repeat similar mistake
- Begin anew
- Make a wish to act in a more caring way
- Dedicate our lives to others
- Do something to redeem the past if necessary
- Forgive ourselves if we are not ready to forgive completely
- Practice forgiving ourselves regularly
- Practice empathy for ourselves
- Open our heart to ourselves fully
- Forgive others
- Forgive the person, not the misdeeds
- Look deeply into the reasons causing the misdeeds
- Look deeply into the life of the person
- Practice empathy for the person
- Release our heart from the grip of anger or hatred
- Free ourselves from the past
- Let go of our judgment
- Do not force forgiveness
- Forgive little by little if necessary
- Open our heart to the person fully
- Do something to change the person skilfully
- Do something to change the world little by little
- Make peace with the past
- Live in the present moment

Gratitude

- Do not take things for granted
- Complain less
- Criticize less
- Judge less
- Gossip less
- Appreciate everyone and everything
- Express our gratitude to our family and friends
- Express our gratitude to our colleagues
- Express our gratitude to patients and their family members
- Express our gratitude to strangers
- Express our gratitude to enemies: they teach us patience
- Keep a gratitude journal
- Write down things you are grateful for daily
- Express thank you daily
- Appreciate and learn from adverse situations
- Praise a colleague
- Give a thank you card to a colleague
- Slow down our pace of life
- Breathe in and out to calm ourselves
- Count our blessing daily
- Start our day with lovely words

Waking up in the morning, I smile,
twenty-four brand new hours are before me,
I vow to live fully in each moment
and to look at all beings with eyes of compassion.

Thich Nhat Hanh

- Appreciate life and all its beauty from moment-to-moment
  - The sleeping faces of our loved ones
  - The first step out of bed
  - The smell of toothpaste
  - The cold running tap water
  - The mentally constructed "me" in the mirror
  - The breakfast
  - The flowers in our garden
  - The morning sun
  - The clouds
  - The swaying trees
  - The road full of cars
  - The rushing pedestrians
  - The ground that we walk as we arrive at work
  - The smile of our colleagues
  - The smile of patients or their family members
  - The tears
  - The silent grief
  - The faces of pain relief
  - The lunch
  - The wind and the falling leafs
  - The dinner
  - The time with our own family
  - The laughters and tears of our own children
  - The television
  - The book
  - The cozy sofa
  - The bed waiting for us for a whole day
- End our day with gratitude
  - Be thankful for every person that we meet that day
  - Be thankful for every little things in our life
  - Realize how blessed we are

Humour

- Practice light-heartedness
- Practice laughing without reasons when nobody is watching
- Learn to laugh at ourselves
- Learn to laugh at our adversities
- Watch a comedy
- Do some research on humour
- Memorize a few jokes every week
- Pay attention when others are joking
- Think three times before joking while breaking bad news
- Tell a patient our pulse is weaker while feeling their pulses
- Prescribe food in the medication chart
- Prescribe smiles from nurses three times a day in the care plan
- Request KY jelly from a nurse during PR, not the edible jelly
- Tell your colleague a correct PR examination can be enjoyable
- Put some jokes on the notice board
- Do not share dirty jokes openly unless boss is not around
- Laugh when others are laughing
- Avoid sarcastic jokes
- Avoid laughing at others unless they are not paying attention
- Avoid laughing when others are grieving
- Stand close to a door to escape when our joke is not funny
- Imagine the joke if it is inappropriate to share
- Look for opportunity to laugh in everyday life
- Learn from children how they laugh
- Hang around more with friends who can understand our jokes
- Type more LOLs in social media, appropriately
- Exaggerate our stories a bit while joking
- Use funny comparisons
- Treat our life as a joke
- Laugh at death, but not in front of patients
- Laugh five seconds before sleeping if we are sleeping alone

The social brain

- Neural networks that synchronize around relating to others
- Sensory stimuli: humans
- Key regions of the social circuitry
    - Amygdala
    - Fusiform gyrus
    - Superior temporal sulcus
    - Prefrontal cortex
- Amygdala
    - Two almond-shaped nuclei within the temporal lobe
    - Part of the limbic system: the emotional brain
    - Functions
        - Attaches emotional significance to sensory stimuli
        - Forms and stores emotional memories
        - Detects threat
        - Shapes social life
            - How we interact with people
            - How we react to people
    - Amygdala volume correlates with social network size
- Fusiform gyrus
    - Spindle-shaped
    - Also called occipitotemporal gyrus
    - Part of occipital lobe and temporal lobe
    - Function: facial recognition
- Superior temporal sulcus (STS)
    - Separates superior temporal from middle temporal gyrus
    - Function: social perception
        - Recognizes voices as opposed to sounds
        - Recognizes stories as opposed to nonsense speech
        - Recognizes moving faces as opposed to objects
        - Detects biological motion

- Prefrontal cortex
  - Orbitofrontal cortex (OFC)
    - Medial OFC: stimulus-reward association
    - Lateral OFC: stimulus-outcome association
    - Functions
      - Judges facial attractiveness
      - Supports the "reward" feelings
- The resonance circuit of empathy
  - Components
    - Mirror-neuron system for reflexive empathy
      - Broca's area
      - Premotor cortex
      - Motor cortex
      - Posterior superior temporal sulcus (STS)
      - Inferior parietal lobule
    - Emotional empathy
      - Amygdala
      - Fusiform gyrus
      - Superior temporal sulcus
    - Cognitive empathy
      - Middle prefrontal cortex
        - Orbitomedial prefrontal cortex
          - Orbitofrontal cortex
          - Medial prefrontal cortex
        - Anterior cingulate cortex
        - Ventrolateral prefrontal cortex
    - Insular cortex
      - Connects mirror neurons to limbic system for the development of emotional empathy
      - Connects limbic system and bodily information to middle prefrontal cortex for the empathic imagination of cognitive empathy

Index

S

Saline laxative 253, 257
savouring 533
Scopolamine patch 108, 238, 322
self-care 468-9, 475, 481, 492
senna 104, 109, 258, 262-3
sensitization 34, 51, 59
Simethicone 233, 272
sleep 113, 159, 198, 274-6, 278-82, 284-9, 292-3, 295, 298, 301, 398, 468, 492
sleep center 275
sleep hygiene 281, 284, 287
The social brain 554
Sodium citrate enema 263
Sodium phosphate enema 263
Sodium picosulphate 259
Sodium valproate 162, 168, 172
Somatic pain 73, 85
spinal cord compression 85, 175, 249
spiritual care 14, 436
spirituality 427-8, 492, 536
Squashed stomach syndrome 214
Steroid 64
Stool lubricant 253, 263
Stool surfactant 253, 255
stress 49, 338, 380, 473, 475-6, 478

Strong opioid 92, 94, 100-1, 117, 124, 130-1, 143, 149-51, 154, 162
sufentanil 128-9, 132, 139, 152, 178-80, 209
Suffering 394-6, 412-13, 460, 515, 517, 525
Suffering pictogram 412-13
syrup morphine 103, 119-20, 122-5, 131, 178-80, 201

T

Tapendatol 147
Tegaserod 261
Terminal agitation 306
terminal breathlessness 210
terminal delirium 305
Terminal restlessness 306
tolerance 107-8, 116, 294
Topiramate 162, 168
The total care model of palliative care stress 478
Tramadol 92, 100-1, 130-1, 147, 150, 154, 162, 180, 249
Trazodone 294, 303
Tropisetron 225

V

Venlafaxine 161, 164-5
Ventilation withdrawal 339-41
Vicarious traumatization 483, 528

Visceral pain   63, 70, 73, 86
Visceral pain syndrome
    63, 70
vomiting   213, 215-17, 219,
    231
vomiting center   216-17

W

Weak opioid   92, 100, 119,
    123, 125, 130, 150
well-being   31, 456

Z

zaleplone   292
Ziprasidone   303
zoledronate   174
Zolpidem   292
Zonisamide   169
zopiclone   292

Printed in the United States
By Bookmasters